ADVANCES IN

Anesthesia

Editor-in-Chief
Thomas M. McLoughlin, MD

ELSEVIER

An Imprint of Elsevier, Inc.

PHILADELPHIA   LONDON   TORONTO   MONTREAL   SYDNEY   TOKYO

ADVANCES IN
Anesthesia

VOLUMES 1 THROUGH 24 (OUT OF PRINT)

Vice President, Continuity Publishing: John A. Schrefer
Associate Developmental Editor: Yonah Korngold

Editorial Office:
Elsevier
1600 John F. Kennedy Blvd,
Suite 1800
Philadelphia, PA 19103-2899

International Standard Serial Number: 0737-6146
International Standard Book Number-10: 1-4160-5728-5
International Standard Book Number-13: 978-1-4160-5728-4

ADVANCES IN
Anesthesia

Editor-in-Chief

THOMAS M. McLOUGHLIN, MD, Chair, Department of Anesthesiology, Lehigh Valley Hospital and Health System, Allentown; and Professor of Clinical Anesthesiology, Penn State College of Medicine, Hershey, Pennsylvania

Associate Editors

JOEL O. JOHNSON, MD, PhD, Professor, Department of Anesthesiology, University of Wisconsin, Madison, Wisconsin

FRANCIS V. SALINAS, MD, Staff Anesthesiologist; Section Head of Orthopedic Anesthesia; and Coordinator of Ultrasound-Guided Regional Anesthesia Education, Virginia Mason Medical Center, Seattle, Washington

ADVANCES IN
Anesthesia

CONTRIBUTORS

SIMON C. BODY, MBChB, MPH, Department of Anesthesiology, Perioperative and Pain Medicine, Brigham and Women's Hospital, Boston, Massachusetts

ASOKUMAR BUVANENDRAN, MD, Associate Professor of Anesthesiology; and Director of Orthopedic Anesthesia, Division of Pain Medicine, Department of Anesthesiology, Rush University Medical Center, Rush Medical College, Chicago, Illinois

CHRISTOPHER C. CAMBIC, MD, Instructor, Department of Anesthesiology, Northwestern University Feinberg School of Medicine, Chicago, Illinois

LAURA CLARK, MD, Professor of Anesthesiology and Perioperative Medicine; Director of Acute Pain and Regional Anesthesia; and Program Director, University of Louisville Hospital, Louisville, Kentucky

TONY J. GAN, MB, FRCA, FFARSC(I), Professor, Department of Anesthesiology, Duke University Medical Center, Durham, North Carolina

ASHRAF S. HABIB, MBBCh, MSc, FRCA, Associate Professor, Department of Anesthesiology, Duke University Medical Center, Durham, North Carolina

SHAILENDRA JOSHI, MD, Assistant Professor of Clinical Anesthesiology, Department of Anesthesiology, College of Physicians and Surgeons of Columbia University, New York, New York

MICHAEL W. KAUFMANN, MD, Professor, Clinical Psychiatry, Penn State College of Medicine; and Chair, Department of Psychiatry, Lehigh Valley Health Network, Bethlehem, Pennsylvania

SEAN D. LAVINE, MD, Director of Endovascular Neurosurgery and Assistant Professor of Neurological Surgery and Radiology, Columbia University, New York, New York

J. BRUCE LEVIS, Jr., MBA, CFP, Managing Director, McQueen, Ball, and Associates, Inc., Bethlehem, Pennsylvania

DAVID S. MARKLE, CPA/PFS, CFP, Financial Planner, McQueen, Ball, and Associates, Inc., Bethlehem, Pennsylvania

EDWARD R. NORRIS, MD, Assistant Professor, Clinical Psychiatry, Penn State College of Medicine; and Vice Chair of Research and Education, Department of Psychiatry, Lehigh Valley Health Network, Bethlehem, Pennsylvania

JARED K. PEARSON, MD, Resident Physician, Virginia Mason Medical Center, Graduate Medical Education, Seattle, Washington

MUHAMAD ALY RIFAI, MD, Associate Professor, Clinical Psychiatry, Penn State College of Medicine; and Medical Director, Behavioral Health Emergency Services, Department of Psychiatry, Lehigh Valley Health Network, Bethlehem, Pennsylvania

MARINA VARBANOVA, MD, Assistant Professor, Department of Anesthesiology and Perioperative Medicine, University of Louisville Hospital, Louisville, Kentucky

CHRISTOPHER VISCOMI, MD, Associate Professor of Anesthesiology, Department of Anesthesiology; and Director, Acute Pain Service, University of Vermont/ Fletcher Allen Healthcare, Burlington, Vermont

BRYAN S. WILLIAMS, MD, MPH, Assistant Professor of Anesthesiology, Division of Pain Medicine, Department of Anesthesiology, Rush University Medical Center, Rush Medical College, Chicago, Illinois

CYNTHIA A. WONG, MD, Professor, Department of Anesthesiology; and Chief, Section of Obstetrical Anesthesiology, Northwestern University Feinberg School of Medicine, Chicago, Illinois

WILLIAM L. YOUNG, MD, Director, University of California San Francisco Center for Cerebrovascular Research; and James P. Livingston Professor and Vice-Chair, Department of Anesthesia and Perioperative Care, University of California San Francisco, San Francisco, California

ADVANCES IN
Anesthesia

CONTENTS

VOLUME 27 • 2009

Perioperative Management of the Opioid-Tolerant Patient
By Christopher Viscomi and Jared K. Pearson

Preoperative Stress Syndromes and Their Evaluation, Consultation, and Management
By Edward R. Norris, Muhamad Aly Rifai, and Michael W. Kaufmann

Genomics: Implications for Anesthesia, Perioperative Care and Outcomes
By Simon C. Body

Retirement Planning for Physicians
By J. Bruce Levis, Jr., David S. Markle

Nonopioid Adjuvants in Multimodal Therapy for Acute Perioperative Pain
By Bryan S. Williams, Asokumar Buvanendran

Evidence-Based Update and Controversies in the Treatment and Prevention of Postoperative Nausea and Vomiting
By Ashraf S. Habib, Tong J. Gan

Impact of Central Neuraxial Analgesia on the Progress of Labor
By Christopher R. Cambic, Cynthia A. Wong

Regional Anesthesia in Trauma
By Laura Clark, Marina Varbanova

Advances in Anesthesia 27 (2009) 1–24

ADVANCES IN ANESTHESIA

ELSEVIER
MOSBY

Anesthetic Management of Interventional Neuroradiological Procedures

Shailendra Joshi, MD[a],*, Sean D. Lavine, MD[b],
William L. Young, MD[c]

[a]Department of Anesthesiology, P&S Box 46, College of Physicians and Surgeons of Columbia University, 630 West 168th Street, New York, NY 10032, USA
[b]Department of Neurological Surgery and Radiology, Columbia University, New York, NY 10032, USA
[c]UCSF Center for Cerebrovascular Research, University of California, San Francisco, CA 94110, USA

R apid advances in endovascular surgery have created new opportunities and challenges for the treatment of brain diseases. There have been advances in catheter technology, imaging techniques, computational methods, new pharmacologic agents, and better understanding of drug delivery. In general, interventional neuroradiological (INR) or endovascular neurosurgical procedures are technically simple, yet they carry a low but significant morbidity. Although 0.2% to 1% of the patients may develop transient or permanent neurologic symptoms after diagnostic cerebral angiography, therapeutic interventions carry significantly greater risks of neurologic complications. The primary goals of anesthesia for INR procedures are to control the level of sedation in a manner that permits prompt neurologic examination, to render the patient immobile, and to manipulate cerebral hemodynamics. Many INR procedures (such as diagnostic angiography, carotid stenting, and embolization of cerebral arteriovenous malformations [AVMs]) can be undertaken with intravenous sedation. However, a growing number of INR procedures (such as aneurysm embolization, intracranial angioplasty, and embolization of some high-flow AVMs), require general anesthesia. General anesthesia is usually required for diagnostic procedures in children, in uncooperative patients, those at risk of aspiration or unable to protect the airway, and for prolonged procedures, such as those on the spinal cord. Often, the choice of anesthetic technique is a collaborative decision by the radiologist and the anesthesiologist, based on individual patient assessment.

Funding support: National Institute of Heath NCI R01 127500 Grant, from the National Institute of Health, Bethesda, Maryland.

*Corresponding author. E-mail address: sj121@columbia.edu (S. Joshi).

0737-6146/09/$ – see front matter
doi:10.1016/j.aan.2009.07.003

NEUROVASCULAR TECHNIQUES

Vascular access

INR procedures typically involve placement of catheters in the arterial circulation of the head or the neck, usually through the transfemoral route. As illustrated in Fig. 1, transfemoral access is accomplished by the placement of a large introducer sheath into the femoral artery, usually 5.0 to 7.5 Fr in size. Through the introducer sheath a 5.0 to 7.5 Fr coaxial catheter is positioned by fluoroscopic control into the carotid or vertebral artery. Finally, a 1.5 to 2.8 Fr superselective microcatheter is introduced into the cerebral circulation. This microcatheter can be used to deliver drugs, embolic agents, or balloons to distal regions of the brain. The transfemoral placement site is usually infiltrated with local anesthetic agent, which can result in femoral nerve block and a temporary weakness of the quadriceps muscle. Transfemoral venous access can be used to reach the dural sinuses and, in some cases, the arterial side of the AVMs. Direct percutaneous puncture is used to access superficial lesions of the head and neck such as tumors, arteriovenous and venous malformations.

Imaging technology

Radiological imaging techniques needed for INR procedures include high-resolution fluoroscopy and high-speed digital subtraction angiography (DSA) with

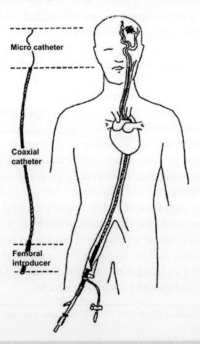

Micro catheter

Coaxial catheter

Femoral introducer

Fig. 1. Typical arrangement of the transfemoral coaxial catheter system showing the femoral introducer sheath, the coaxial catheter, and the microcatheter. (*From* Young WL. Clinical neuroscience lectures. Munster (IL): Cathenart Publishing; with permission.)

road mapping functions. The road mapping function enables the radiologist to observe the advance of the catheter against the background map of the patient's cerebral vessels in real time. DSA enables visualization of only those vessels that are opacified by contrast injection. DSA involves subtraction of images obtained before and after injection of radiocontrast. Any displacement of the cerebral vessels because of movement of the head profoundly degrades DSA images. Hence, it is critical that the patient remains immobile during the procedure. There have been many recent advances in angiography. These include the three-dimensional reconstruction of angiographic images with spin angiography. Stereoscopic examination of angiographic images that can be further manipulated on the screen in 3 dimensions can help to precisely define the anatomy of the lesions. Mechanized injections of radiocontrast with high-quality imaging can determine flow patterns within the vascular lesions. These advances combined with other conventional techniques, such as pressure measurements in distal regions of the brain through small 1.2 to 1.5 Fr micro-catheters or flow velocity measurements with intravascular Doppler ultrasound probes, can be used to characterize the neurovascular lesions. Definition of anatomic characteristics is a critical component in therapeutic decision-making and, in the future, is likely to advance the understanding of underlying vascular pathology.

Embolic materials

Factors that affect the choice of embolic agent include the nature of the disease, the purpose of embolization, the size and penetration of vessels that are being embolized, and the permanency of occlusion. The ideal choice and the combination of agents remain controversial. Embolic agents include balloons, coils, polyvinyl alcohol particles, gelatinous embolization spheres, and glue. N-butyl cyanoacrylate (NBCA) glue, used for embolization, is available as a liquid monomer that rapidly polymerizes in contact with ionic solutions such as blood and saline.

Anesthetic considerations

The objectives of anesthesia are to: (1) provide a level of sedation to a patient that permits prompt neurologic assessment when needed; (2) provide a physiologically stable and immobile patient; (3) optimally manipulate systemic blood pressure as dictated by the needs of the procedure; and (4) provide emergent care of catastrophic complications.

Preoperative assessment

Ability to communicate effectively with the patients is critical for INR procedures. The patients must be able to follow instructions during procedures for neurologic testing, such as hold their breath and remain immobile to reduce image artifacts. A careful assessment of the airway has to be made. A history of snoring may suggest that partial airway obstruction might occur with sedation. Snoring results in movement artifacts that may degrade the quality of images during cerebral angiography. If there is a history of significant snoring or obstructive sleep apnea, consideration must be given to the placement of a nasal trumpet. The placement of nasal trumpet has to be atraumatic. It should be lubricated with a local anesthetic-vasoconstrictor mixture, before the start of the procedure to minimize the chances of bleeding at placement, and after the patient is anticoagulated for the procedure. Patients with a history of adverse reaction to radiocontrast drugs require pretreatment with steroids and antihistaminic drugs. In the population with occlusive cerebrovascular disease, patients might require adequate treatment of hypertension, heart failure, or angina. Preoperative communication should exist with the INR team to develop a clear strategy for sedation and hemodynamic interventions that might be needed during the procedure.

Preoperative investigations
Routine guidelines for laboratory investigations before surgery are applicable to INR procedures. Of particular interest is the baseline coagulation screen, because anticoagulation will be required for the procedure.

Premedication
As in general anesthetic practice, premedication is seldom used for anesthesia for INR. Minimal premedication, generally with anxiolytics, is required for INR procedures, although oral nimodipine or transdermal nitroglycerin is sometimes used to decrease intraoperative vasospasm.

Room preparation
The INR suite should be equipped exactly like a standard anesthesia operating room. Suction, gas evacuation, oxygen, and nitrous oxide should be available from the wall outlets. Ideally, the anesthesia machine should have the capacity to provide carbon dioxide for deliberate hypercapnia. An extended anesthetic breathing system is necessary to reach the remotely located patient's airway. Rapid access to all critical equipment should be possible at all times during the procedure. Induction and emergency drugs must be prepared for immediate use.

Patient positioning
Because INR procedures may last for several hours, it is essential that the patient be made as comfortable as possible before the start of sedation. An inflatable air mattress and warm blankets are usually sufficient to ensure patient comfort. Soft padded restraints to secure the hands alongside the patient are necessary to avoid any inadvertent contamination of the arterial puncture site, which is usually the groin.

Intravenous access
During INR procedures the patients are often moved cephalad by as much as 60 to 90 cm (2–3 feet) to image the groin. Multiple imaging monitors and transparent lead screen (to decrease radiation exposure) are interposed between the patient and the anesthesiologist. Therefore access to venipuncture sites and injection ports is limited during the procedure. Adequate vascular access and sufficient length of tubing should be in place before the start of the procedure.

In adults, 2 intravenous cannulae are usually placed for this purpose; 1 cannula is at least 18 gage. The anesthetic and vasoactive agents should be in line before the patient is draped.

MONITORING
Arterial pressure
Because of the need for manipulating systemic hemodynamics and, at times, the emergent need for hemodynamic interventions, it is usually desirable to obtain direct systemic arterial pressure measurements during INR procedures. This requirement is most conveniently achieved by transducing the side arm of the femoral introducer sheath. It must be realized that, if a large coaxial catheter passes through the introducer, the arterial pressure trace will be "damped." Despite damping, the mean pressure will still be reliable in such a situation. To avoid excessive damping of the femoral arterial trace, the introducer sheath should be at least 1/2 Fr larger than the coaxial catheter. Radial artery cannulation may be desirable when systemic pressures are to be monitored before the femoral introducer sheath is placed, such as during induction of general anesthesia for coiling of intracranial aneurysms or when postoperative blood pressure monitoring is necessary.

For a typical intracranial procedure, in addition to the systemic arterial pressure, 2 other pressures may be measured in real time: the internal carotid artery (ICA) or vertebral artery pressure through the coaxial catheter, and the distal cerebral arterial pressure through the microcatheter or a balloon-tipped catheter. The coaxial catheter pressure is monitored to detect any thrombus formation or vasospasm at the catheter tip as shown by a damped arterial trace. A high volume of heparinized flush is passed continuously through the coaxial tip to discourage thrombus formation; hence, the pressure reading characteristically increases by 10 to 20 mm Hg when recorded through the coaxial catheter. The setup for measuring arterial pressures is shown in Fig. 2. The pressure transducers and access stopcocks for blood withdrawal and zeroing are mounted, depending on the institutional preferences, either on the sterile field or toward the anesthesiologist. The distal cerebral arterial pressure measurements made through the microcatheter are useful during embolization of AVMs (see section on Superselective Angiography and Therapeutic Embolization of AVMs). When a balloon catheter is used for ICA occlusion, pressure measurements at the tip of the catheter provide the stump pressure (see section on Carotid Test Occlusion and Therapeutic Carotid Occlusion).

Other systemic monitoring
Other monitors include 5-lead electrocardiogram, preferably with ST segment trending and respiratory trace, automated blood pressure cuff, end-tidal carbon dioxide, and peripheral temperature monitors. Loss of end-tidal carbon dioxide trace despite adequate respiratory excursion, as detected by thoracic impedance, can be a result of the displacement of the sampling cannula or upper

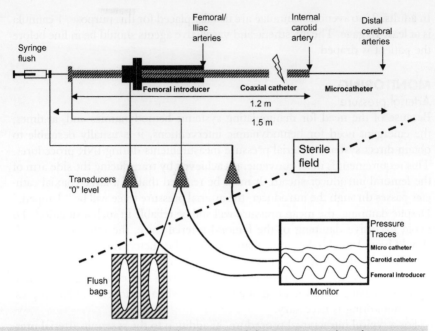

Fig. 2. Schematic representations of catheters used during INR procedures for monitoring arterial pressures in regions of cerebral arterial system. (*From* Young WL. Clinical neuroscience lectures. Munster (IL): Cathenart Publishing; with permission.)

airway obstruction. Thus, the 2 respiratory monitors complement each other. Pulse oximeter probes are placed on each of the great toes and are useful for qualitatively comparing distal pulses in the lower limbs. Loss of oximeter pulse trace on the side of the femoral introducer sheath might give an early warning of thromboembolism, vasospasm, or mechanical obstruction.

Central nervous system monitoring

During many procedures, neurologic examination provides adequate monitoring of central nervous system (CNS) integrity. Adjuncts that are especially useful during general anesthesia or planned proximal occlusions include electroencephalogram, somatosensory and motor evoked potentials, transcranial Doppler (TCD) ultrasound, and ^{133}Xe cerebral blood flow (CBF) monitoring.

Urinary output

Most patients undergoing INR procedures will require bladder catheterization to assist in fluid management and to increase patient comfort. Increased diuresis might occur during the procedure as a result of an increase in intravascular volume after continuous flushing of the intravascular lines and osmotic load due to radiocontrast or mannitol injection. The timing and volume of contrast injected should be monitored, especially during prolonged procedures.

Laboratory tests

A baseline arterial blood gas (ABG) at the time of arterial puncture is useful to assess the gradient between PaO_2 and arterial oxygen concentration (SaO_2) and the $PaCO_2$ to end-tidal pressure of CO_2 ($PETCO_2$) gradient. Activated clotting time (ACT) is used to monitor coagulation. The patients are given large quantities of fluids and dye, and can diurese considerably, so a baseline hematocrit determination is helpful.

ANESTHETIC TECHNIQUES
Dynamic sedation

Primary goals of anesthetic choice for conscious sedation are alleviating pain and discomfort, anxiolysis, and patient immobility. At the same time, one must allow a rapid decrease in the level of sedation when neurologic testing is required. The procedures are not generally painful, with the exceptions of sclerotherapy and chemotherapy. There is an element of pain associated with distention or traction on the vessels; contrast injection into the carotid artery is frequently described as "burning." Discomfort might be a result of prolonged periods of lying still, bladder catheterization, and, to a lesser extent, the femoral puncture site. The procedure might be psychologically stressful because of the potential risk of stroke during the procedure. Patient immobility, whether by conscious effort or by deep sedation, is essential. Movement not only can degrade the quality of images but can also result in vascular injury.

Sedation scores

It is critical to quantify the level of sedation during interventional radiological procedures to carefully control drug delivery. A variety of sedation scores are available. A popular one is the Ramsay score, which grades sedation at 6 levels, as shown in Table 1. Most of the sedation scores require eliciting responses to verbal commands or noxious stimuli. Because of the remote location of the head, communication with the patient may be limited and it might be difficult to elicit the glabellar tap. Thus, close monitoring of the patient for movements and respiratory functions is critical. The surgeons, who are often located closer to the patient, could assist in eliciting a verbal response when needed. However, close observation of respiratory parameters, such as the capnographic trace, respiratory excursion by thoracic impedance, and adequate oxygen saturation, is critical, with deeper levels of sedation in the absence of verbal response.

Anesthetic agents are selected to provide sedation, analgesia, and anxiolysis, and to ensure comfort and relative immobility. Our primary approach to conscious sedation is to establish a base of neurolept anesthesia by titration of 1 to 2 µg/kg of fentanyl, and 1 to 2 mg of midazolam after intravenous access and monitoring have been established and oxygen administration has begun. A small bolus of propofol can be useful just as the bladder catheter is passed in men. The bolus dose of propofol also helps the anesthesiologist assess the airway under deep sedation and determine when a nasopharyngeal airway is

Table 1
Ramsay sedation score

Sedation score	Awake or asleep	State/response
1	Awake	Restless
2	Awake	Cooperative
3	Awake	Responds to verbal commands
4	Asleep	Response to glabellar tap brisk
5	Asleep	Response to glabellar tap sluggish
6	Asleep	No response to glabellar tap

required. Placement of the nasopharyngeal airway after anticoagulation can result in troublesome bleeding and is best avoided.

When the patient is in the final position, draping is begun and a propofol infusion is started at low doses (10–20 µg/kg/min) and then increased slowly to render the patient immobile yet breathing spontaneously. The availability of the α-2 agonist, dexmedetomidine, offers an alternative to propofol. The airway is better maintained during sedation with dexmedetomidine. Dexmedetomidine (0.5–1 µg/kg over 10–20 min loading dose, with an infusion of 0.2–0.7 µg/kg/h) permits neurologic examination during awake craniotomy. Patients sedated with this agent tend to have lower blood pressures in the recovery period, which may not be desirable in patients who are critically dependent on maintaining adequate collateral perfusion pressure. Thus, the choice must be based on the experience of the practitioner and the requirements of the procedure (Table 2).

Dexmedetomidine
Dexmedetomidine is a selective α-2 adrenoreceptor agonist. It is an exceedingly short-acting drug with minimal respiratory depression in sedative doses. Hemodynamic depression manifesting as hypotension and bradycardia can occur, and the drug has to be used with caution in patients with advanced heart blocks or severe ventricular dysfunction. Dexmedetomidine is highly protein bound and can potentially have interactions with other protein bound drugs. It is metabolized in the liver by glucuronide formation and by cytochrome P-450. Most of the drug is eliminated in the urine. Liver dysfunction affects clearance of dexmedetomidine: mild, moderate, and severe hepatic dysfunction decreases clearance to 74%, 64%, and 53% respectively.

Propofol
Propofol is a sterile oil-in-water emulsion of 2,6-diisopropopylphenol. It is available as a 1% or 2% solution. Propofol is a highly lipid soluble and protein bound compound. High initial volume of distribution of propofol results in rapid redistribution of the drug after bolus injection. It is principally metabolized in the liver, and inactive glucuronide is eliminated in the urine. There is sufficient hepatic reserve to metabolize propofol in patients with mild to moderate liver failure, although caution is warranted in patients with severe

Table 2
Pharmacokinetics of sedative hypnotics

	Dexmedetomidine	Propofol	Midazolam
Commercial name	Precedex	Diprivan	Versed
Vd ss (L)	120	250–300	80–120
T1/2 α (min)	6	2–4	6–15
T 1/2 β	2 h	30–60 min	100–150 min
Protein binding (%)	94	97–99	95
Metabolism	Liver	Liver	Liver
Cl (L/min)		1.5–2	0.5–0.8
			1–2 mg bolus
Loading dose	0.5–1 μg/kg over 10–20 min	Optional for sedation	
Maintenance dose	0.2–0.7 μg/kg/h	0.3 mg/kg/h	

liver failure. Renal failure does not significantly alter the pharmacokinetics of propofol.

Midazolam
Midazolam is a short-acting benzodiazipine. It has an aqueous soluble ring structure that is open when stored at a pH of 4, but after injection it cyclizes at a pH of 7.4 to enhance its lipid solubility. Midazolam with its sedative and anxiolytic properties is a useful premedication. It is to be used with caution if memory tests are planned as a part of diagnostic or therapeutic procedures. Small doses of midazolam (1–2 mg) are unlikely to impair memory tests if given 20 minutes or more before the test. Use of midazolam for procedures that involve memory tests should be discussed with the surgical team.

Narcotics
Most INR procedures are not associated with long lasting pain, therefore phenylpiperidine narcotics have become the mainstay for pain management in the INR suite. Fentanyl, sufentanil, alfentanil, and remifentanil belong to this class of drugs (Table 3). Although fentanyl, with its long duration of action, is the most frequently used narcotic, remifentanil, with its exceedingly short half-life, offers greater titratability. Remifentanil has a short elimination half-life as a result of hydrolysis by nonspecific esterases in the blood. Respiratory depression, pruritus, and vomiting are some of the side effects relevant to INR procedures. Because of the remote location of the airway, the use of narcotics has to be judicious. Careful attention has to be paid to respiratory monitoring, and the use of narcotics has to be curtailed if the respiratory rate drops below 10 to 12 breaths/min.

General anesthesia with tracheal intubation
General anesthesia with endotracheal intubation in the INR suites is similar to that in other operating rooms, whether for adult or pediatric cases. A theoretical argument can be made for eschewing the use of nitrous oxide because of

Table 3
Pharmacokinetics of narcotics

	Sufentanil	Fentanyl	Alfentanil	Remifentanil
Potency relative to fentanyl	7–10×	1×	0.1–0.2×	0.8×
Vd ss (L)	98	375	36	35
$T_{1/2}\ \alpha$ (min)	1	3	2	1
$T_{1/2}\ \beta$	2.5 h	4 h	1.5 h	5–8 min
Cl (L/min)	0.75	1	0.3	0.3
Octanol/water partition coefficient	1800	810	130	18
Sedation doses	5–10 µg bolus	50–100 µg bolus	250–500 µg bolus	0.03–0.05 µg/kg/min

the possibility of introducing air emboli into the cerebral circulation. The primary reason for using general anesthesia is to reduce motion artifacts and to improve the quality of images. This reason is especially pertinent in the INR treatment of spinal pathology, in which extensive multilevel angiography must sometimes be performed. Because chest excursion during positive pressure ventilation can interfere with road mapping, radiologists frequently request apnea for DSA for certain procedures.

ADJUVANT TECHNIQUES FOR SEDATION AND GENERAL ANESTHESIA

Anticoagulation
Careful management of coagulation is required to prevent thromboembolic complications as a result of the presence of foreign bodies (catheters) and endothelial injury as a result of the passage of microcatheters (Table 4). After placement of the femoral introducer sheath, a baseline ACT is obtained. Heparin (2000–5000 U/70 kg) is given and another ACT obtained approximately 3 to 5 minutes later. The target ACT depends on the clinical needs, and could be 2 to 3 times the baseline value. Additional heparin may be required throughout the procedure to maintain adequate anticoagulation.

On occasion, when the INR procedure is completed, the anticoagulant effect of heparin is reversed with protamine and the femoral artery catheter is removed in the angiography suite. The proliferation of percutaneous closure devices has improved hemostasis at the arteriotomy site, particularly in patients receiving thrombolytics and antiplatelet agents.

Deliberate hypotension
Two primary indications for deliberate hypotension are to decrease flow through an arteriovenous fistula during injection of glue, and to test the cerebrovascular reserve of the patient undergoing carotid occlusion. In most

Table 4
Anticoagulant therapy

	Heparin	Low Molecular Weight Heparin (Lovenox)	Fondaparinux	Lepirudin
Mechanism of action	Inhibits antithrombin	Inhibits antithrombin	Synthetic, specific to the binding region of heparin	Bind to thrombin exosite I
Dose	50–100 U/kg guided by ACT	Acute: 30 mg IV followed by 1 mg/kg subcutaneous	2.5–10 mg subcutaneous	0.1–0.4 mg/kg
Half-life	Dose dependent 1–5 h		17–21 h	1.3 h
Thrombocytopenia	Yes	Yes	Yes	No
Monitoring	ACT, APTT	PT and APTT insensitive needs antifactor Xa assay	PT and APTT insensitive, INR	APTT

Abbreviations: APTT, activated partial thromboplastin time; IV, intravenous; PT, prothrombin time.

instances, the level of sedation is decreased to permit neurologic examination during deliberate hypotension. Induction of hypotension in awake or minimally sedated patients can be fairly challenging. Large doses of hypotensive drugs might be required to reduce the blood pressure in minimally sedated patients. Adrenergic blocking drugs that do not directly affect CBF might be preferable to drugs that are potential cerebral vasodilators. Typically, high doses of esmolol (1 mg/kg bolus followed by an infusion approx 0.5 mg/kg/min) are required in these patients. Supplemental labetalol might be required during esmolol infusion. Agents such as sodium nitroprusside and nitroglycerin may also be used. Hypotension may lead to nausea and vomiting. Supplemental doses of antiemetic drugs (eg, ondansetron 4 mg, or dolansetron 12.5 mg) may be given before decreasing the blood pressure.

Flow arrest

Transient flow arrest has been used successfully for treating high-flow cerebral AVMs in healthy (ASA I and II) patients with NBCA glue embolization. If flow arrest is planned, the patient is prepared for general anesthesia. In addition to usual preparation, a central venous line is placed for injecting drugs. Intravenous adenosine (10–90 mg bolus) has been used for this purpose. External pacing pads or a transvenous pacing line is placed for the treatment of any persistent arrythmias. The procedure is generally conducted in 2 parts. In the first part the target feeding artery is identified and the safety of embolizing the vessel is assessed by a superselective Wada test under minimal anesthetic concentration (MAC) sedation. Once the catheter is placed in the desired location the general anesthesia is induced. The authors recommend conducting a dose response study to determine the optimal dose of adenosine. The dose of intravenous adenosine is aimed to produce 5 to 15 seconds of asystole and ranges between 10 and 90 mg. Small amounts of esmolol or nitroprusside might be necessary to treat rebound hypertension or tachycardia.

Deliberate hypertension

During cerebral arterial occlusion, planned or inadvertent, systemic blood pressure might need to be increased to augment collateral blood flow. The extent to which blood pressure has to be raised depends on the condition of the patient and the nature of the disease. Typically, during deliberate hypertension the systemic blood pressure is increased by 30% to 40% above the baseline, or until ischemic symptoms resolve. Electrocardiogram and ST segments should be inspected for myocardial ischemia. Phenylephrine is the first-line agent for deliberate hypertension. Dopamine might be useful in patients who have a low heart rate.

Deliberate hypercapnia

Deliberate hypercapnia ($PaCO_2$ 50–60 mm Hg) may be used during the treatment of venous malformations of the head and neck. The rationale for using hypercapnia is to increase cerebral venous outflow relative to extracranial venous drainage and to create a pressure gradient that would divert sclerosing agents away from the intracranial veins. Hypercapnia is usually achieved by decreasing minute ventilation. Alternatively, carbon dioxide may be added to inspired gases.

Radiation safety

There are 3 sources of radiation in the INR suite: direct radiation from the x-ray tube, leakage (through the collimator's protective shielding), and scattered (reflected from the patient and the area surrounding the body part to be imaged). The amount of exposure drops off in proportion to the square of the distance from the source of radiation (inverse square law). DSA delivers considerably more radiation than fluoroscopy. While working in the INR suite all persons should wear lead aprons and thyroid shields and have exposure badges.

Management of procedural catastrophes

Complications arising from cerebrovascular instrumentation can be rapid and dramatic, and require a multidisciplinary approach. A catastrophe plan should be clearly defined by the anesthesia team for every INR procedure. Drugs and equipment required to secure the airway should be available without any delay. Protamine should be available for immediate injection if the decision is made to reverse heparin. There should be effective communication between the INR team and the anesthesiologist. Appropriate neurology and neurosurgical consultants should be contacted as soon as possible. It is the primary responsibility of the anesthesia team to secure the airway and ensure adequate ventilation. Simultaneously with airway maintenance, it is essential to communicate with the INR team to determine if the problem is occlusive or hemorrhagic.

Occlusive catastrophes

In case of vascular occlusion, the primary approach is to augment distal perfusion. Restoring vascular patency is the immediate surgical goal, and may require intra-arterial vasodilators to treat arterial spasm, thrombolysis, mechanical clot retrieval, angioplasty or stent placement to treat emboli, or arterial dissection. Simultaneously, systemic interventions such as induced hypertension, hypercapnia, and volume expansion can be used to increase primary and collateral blood flow. Local and systemic interventions are required to prevent ischemic injury.

Hemorrhagic catastrophes

Intracranial hemorrhage might be heralded by headache, nausea, vomiting, and vascular pain related to the area of vascular perforation. The radiologist might see the contrast extravasate seconds before the patient becomes symptomatic. In the case of vessel puncture, heparin reversal before withdrawing the offending wire or the catheter back into the lumen of the vessel will keep the perforation partially blocked until the hemostatic function is restored. As soon as an intracranial hemorrhage is diagnosed, immediate reversal of heparin is indicated. Protamine (1 mg for every 100 U of heparin) is given without undue regard to systemic blood pressure. Later, an ACT may be done to adjust the final dose. With active bleeding, the blood pressure should be kept as low as possible. Once bleeding is controlled, the target blood pressure should be discussed with the radiology team. If vascular occlusion has been used to control hemorrhage, the INR team may ask for deliberate hypertension. Allergic reactions to protamine are rare, but may occur.

Transport and postprocedural considerations

After intracranial and spinal procedures, patients are usually observed in the intensive care unit for the first 24 hours. The groin should be monitored for bleeding from the puncture site. In general, INR procedures have their own inherent potential complications, and require frequent neurologic, metabolic, and hemodynamic monitoring. For example, after AVM embolization there might be minimal tissue edema that could lead to some deterioration in the neurologic status during the course of the first evening after the procedure.

SPECIFIC PROCEDURES

Superselective anesthesia and functional examination (SAFE) or superselective Wada is routinely performed before therapeutic embolizations to minimize the risk of occluding a nutritive vessel to eloquent regions, either in the brain or the spinal cord, which may happen if the microcatheter tip is proximal to the origin of nutritive vessels. However, not all investigators recognize the need for SAFE before embolization. The level of sedation should be decreased before testing by stopping the propofol infusion. In rare instances it might be necessary to use naloxone or flumazenil to antagonize other intravenous agents. Before the start of the embolization procedure when the catheter is in situ, sedation is stopped and a baseline neurologic examination is undertaken. In our experience small doses of midazolam (1–2 mg) or propofol (10–20 µg/kg/min) do not interfere with neurologic testing if they are withheld 20 minutes before the examination.

Sodium amobarbital (30 mg/mL) or lidocaine (30 mg/mL) mixed with contrast is injected through the superselective catheter and an angiogram of the drug/contrast mixture is obtained. Sodium amobarbital is used for investigating the gray matter. Lidocaine can be used to evaluate the integrity of the white matter tracts, especially in the spinal cord. Injection of lidocaine into cortical areas, particularly close to the motor strip, can cause seizures. Seizure activity can result in transient neurologic deficit. Postictal paralysis may confuse interpretation of the test. For this reason the barbiturate is usually given first, followed by lidocaine. If the amobarbital test is negative, it can protect against seizure but will not interfere with the assessment of lidocaine's effect on white matter tracts.

Superselective angiography and therapeutic embolization of AVMs

Typically, patients who present for embolization have large, complex, parenchymatous AVMs, which are composed of several discrete fistulae with multiple feeding arteries. The goal of the therapeutic embolization is to obliterate as many of the fistulae as possible. Although in rare cases INR treatment is aimed at total obliteration, embolization is usually used as an adjunct in preparation for surgery or radiotherapy, and can be beneficial in several ways. First, embolization may facilitate surgery by obliterating deep feeding arteries that are difficult to approach surgically and thereby reduce the surgical risk. Second, staging obliteration of arteriovenous shunts also theoretically allows the surrounding brain to accommodate the alterations in hemodynamics and may prevent normal perfusion pressure breakthrough. Third, obliteration of high-flow feeders can be of benefit in patients with progressive neurologic deficits or intractable seizures, ostensibly by diminishing steal but more likely by decreasing mass effect. Finally, approximately 10% of AVM patients harbor intracranial aneurysms. Such aneurysms seem to increase the risk of spontaneous hemorrhage from AVMs. Obliteration of intranidal aneurysms during the initial embolization may decrease the rate of recurrent hemorrhage during the course of treatment. The procedure can last 4 to 5 hours depending on the complexity of the lesions. A variety of embolic materials have been used to obliterate AVM fistulae, such as polyvinyl alcohol particles. More durable results are achieved with NBCA glue (Fig. 3).

When the catheter is placed in position for potential glue injection, SAFE is performed. If SAFE is positive (ie, if focal neurologic deficits develop), then the catheter is repositioned or embolization of that pedicle is aborted. If the test is negative, glue or another embolic material can be injected. Controlled deposition of glue is necessary to decrease complications from obstruction of AVM venous drainage or pulmonary embolism. Flow arrest through the fistula is desired during glue injection to permit polymerization and solidification of NBCA glue. Techniques for flow arrest include deliberate hypotension, balloon occlusion of the proximal vessel, or circulatory pause with adenosine or controlled ventricular fibrillation. In most instances deliberate hypotension suffices to achieve flow arrest. Typically the mean systemic blood pressure is reduced to approximately 50 mm Hg to achieve such a flow arrest. Flow arrest is usually not needed for polyvinyl alcohol embolization.

Measurement of immediate postembolization pressure has been suggested as a means of following the course of hemodynamic changes and predicting postprocedure complications. A large increase in feeding artery pressure after embolization may be associated with intracranial hemorrhage. Because AVM feeding arteries supply normal vascular territories to a variable degree, abrupt restoration of normal perfusion pressure to a chronically hypotensive vascular bed might overwhelm the autoregulatory capacity and result in hemorrhage or swelling (normal perfusion-pressure breakthrough). It is for this reason that the target range for post-treatment blood pressure is at or slightly below the patient's normal blood pressure.

Embolization of spinal sord lesions

Embolization can be used for intramedullary spinal AVMs, dural fistulae, or tumors invading the spinal canal. For cases performed under general anesthesia with endotracheal intubation, an intraoperative "wake-up test" may be requested. The wake-up test must be explained to the patient the night before

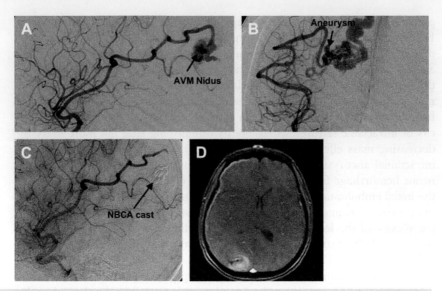

Fig. 3. A 29-year-old woman presented with acute onset headache and visual disturbances, which was diagnosed as being due to a ruptured occipital AVM (*A*) with intranidal aneurysm (*B*). It was treated under MAC anesthesia with NBCA embolization (*C*). Postoperative MRI shows a complete obliteration of the lesions (*D*).

and on the day of surgery. A nitrous oxide/narcotic anesthetic technique with concurrent propofol may be used for the procedure. Neuromuscular block, if required, should be readily reversible for the wake-up test. For selected lesions, somatosensory and motor evoked potentials can be helpful in anesthetized and sedated patients. When motor evoked potentials are monitored, the neuromuscular block should be titrated to the monitoring needs.

Carotid test occlusion and therapeutic carotid occlusion

Test occlusion of the carotid artery is undertaken before anticipated sacrifice of the vessel or when temporary carotid ligation might be required during surgery. During test occlusion, a catheter with a distal balloon and a lumen is placed in the ICA. A baseline neurologic examination is done. Flow velocity can be measured over the middle cerebral artery (MCA) by TCD ultrasound, if available, and the CBF can be measured by the intracarotid ^{133}Xe injection technique. Baseline femoral and carotid artery pressures are noted. The balloon is then inflated and the pressure in the carotid artery distal to the balloon recorded. Inflation of the balloon might cause headache and at times an increase in the systemic blood pressure. Aggressive treatment of hypertension is probably not warranted as it may decrease collateral perfusion pressure. The anesthesiologist should be prepared to treat bradycardia with atropine. The neurologic examination is repeated a few minutes after occlusion, and TCD and ^{133}Xe CBF measurements are also repeated. After ^{133}Xe washout data have been obtained, radioactive tracer for single-photon emission computerized tomography (SPECT) studies may be injected. This procedure provides a snapshot measurement of regional CBF during ICA occlusion. Because SPECT tracers usually have a long half-life and bind avidly to cerebral tissues, the imaging part of a SPECT study may be undertaken in the nuclear medicine department after the patient leaves the INR suite.

To assess the cerebrovascular reserve, if the patient does not demonstrate any neurologic impairment during the initial ICA occlusion, the systemic blood pressure is decreased. During reduction of the systemic blood pressure, neurologic examination is repeated at frequent intervals. The distal ICA (stump) pressure at which neurologic deterioration occurs, or whether the patient starts yawning (which is often a sign of impending cerebral ischemia), is noted, along with the corresponding TCD flow velocity. Depending on the clinical condition of the patient, another ^{133}Xe measurement is obtained. If overt neurologic symptoms develop, the balloon is immediately deflated, hypotensive agents are discontinued, and, depending on the clinical situation, vasopressors might be required to increase the blood pressure to normal levels.

Although a uniform guideline for interpreting the results of test occlusion has yet to be formulated, occurrence of a new neurologic deficit, a significant asymmetry on SPECT imaging, or a 25% to 30% reduction in ^{133}Xe CBF or TCD after occlusion may be considered as relative indications for an extracranial-to-intracranial bypass procedure before sacrifice of the carotid artery.

Aneurysm ablation

Many intracranial aneurysms are amenable to endovascular treatment, and, as interventional therapy has continued to evolve, it has increasingly become the primary treatment modality for ruptured and unruptured intracranial aneurysms. The choice of open surgical versus endovascular treatment is currently a topic of vigorous discussion. There are 2 basic approaches for endovascular obliteration of intracranial aneurysms: (1) the occlusion of the proximal parent artery, such as the carotid artery, which has been discussed earlier; and (2) obliteration of the aneurysmal sac. Endovascular obliteration of the aneurysmal sac is usually done using detachable coils by a wide variety of vendors (Fig. 4). Complicated aneurysms with wide necks and large sacs may require advanced techniques involving temporary balloon remodeling or intracranial stent placement. These procedures may be prolonged and require general anesthesia with endotracheal intubation. The anesthesiologist should be prepared for aneurysmal subarachnoid hemorrhage (SAH) spontaneously or as a result of intravascular manipulations. Occlusive complications may also develop, requiring additional maneuvers to enhance CBF and initiate revascularization. In the setting of an aneurysm, hemodynamic manipulation, either for ischemic or hemorrhagic complications, has to be rigorously controlled. Unlike surgical clipping, aneurysm occlusion and thrombosis may be ongoing immediately following endovascular interventions, therefore careful attention to

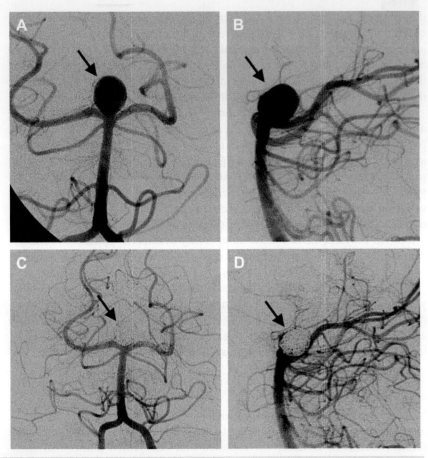

Fig. 4. A 59-year-old woman complained of severe headache and became unconscious. Angiography revealed a large basilar tip aneurysm (*arrows*); (A) Anterior-posterior image; (B) lateral images. Complete aneurysm embolization was achieved with Guglielmi detachable coil (GDC) embolization under general anesthesia; (C) anterior-posterior; (D) lateral images.

postprocedure blood pressure control remains critical, especially in patients presenting with SAH.

Angioplasty
Mechanical angioplasty or pharmacologic dilation may be indicated for vasospasm after SAH and for atherosclerotic cerebrovascular disease.

Angioplasty for cerebral vasospasm is usually undertaken in patients who, despite maximum medical management, continue to have ischemic neurologic symptoms. These patients are often in extremis and are therefore frequently intubated, receiving vasopressor agents, and have either an external ventricular drain or other intracranial pressure monitoring devices in place. Angiography is first undertaken to demonstrate that there is a significant degree of spasm in large proximal vessels (anterior, middle, and posterior cerebral arteries). A balloon catheter is guided under fluoroscopy into the spastic segment and inflated to distend the constricted area mechanically. If deliberate hypertension is being used to ameliorate a focal neurologic deficit before angioplasty, after angiographic demonstration of a significantly widened spastic segment, blood pressure should be reduced to the normal range.

Pharmacologic dilation is also used for the treatment of cerebral vasospasm by direct intra-arterial injection of vasodilators under fluoroscopic guidance. Originally described for papaverine, the use of vasodilators has now expanded to more frequent use of calcium channel blockers such as verapamil and nicardipine. The anesthesiologist should monitor for systemic side effects of these agents during recirculation, such as hypotension and bradycardia with calcium channel blockers (Fig. 5).

Angioplasty for atherosclerosis

At present, patients with high risk factors for carotid endarterectomy are considered favorable candidates for cervical carotid angioplasty and stenting (CAS; SAPPHIRE Trial). Studies evaluating the safety and efficacy of carotid stenting in traditional low-risk patients are ongoing (CREST), with encouraging preliminary results. These patients generally require balloon dilatation and placement of a vascular stent. In many cases, the placement of a cerebro-protective device may be used to decrease the risk of distal thromboembolism. Angioplasty of the ICA is usually undertaken with minimal sedation. General anesthesia is required for treating segments of intracranial arteries.

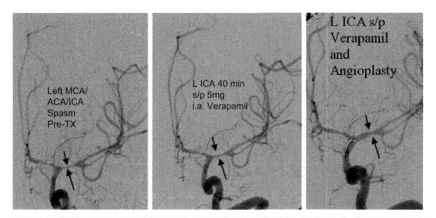

Fig. 5. A 29-year-old woman with right posterior communicating artery aneurysm that was treated with coil embolization 7 days after SAH developed new-onset aphasia and right-sided weakness. Angiography revealed a severe vasospasm in the left ICA, MCA, and anterior cerebral artery (ACA). It was treated with a combination of verapamil and balloon angioplasty under general anesthesia, with good clinical response. Arrows show change in diameter of the M-1 segment of the MCA in response to verapamil and balloon angioplasty.

Intracranial angioplasty and stenting procedures for atherosclerosis have a higher level of risk secondary to the inherently more delicate nature of intracranial vessels. Intracranial arteries have thinner media, therefore are more prone to dissection, or perforation. The selection of anesthetic techniques also depends on the patient's medical condition, his or her ability to cooperate during the procedure, or if there is an anticipated technical difficulty in negotiating the stenosed segment. Deliberate hypertension might be required for augmenting collateral blood flow. Considerations for general anesthesia are similar to those for carotid endarterectomy. A range of antiplatelet drugs are now available to prevent stroke and consolidate the results of therapeutic interventions (Table 5).

Thrombolysis for acute stroke

It is possible to recanalize the occluded vessel in acute thromboembolic stroke by mechanical means or by superselective intra-arterial delivery of thrombolytic agents such as rTPA, streptokinase, or urokinase (Table 6). Significant improvements in neurologic outcomes have been demonstrated if pharmacologic thrombolysis is completed within 6 hours of the onset of ischemic symptoms (PROACT II), or if mechanical thrombolysis is performed within 8 hours (MERCI trial). Mechanical means of clot retrieval, balloon angioplasty, and laser ablation are also being developed. These methods can rapidly restore arterial flow in contrast to intra-arterial thrombolysis, which may require up to 2 hours. In the vertebrobasilar circulation, treatment may be effective if delayed as long as 24 hours from the onset of symptoms. The main risk of intra-arterial thrombolysis is hemorrhagic conversion of ischemic infarcts, which has a high mortality.

Anesthetic considerations in these patients include those for the elderly and for patients with widespread arterial disease. Patients with acute thromboembolic stroke are spontaneously hypertensive and, in the face of nonhemorrhagic focal neurologic deficits, should not have their blood pressure aggressively treated. After clot lysis, blood pressure should be maintained in the normal range and, ideally, titrated to some index of CBF to prevent hyperperfusion injury.

TREATMENT OF OTHER CNS VASCULAR MALFORMATIONS

Dural AVMs

Dural AVMs induce venous hypertension and, when cortical venous drainage is involved, may cause intracranial hemorrhage. Multiple intracranial and extracranial arteries may feed them, and multistage embolization is usually performed. SAFE is usually performed, as in the case of intracranial AVMs. Transarterial NBCA embolization is a commonly used technique, as is transvenous coil occlusion of pathologic venous pouches.

Carotid cavernous fistulae

Skull base trauma is the most common cause of carotid cavernous fistula. Traumatic fistulae can also occur between the vertebral artery and the paravertebral

Table 5
Antiplatelet drugs

	Aspirin	Clopidogrel (Plavix)	Antiplatelet Antibodies (Abciximab)
Mechanism of action	Inhibition of prostaglandin synthesis by cyclo-oxygenase inhibition	Prevent ADP binding to glycoprotein receptor IIb and IIIa, inhibiting platelet activation	Antibody to glycoprotein receptor IIb and IIIa
Dose	50–325 mg/d	300 mg loading dose +75 mg/d	0.15–0.25 mg/kg, followed by an infusion 0.125 mg/kg/min
Half-life	1–2 h	Rapidly metabolized, main metabolite has elimination half-life of 8 h	10–30 min
Correction strategy	Platelet transfusion	Withhold for at least 5–7 days, platelet transfusions	Platelet transfusion
Contraindication	Renal and hepatic failure, drug interactions	Allergic reactions	Allergic reactions

veins. Such arteriovenous fistulae can lead to chronic hypotension of the surrounding normal vascular territories. Treatment may include transarterial detachable balloon occlusion or transvenous occlusion of the involved cavernous sinus. Their obliteration might result in normal perfusion-pressure breakthrough. Therefore, after obliteration of these lesions the blood pressure should be maintained at 10% to 20% below the patient's normal pressure.

Vein of galen malformation

These are uncommon, but complicated, lesions that usually present in infancy and childhood. These patients may have congestive heart failure, intractable seizures, hydrocephalus, and mental retardation. Several approaches have been attempted, including transarterial and transvenous methods. Concerns during general anesthesia for INR therapy are the same as for surgical treatment. In the setting of congestive heart failure, pre-existing right-to-left shunts, and pulmonary hypertension, a small glue embolus can be fatal.

Table 6
Antithrombolytic therapy

	Prourokinase	Tissue Plasminogen Activator (TPA) Alteplase	Reteplase	Streptokinase[a]
Mechanism of action (specific features)	Plasminogen activation	Activates fibrin associated plasminogen (527 amino acids)	Activates fibrin associated plasminogen (355 amino acids)	Forms activator complex with plasminogen
Dose[b]	4 mg in clot, 2–8 mg/h	0.05 mg/kg/h	5 units, 0.5–1 units/h infusion	1–1.5 million U/60 min
Half-life (min)	11–16	4–6	15	10–20
Antidote	Amicar	Amicar	Amicar	Amicar
Contraindication	Allergic reaction	Allergic reaction	Allergic reaction	Allergic reaction

[a]Not available in the United States.
[b]Doses vary based on route and clinical circumstances.

Intra-arterial chemotherapy and embolization of tumors

Endovascular surgery for the treatment of brain tumors has made little progress in the last decade. The exception, perhaps, is preoperative embolization before surgical resection, as a means of decreasing blood loss for vascular intracranial or spinal tumors. Superselective administration of chemotherapeutic agents can be used for treating neoplasms refractory to conventional treatment, and a variety of germ cell tumors and CNS lymphomas respond well to intra-arterial chemotherapy. However, the inability of most chemotherapeutic drugs to penetrate the blood-brain barrier limits the use of intra-arterial drug treatments. Disruption of the blood-brain barrier with intra-arterial injection of mannitol is often undertaken. Because of the pain and potential neurologic complications, the procedure is undertaken under general anesthesia. Intravenous atropine is sometimes given to increase cardiac output and thereby blood flow to the brain. To test for the effectiveness of the procedure, radiocontrast and computed tomography (CT) imaging may be undertaken after the procedure, and hence the anesthetized patient might have to be transported from the angiographic to the CT scan room. Complications of blood-brain barrier disruption include focal and generalized seizures, arrythmias, postoperative nausea and vomiting, transient neurologic deficits, and, rarely, significant brain edema.

Vertebral body compression fracture therapy

Vertebroplasty and kyphoplasty procedures involve the intravertebral body administration of acrylic bone cement compounds via a percutaneous, often transpedicular, approach. Many of these patients report significant pain relief following these procedures. The demographics of this population (elderly, frail, osteoporotic) and prone positioning require extra care during the preparation process. Most of these procedures can be performed, and are well tolerated, with mild sedation (Fig. 6).

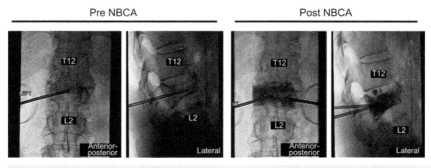

Fig. 6. A 65-year-old man with Parkinson disease fell while climbing rocks on a beach. Investigations revealed increased uptake of isotope on bone scan and a collapsed L1 vertebra. He complained of intractable pain in the upper lumbar region that was refractory to oral narcotics. Percutaneous vertebroplasty with NBCA glue was successfully undertaken to alleviate the pain.

SUMMARY

INR procedures offer a new approach to several intracranial and spinal diseases. To some extent, the risk/benefit ratio of INR procedures remains to be elucidated against traditional surgical approaches. Anesthetic management of these lesions, although similar to traditional operative approaches, is beset with hazards and requires careful management.

Acknowledgments

We thank Ms. Mei Wang, MPH, Staff Researcher, and Cryus Mintz, MD, Resident, Department of Anesthesiology, for their help in preparing this manuscript.

Suggested Readings

Pile-Spellman J, Young WL, Hacein-Bey L. Perspectives on interventional neuroradiology. In: Maciunas RJ, editor. Endovascular neurological intervention. Park Ridge (IL): AANS; 1995. p. 279–84.

Young WL, Pile-Spellman J, Hacein-Bey L, et al. Invasive neuroradiologic procedures for cerebrovascular abnormalities: anesthetic considerations. Anesthesiol Clin North America 1997;15(3):631–53.

Duong H, Hacein-Bey L, Vang MC, et al. Management of cerebral arterial occlusion during endovascular treatment of cerebrovascular disease. In: Donals S, Zornow MH, editors. Problems in anesthesia: controversies in neuroanesthesia. Philadelphia: Lippencott Raven; 1997. p. 99–111.

Schell RM, Cole DJ. Cerebral protection and neuroanesthesia. Anesthesiol Clin North America 1992;10:453–69.

Young WL, Pile-Spellman J. Anesthetic considerations for interventional neuroradiology [review]. Anesthesiology 1994;80:427–56.

ISAT investigators ISAT investigators. International Subarachnoid Aneurysm Trial (ISAT) of neurosurgical clipping versus endovascular coiling in 2143 patients with ruptured intracranial aneurysms: a randomised trial. Lancet 2002;360:1267–74.

Gobin YP, Starkman S, Duckwiler GR, et al. MERCI 1: a phase 1 study of mechanical embolus removal in cerebral ischemia. Stroke 2004;35(12):2848–54.

Yadav JS, Wholey MH, Kuntz RE, , et alStenting and Angioplasty with Protection in Patients at High Risk for Endarterectomy Investigators. Protected carotid-artery stenting versus endarterectomy in high-risk patients. N Engl J Med 2004;351(15):1493–501.

Joshi S, Ornstein EO, Bruce JN. Targeting the brain. J Neurocritcal Care 2007;6(3):200–12.

Joshi S, Meyers PM, Ornstein EO. Intracarotid drug delivery: the pitfalls and the potentials [review]. Anesthesiology 2008;109(3):543–64.

Advances in Anesthesia 27 (2009) 25–54

ELSEVIER
MOSBY

ADVANCES IN ANESTHESIA

Perioperative Management of the Opioid-Tolerant Patient

Christopher Viscomi, MD[a,b,*], Jared K. Pearson, MD[c]

[a]Department of Anesthesiology, University of Vermont/Fletcher Allen Healthcare, ACC WP2 GME, 111 Colchester Avenue, Burlington, VT 05401, USA
[b]Acute Pain Service, University of Vermont/Fletcher Allen Healthcare, ACC WP2 GME, 111 Colchester Avenue, Burlington, VT 05401, USA
[c]Virginia Mason Medical Center, Graduate Medical Education, H8-925 Seneca Street, Seattle, WA 98101, USA

There is no symptom more treated in the history of medicine than pain. As early as 3400 BC, the Sumerian civilization in Mesopotamia cultivated the opium poppy, and 2000 BC writings indicate that doctors crushed opium pods into sap, mixing several concoctions to treat a variety of ailments including pain. Further extraction and purification of opium eventually led to the isolation of morphine to aid in the treatment of pain [1]. In modern medicine, acute or chronic pain is the chief complaint in nearly 80% of outpatient physician visits, representing the primary reason why Americans visit their doctor [2,3]. Furthermore, it is believed that the economic burden of pain in the United States alone is as high as $100 billion per year [2]. Of course, the problem of pain is not unique to North America. According to a recent meta-analysis of international studies, the prevalence of chronic pain in adults is greater than 10% [4]. Perhaps for this reason some physicians have called modern health care an epidemic of pain [5,6].

In efforts to improve the treatment of pain, the American Pain Society (APS) began in 1995 to develop guidelines for the assessment and recording of pain [7]. In James Campbell's 1996 APS presidential address, he stated that "If pain were assessed with the same zeal as other vital signs are, it would have a much better chance of being treated properly [8]." Such sentiments led to the "Pain as the Fifth Vital Sign" movement, originally coined by the Veteran's Health Administration in 1999, and paved the way for the establishment of pain measurement standards [9]. Standardized pain scoring systems were fully implemented by the Joint Commission for Accreditation of Health Organizations (now named The Joint Commission) in 2001 [10].

*Corresponding author. Department of Anesthesiology, University of Vermont/Fletcher Allen Healthcare, ACC WP2 GME, 111 Colchester Avenue, Burlington, VT 05401. E-mail address: christopher.viscomi@vtmednet.org (C. Viscomi).

0737-6146/09/$ – see front matter
doi:10.1016/j.aan.2009.07.004

Opiates have been a mainstay in pain management from ancient through modern times. As the most commonly prescribed class of medication, it is estimated that the prevalence of opiate use is as high as 4.9%, and that 2.7% of Americans use opiates chronically [11–13]. The incidence of opioid use in patients presenting for surgery is undoubtedly higher than in the general population. The number of opioid prescriptions per year has more than doubled since the years just before the "Pain as the Fifth vital sign" era. However, treating pain in this way has not come without personal and societal risks. Opiates have many common side effects, such as nausea and constipation, and more serious consequences such as respiratory depression. Over time, opioids become less effective, and some patients become more pain sensitive. Addiction is a well-recognized risk of long-term use. As a result of the myriad of opioid ill effects, many practitioners have begun to question if the fifth vital sign's mandate of more aggressive use of opioids to control pain has actually caused more harm than good [14,15].

As alluded to in the previous paragraph, intermediate- or long-term opiate use may also paradoxically cause pain, termed opioid-induced hyperalgesia (OIH). Given the widespread use and reliance of opioids for pain control, the existence of OIH has a profound impact on the current practice of anesthesia and perioperative pain control. To discuss its impact, this article briefly reviews concepts of nociception, compares and contrasts OIH with opiate tolerance, and discusses the literature from animal and human studies to aid in a better understanding of OIH. In addition, the authors explore adjunctive therapies to aid the anesthesiologist in treating acute pain in the opioid-tolerant individual, and provide several case examples to reinforce the information and suggest treatment regimens.

NOCICEPTION: A NEUROANATOMICAL REVIEW

The process of nociception involves 4 basic components: nociceptors (transduction and conduction), ascending nociceptive tracts (transmission), central nervous system (CNS) higher centers (pain interpretation), and descending systems (modulation or facilitation) (Fig. 1). In response to mechanical, thermal, or other noxious stimuli, sufficient nociceptor activation generates an action potential conducted along thinly myelinated Aδ fibers, or along unmyelinated C fibers to the dorsal horn of the spinal cord. These nociceptive afferent signals then undergo continued processing and modulation through multiple mechanisms while ascending the spinal cord to the thalamus and other higher centers for interpretation.

Mechanisms of modulation can be classified as pronociceptive or antinociceptive [16]. Antinociception dampens the incoming pain signals through local and distal inhibitory pathways. On the other hand, pronociception heightens the body's awareness to pain in an effort to reduce further potential tissue damage, and may include central and peripheral sensitization. Each of these processes can involve temporary or permanent neuronal changes, termed "plasticity," as the nociceptive system adapts to the environment [17].

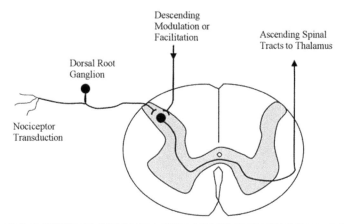

Fig. 1. Afferent signals from peripheral stimuli undergo modulation and processing, often by descending pathways, before ascending to supraspinal structures.

Analgesia can be achieved by increasing antinociceptive or decreasing pronociceptive mechanisms at various locations along the nociceptive pathway. Opioids, for example, activate μ-opiate receptors, which decrease nociceptive signal transduction and neurotransmitter release. However, the pain signaling mechanisms are not static. The use of opioids to treat pain will eventually alter pain processing, and may shift the overall impact of opioids from anti- to pronociceptive.

TOLERANCE AND HYPERALGESIA

It is well understood that with repeated use, the opioid effect will be of lesser magnitude. This phenomenon is termed "tolerance." These time- and dose-related analgesic effects may be caused by cellular changes, resulting in increased drug elimination or reduced activation of antinociceptive pathways. This resulting rightward shift in the opioid analgesia dose-response curve may be addressed by increasing the dose of the opiate to once again obtain adequate pain relief (Fig. 2) [18].

In addition to tolerance, persistent pain with opioid therapy can also result from sensitization of pronociceptive pathways, known as opioid-induced hyperalgesia [19]. This results in a downward shift in the dose-response curve. The distinction between the two is important because unlike tolerance, hyperalgesia can be exacerbated by increasing opioid consumption. Therefore, some investigators have offered recommendations to assist the physician in distinguishing between the two clinically [20,21]. Hyperalgesia pain, unlike tolerance, in comparison to preexisting pain may be characterized by

(a) Increased intensity in the absence of worsening disease progression
(b) Poorly defined quality and location

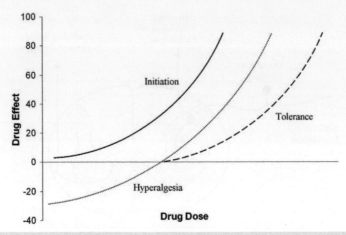

Fig. 2. Opioid analgesia dose-response curves at drug initiation (*solid line*), and after the development of tolerance (*hashed line*) or hyperalgesia (*gray line*).

    (c) Changed threshold, tolerability, and pattern of distribution
    (d) Worsened pain following trial of dose escalation

In addition, Table 1 illustrates a few simple questions that may alert the clinician to consider the possibility of OIH.

OPIOID-INDUCED HYPERALGESIA: ESSENTIALS OF CURRENT KNOWLEDGE
Opioid-induced hyperalgesia in animal studies
Many rodent studies report the existence of OIH and attempt to characterize it. The following review of animal studies is not intended to be exhaustive, but to provide the reader with an overview of past and current areas of focus. Most studies have attempted to further define OIH by investigating the pain stimulus type (ie, mechanical, thermal, or chemical), the time course for development and resolution of OIH depending on varying dosing schedule, or the specific receptors and neuroanatomical structures purportedly involved in OIH development.

Table 1
Screening questions when considering the possibility of opioid-induced hyperalgesia

1	Has my patient ever used opiates for an extended period of time?
2	Has the pain changed in quality, location, or pattern of distribution since being treated with opiates?
3	Has the original pain become more intense with no explanation of worsening disease?
4	Is my patient experiencing intense pain despite a routine surgical procedure?
5	Has the pain become acutely worsened following an opioid dose increase?
6	Are activities previously tolerated since using opioids now causing the patient new pain?

OIH in animal studies: type of pain stimulus

Many studies investigate the existence of OIH by varying the type of pain stimulus. Most studies are based on behavioral models of pain, such as rat-tail flick when exposed to heat or cold, or hind paw withdrawal in mechanical pain models using hind-paw pressure or incision. Less common are studies that use chemical or electrical pain stimuli. A recent systematic review of the literature suggests that rats are more susceptible to mechanical pain than thermal stimuli [19].

Opioid-induced hyperalgesia in animal studies: time course and dosing regimen

The development of OIH when exposed to single, continuous, or intermittent dosing of opioids has been an area of extensive investigation (Table 2). A recent literature review summarizes that rats exposed to a dose of opioids usually demonstrate antinociception followed often by a period of mechanical hyperalgesia that can last for 2 to 3 hours [19]. Other studies using high-dose fentanyl before hind-paw mechanical or chemical-induced pain demonstrate periods of hyperalgesia lasting several days [22,23]. Because it seems that the duration of acute OIH may be dose dependent, others have studied how dosing regimens affect the occurrence of OIH with continuous or prolonged opioid administration. These studies often report a short period of antinociception, followed by mechanical and thermal hyperalgesia throughout ongoing opioid administration [24–26]. Angst and Clark [19] noted that the time course for hyperalgesia resolution is similar to that for its development. A recent study by Zissen and colleagues [27] further attempted to characterize whether the dosing schedule and the development of OIH is dependent on rat developmental age. Zissen and colleagues [27] report that thermal hyperalgesia and mechanical hyperalgesia were observed only in young rats exposed to intermittent and continuous dosing, respectively, and postulate that age of exposure and drug schedule are important factors in the development of hyperalgesia.

These apparent changes in pain sensitization may also last well beyond the period of exposure and recovery. Celerier and colleagues [28] reported that rats, having appeared to recover from the hyperalgesic effects, once again develop hyperalgesia when given a single bolus of either an opiate agonist or antagonist. Perhaps animals that recover from the initial hyperalgesia retain some hyperalgesia memory, given that OIH quickly recurs following agonist or antagonist administration [19].

Table 2
Summary of animal studies: time course and dose schedule

1	Degree of OIH and time to resolution is dose dependent
2	Other factors may include age and dosing schedule (single, intermittent, continuous)
3	"Memory" of prior OIH episodes can occur and be once again precipitated by opiate agonist or antagonist administration

Abbreviation: OIH, opioid-induced hyperalgesia.

Opioid-induced hyperalgesia in animal studies: neuroanatomical structures and receptors

Peripheral mechanisms

There is a great deal of recent investigative work centered on peripheral mechanisms of opioid effects (Table 3). Previous studies seem to demonstrate that neuronal changes related to m-agonist mechanical hyperalgesia are mediated by peripheral G protein and protein kinase C (PKC) cellular mechanisms [29–31]. A more recent study looking at the peripheral milieu following hind paw incision observes that higher levels of inflammatory cytokines and chemokines (interleukin [IL]-1β, IL-6, granulocyte colony-stimulating factor, tumor necrosis factor-α, and keratinocyte chemoattractant) are present with escalating doses of systemic morphine. The investigators report that pentoxifylline administration, which is believed to attenuate cytokine release, decreased local incisional cytokine levels and decreased OIH [32].

Other investigators have examined specific pain receptor types. For example, given evidence that opiates may induce thermal hyperalgesia, Vardanyan and colleagues recently used gene knockout methods to explore the role of the transient receptor potential vanilloid 1 (TRPV1) receptor, a nociceptor believed to be responsible for noxious heat transmission. These investigators report that morphine elicits thermal and mechanical hyperalgesia in wild-type mice, but not TRPV1 receptor knockout mice. Furthermore, immunohistochemical analysis of TRPV1 labeling in the dorsal root ganglion of morphine rats shows increased signal intensity [33]. These findings suggest that TRPV1 receptors may play an important role in OIH.

A new and robust method for discovering the genetic underpinnings of disease is called in silico genetic analysis. In silico methods use computational algorithms to compare a phenotypic trait (such as OIH) with minor variations

Table 3
Opioid-induced hyperalgesia in animal studies: neuroanatomical structure and receptor

Peripheral	– G-proteins and PKC
	– Inflammatory cytokines (IL-1β, IL-6, G-CSF, TNF-α, KC)
	– TRPV1 receptor
	– β2 adrenergic receptor
	– Glycoprotein Abcb1b
Neuraxial	– NMDA receptor
	– PKC
	–Cytokines—IL-1, NK-1
	–Calcium channels
Supraspinal	– Thalamus
	Ventrolateral orbital complex
	Submedial nucleus
	– Amygdala and c-Fos expression
	– CCK and rostral ventral medulla

Abbreviations: CCK, cholecystokinin; G-CSF, granulocyte colony-stimulating factor; IL, interleukin; KC, keratinocyte chemoattractant, NK, neurokinin, NMDA, N-methyl-D-aspartate; PKC, protein kinase C; TNF, tumor necrosis factor; TRPV, transient receptor potential vanilloid.

in related gene alleles (single nucleotide polymorphisms, or SNPs) across different mouse strains to determine associations much more quickly than traditional molecular biology techniques. For example, previous studies suggest that peripheral β2-adrenergic receptor (β2-AR) stimulation is related to hyperaglesia [34]. Using in silico methodology in sixteen different mouse strains, Liang and colleagues identified different haplotypes (possible combinations of SNPs in gene alleles) that encode the β2-AR, and determined which haplotypes were causative in OIH. These investigators demonstrated mechanical OIH, and dose-dependent reversal, by locally injecting the β2-AR antagonist butoxamine [35]. Powerful use of this in silico technique additionally suggests an association between OIH and Abcb1b, a specific glycoprotein drug transporting gene [36]. Discoveries from these sophisticated methods suggest that OIH is predictable given a particular genetic screen. Application of these specific genetic techniques to humans may accurately predict individuals who are more susceptible to developing OIH.

Neuraxial mechanisms
Given that much of the pain modulation occurs in the spinal cord, many studies have focused on this area. One of the first spinal cord studies by Mao and colleagues [37] discovered that excitatory neurotransmitter systems and the dorsal horn *N*-methyl-D-aspartate (NMDA) receptors play an important role in the development of OIH. A recent study using remifentanil measured a dose-dependent increase in NMDA receptor current from cultured rat dorsal root ganglion. These currents were attenuated by naloxone. Mao and colleagues report that these currents are inducible by activation of δ-opioid receptors alone, and suggest that selective inhibition of δ receptors might prevent OIH [38]. NMDA receptor activation is consistent with data that suggest its role in spinal cord windup and potentiation with long-term opiate use. Furthermore, the NMDA receptor antagonist ketamine has been shown to prevent spinal cord windup [39]. In addition, PKC plays an important role in spinal cord potentiation, as rats lacking the PKC-γ gene do not seem to develop OIH [40,41]. Cytokines, such as IL-1 and neurokinin-1 (NK-1), also seem to be involved in OIH development [42]. A recent study found that mechanical and thermal hypersensitivity was prevented in rats by spinal dorsal horn ablation of NK-1 expressing cells [43]. Finally, voltage-gated calcium channels may also be involved as administration of gabapentin in fentanyl rats seems to prevent the development of OIH [44].

Supraspinal mechanisms
Several investigators are examining supraspinal mechanisms involved in OIH. Various opiate receptors located in the ventrolateral orbital complex [45] and submedian nucleus of the thalamus [46] have been implicated. In addition, c-fos expression in the amygdala has been found to be induced by morphine, and reduced or blocked by naloxone [47]. Finally, it is believed that prolonged opiate exposure enhances neurotransmitter cholecystokinin (CCK) effects on descending pathways from the rostral ventral medulla, resulting in increased

pronociception and diminished antinociception [21]. These studies suggest that supraspinal areas may be involved in long-term or more permanent changes relating to hyperalgesia following chronic opiate use.

Opioid-induced hyperalgesia in humans: methods and settings of evaluation

Unlike laboratory animal models, which measure nociceptive changes in controlled settings, human studies are more variable and subjective. However, a strong body of evidence is developing that allows for better characterization of hyperalgesia in humans. Methods to evoke and study pain and hyperalgesia in humans similarly include thermal (cold pressor and heat), electrical, and mechanical models. In a cold pressor test, a participant submerges his or her hand up to the wrist in a continuously circulating bucket of ice water. The time the patient first reports pain is recorded as latency to pain onset (threshold), and tolerance is defined by measuring the time until the patient withdraws the hand. At the time of withdrawal, a numerical pain scale is used to measure pain intensity [48]. For heat pain, a temperature probe placed on the participant's arm raises the temperature 1°C per second with a preset upper limit to prevent damage, and heat pain threshold is measured and intensity reported [49]. For electrical stimulation tests, an electrical impulse can be transmitted through the ear lobe with incrementally increasing voltage [50]. Finally, for mechanical pain assessment the von Frey hairs test is frequently used, whereby a calibrated and graduated force is applied to a sensory field until a patient reports pain. Whereas an in-depth discussion of the limitations of such methods is beyond the scope of this review, much of what the authors know regarding OIH in humans is derived from these experimental designs.

In addition to varying experimental designs, there are differences in patient populations that participate in opioid therapy research. In particular, research evaluating hyperalgesia in humans can be categorized into 3 broad subpopulations: chronic opiate users, perioperative opiate exposure, and opiate-naïve patients who receive opiates followed by pain testing.

Opioid-induced hyperalgesia in humans: chronic opiate users

Many investigators study pain sensitivity in former opiate addicts who are maintained on methadone therapy versus former opiate addicts not taking methadone (Table 4). Methadone is relatively novel as an opioid: in addition to opiate receptor binding, NMDA receptors are also moderately bound. Given the NMDA receptor's role in attenuating OIH, it was believed that patients on methadone may be more resistant to OIH. Indeed, in several case reports of purported OIH, patients demonstrate improvements when switched to methadone [51,52]. However, there seems to be pain hypersensitivity differences in these 2 groups depending on the type of pain stimulus. For example, although there seems to be no increased pain sensitivity to electrical [53] or mechanical stimulation [54], several studies suggest that former addicts on methadone seem to be more sensitive to cold pressor pain than former addicts not taking

Table 4	
Summary of opioid-induced hyperalgesia in humans: chronic opiate population	
1	Patients on methadone for opiate addiction may be more susceptible to cold unpleasantness rather than pain intensity compared with former addicts not maintained on methadone
2	OIH is manifested differently in patients on methadone for opiate addition versus methadone for chronic pain
3	These differences may be explained by altered dopamine receptor alleles in former opiate addicts
4	Patients on methadone for chronic pain may experience altered pain modulation and mechanical pain

methadone [50,53,55]. These studies are cross-sectional and not prospective, therefore it is difficult to establish cause and effect.

A recent prospective study evaluated cold pressor pain in opiate addicts undergoing 4-week detoxification versus controls. Although the investigators reported no significant differences along the different time points, and that unexpectedly the opiate addicts had a higher pain threshold and lower reported intensity, opiate users were less tolerant to cold pressor testing [48]. Commenting on these mixed results, some believe that in this subpopulation of patients, perhaps the unpleasantness of cold pain becomes exaggerated and not the actual intensity [56].

This theory may be related to the findings by Pud and colleagues, who report no statistical cold pressor difference between opiate and nonopiate patients with chronic pain. Instead, they suggest that chronic oral opiate use seems to alter pain modulation. Study participants underwent baseline heat stimulation, then repeated heat testing with a concurrent cold-conditioning stimulus in the opposite hand. Minimal variation from baseline with the additional cold stimulus was defined as diffuse noxious inhibitory control (DNIC). Pud and colleagues found a significant decrease in DNIC in opiate users compared with nonopiate users. Of note, a subset analysis found statistical significance in men only [57].

These studies may simply point out the different manifestations of OIH in humans receiving opiates to control addiction versus those taking opiates for chronic pain. For example, despite a lack of evidence for mechanical hyperalgesia in the former opiate addict population, a recent study found that compared with controls, in the chronic pain population opioid dose and duration correlates with increased pain intensity and unpleasantness following lidocaine injection before a regional procedure [58]. Even more compelling data are genetic studies that suggest possible differences in these populations, and therefore may explain different results in these groups. For example, it seems that the same dopamine receptor allele genes related to becoming an opiate addict may actually be associated with an elevation in cold pain thresholds and reduced pain sensitivity [59].

Opioid-induced hyperalgesia in humans: perioperative exposure

The existence of OIH has many implications in patients undergoing surgery (Table 5). In many studies, however, it may be difficult to differentiate between analgesic tolerance and OIH, as most of the data are derived from recorded postoperative opiate consumption and subjective pain scores, which can be influenced by either. For example, patients who received fentanyl intraoperatively were found to have increased postoperative opioid consumption without improved analgesia [60]. More convincing of hyperalgesia, however, is that an apparent fentanyl-induced postoperative consumption increase could be diminished if ketamine or lornoxicam (nonsteroidal anti-inflammatory) was also administered [61].

A similar increase in postoperative opioid consumption was observed in patients receiving high-dose intraoperative remifentanil [62,63]. In these studies patients reported increased pain, peri-incisional wound allodynia, and hyperalgesia compared with low-dose groups, indicating perhaps more of a hyperalgesia than tolerance effect. Of note, however, there are some studies comparing high- and low-dose remifentanil that report no difference in pain sensitivity and opioid consumption [64,65]. The differences in results may be partially explained by variability in drug dosages used (0.3 mg/kg/min vs <0.23 mg/kg/min). No studies to date have used genetic modeling among the study participants to determine associations between genetic characteristics and OIH or tolerance.

Opioid-induced hyperalgesia in humans: pain testing opiate-naïve individuals following acute opiate exposure

There is increasing evidence documenting hyperalgesia in previously opiate-naïve patients who undergo pain testing following acute opiate exposure, although many studies are limited by small sample size (Table 6). The preponderance of evidence suggests that acute exposure to opiates induces cold, mechanical, electrical, and chemical pain hypersensitivity [49,66–69]. One example of the literature in this area is a prospective study assessing tolerance and hyperalgesia following 1 month of oral morphine in 6 patients with chronic back pain. Of note, the median dosage was 75 mg of morphine daily, and 2 of the participants were on 15 to 30 mg daily for longer than 6 weeks before the beginning of the study. Despite the study limitations, the results suggest that oral morphine use may lead to the development of cold, but not heat,

Table 5
Summary of opioid-induced hyperalgesia in human studies: perioperative exposure

1	Intraoperative opiate exposure may result in increased wound allodynia, and postoperative opiate consumption without improved analgesia
2	This increase may be attenuated with multimodal therapy (such as ketamine or NSAIDs)
3	Presence of OIH with remifentanil may be dose dependent

Table 6	
Summary of opioid-induced hyperalgesia in human studies: pain testing	
1	Acute exposure to opiate-naïve induces cold, mechanical, electrical, and chemical pain hypersensitivity
2	Oral morphine may be associated with cold pain hyperalgesia
3	Remifentanil induces mechanical hyperalgesia that may be attenuated by multimodal therapy (ie, ketamine or clonidine)

hyperalgesia [49]. This study also supports previous data suggesting the presence of cold pain hyperalgesia with withdrawal following induction of acute opioid dependence [70].

Studies looking at mechanical, electrical, and chemical pain often use remifentanil in the study methodology. Remifentanil is useful because it can be reliably administered to maintain target receptor concentrations of the drug, and elimination of remifentanil is extremely rapid. A recent double-blind, placebo-controlled study suggested that short-term administration of clinically useful remifentanil doses is not associated with development of significant analgesic tolerance [71]. This finding may therefore aid investigators in looking for hyperalgesic effects without the confounding effects of tolerance. A strong double-blind, randomized, crossover, and placebo-controlled study suggests remifentanil induces mechanical hyperalgesia. Following a 90-minute remifentanil infusion, skin areas of mechanical hyperalgesia were significantly enlarged. Furthermore, this study is congruent with prior animal studies in suggesting that the mechanism of hyperalgesia is related to the NMDA receptor, as coadministration of ketamine prevented pain area enlargement [66]. Another study indicates that whereas ketamine may prevent hyperalgesia when defined as an enlarged area of pain, clonidine actually decreases hyperalgesia defined by pain ratings [67]. These data, together, suggest the need for a multimodal approach to achieve better pain control and prevent opioid-induced hyperalgesia.

MULTIMODAL ANALGESIA
The "concept" of multimodal analgesia has become a mainstream clinical practice [72], and is essential to the care of the opioid-tolerant patient. The pharmacologic underpinnings of this technique involve attacking pain signaling at as many different neuroanatomic locations as possible (Table 7). This method should decrease the dependence of the patient on opioids for acute pain control in the perioperative period. In addition, it is theorized that lower doses of several nonopioid analgesics are less likely to cause toxicity than high doses of opioids used alone.

It is important to implement multimodal analgesia before the surgical trauma if at all possible. At the University of Vermont, the authors' perioperative protocols for total joint arthroplasty, major spine surgery, and major colorectal surgery all involve initiation of analgesic clinical pathways several hours before

Table 7
Analgesics and sites of action

Acetaminophen	Suppresses peripheral PGE2 release and IL formation; CNS: binds cannabinoid-1 receptor
NSAIDs	COX inhibition with decreased PGE2 centrally and peripherally
Ketamine, memantine, dextromethorphan	Inhibits glutamate binding of NMDA receptors in dorsal horn of spinal cord
Gabapentinoids	Locus coeruleus (brainstem): enhanced descending inhibitory pathways; spinal and afferent peripheral nerves: α2 subunits of calcium channels
Dexamethasone	Decreased peripheral and central inflammatory mediators
Opioids	Peripheral: reduced Ca^{2+} entry into primary nociceptive afferents; spinal cord: hyperpolarization of dorsal horn neurons; supraspinal: enhanced efferent inhibitory neuron activity
Tricyclic antidepressants	CNS: enhance descending inhibitory pathways via increased synaptic norepinephrine
Local anesthetics	Peripheral: decreased interleukin release; CNS: inhibition of DRG and frequency-dependent conduction

The concept of multimodal analgesia involves targeting multiple points of pain processing.
Abbreviation: DRG, dorsal root ganglion.

surgery (Table 8). This method enables dampening of the inflammatory surgical cascade, lower intraoperative opioid requirements, and a more subjectively comfortable patient on awakening from general anesthesia. In turn, these effects translate into real clinical benefits. At the authors' institution, after initiation of the analgesic pathway for total joint arthroplasty, a dramatic decrease in the need for parenteral opioids, earlier achievement of physical therapy goals, a decreased need for acute pain management consults, and a nearly 30% decrease in average hospital length of stay were realized (Table 9).

SPECIFIC AGENTS

Acetaminophen

Acetaminophen is often overlooked as a perioperative analgesic due to perceived weak analgesic effects; however, multiple studies have demonstrated a 25% to 35% decrease in opioid requirements when it is administered [73]. Acetaminophen's mechanism of action involves multiple sites of action, and it remains unclear which of these effects is quantitatively most important in human pain processing. Acetaminophen has peripheral effects, including suppression of peripheral prostaglandin E2 (PGE2) release and downregulation of inflammatory IL-2 production. Acetaminophen centrally activates

Table 8
Preoperative medications before major surgery

1–2 hours before surgery:
    Acetaminophen, 1000 mg PO
    Dexamethasone, 4–8 mg IV
    Celecoxib, 200 mg PO
    Gabapentin, 1200 mg PO
Before incision:
    Ketamine, 0.1–0.3 mg/kg IV
    Lidocaine, 1.5 mg/kg IV bolus, consider infusion for bowel resection cases
    Total joints: periarticular infiltration: ropivacaine, ketamine, epinephrine
Postsurgery:
    Gabapentin, 300 mg PO TID
    Acetaminophen, 1000 mg every 8 h PO or PR
    Celecoxib, 200 mg PO daily for up to 5 days
Total knee replacements: femoral nerve block: ropivacaine + clonidine

University of Vermont pain management pathways: common elements. Minor variations on this approach are used in lower extremity joint replacements, major spine surgery, and major intra-abdominal surgery.
Abbreviations: IV, intravenous; PO, by mouth; PR, per rectum; TID, three times per day.

cannabinoid-1 receptors and the serotonergic pathways, and decreases CNS cyclooxygenase-1 (COX-1) expression [74–76].

In comparison with nonsteroidal anti-inflammatory drugs (NSAIDs) and COX inhibitors, acetaminophen does not damage gastric mucosa, inhibit platelets, or trigger asthma in susceptible patients. However, acetaminophen can cause hepatotoxicity and rarely causes renal impairment. Hepatotoxicity with acetaminophen is typically noted with adult dosages exceeding 4 g/d, or in patients with significant preexisting or evolving liver disease. Caution should therefore be exercised in prescribing acetaminophen in patients with known or suspected liver disease (eg, alcohol abuse), in patients receiving medications noted for hepatotoxicity (eg, methotrexate), and suicidal patients. Acetaminophen can be administered by mouth or rectum and, outside of North America, intravenous paracetamol is available.

On a practical note, the authors have observed that acetaminophen is rarely administered by surgical ward nurses if it is ordered on a "prn" or as-needed

Table 9
Total joint arthroplasty pain pathway benefits

	Before pathway	After pathway
Systemic opioids on ward	89%	11%
Length of stay	3.5 days	2.6 days
Physical therapy goals achieved on postop day 1	36%	80%
Pain management consults/month	11	3

Benefits achieved with the University of Vermont total joint arthroplasty pain management pathway.

basis. The authors therefore order acetaminophen on a scheduled basis, most frequently 1 g every 8 hours.

Nonsteroidal anti-inflammatory drugs

Nonsteroidal anti-inflammatory drugs (NSAIDs) are a diverse group of medications that have in common inhibition of the cyclooxygenase (COX) enzyme, resulting in decreased production of PGE2. PGE2 causes inflammation and pain, and inhibition of PGE2 results in both central and peripheral anti-inflammatory and analgesic effects. NSAIDs have most commonly been used for joint and other musculoskeletal pain.

NSAIDs have been categorized as either nonselective COX inhibitors or COX-2 specific inhibitors. The COX-2 enzyme is primarily involved in inflammation, whereas the COX-1 enzyme is involved in gastric mucosal and platelet inhibitory side effects of NSAID therapy. The use of COX-2 selective NSAIDs did indeed lower the rate of gastrointestinal (GI) complications of NSAID therapy [77,78]. Unfortunately, the lack of antiplatelet effects of COX-2 inhibitors also resulted in an increase in acute thrombotic events, principally acute myocardial infarction and stroke. As a result of this increase in thrombotic events, most selective COX-2 inhibitors have been withdrawn from the U.S. market. Celecoxib remains available as a selective COX-2 inhibitor available for analgesic therapy.

There are several factors involved in the decision to employ NSAIDs (Tables 10 and 11). For nonselective COX inhibitors, the risk of GI toxicity merits consideration. According to the United States Food and Drug Administration (FDA) labeling guidelines, clinicians should be particularly cautious in patients with a history of ulcers or GI bleeding (10-fold increased risk), those taking other anticoagulants, tobacco or alcohol abuse, and those who are elderly.

Renal toxicity is another issue with NSAIDs, and both selective and nonselective NSAIDs place patients at risk. Renal toxicity results from decreased glomerular blood flow, and can cause acute tubular necrosis and inappropriate fluid retention. Risk factors for renal toxicity include preexisting renal dysfunction, old age, diabetes, and hypovolemia [79].

Table 10
Patients at high risk of gastrointestinal bleeding with nonselective COX inhibitors

Previous GI bleed or known ulcer (1000% increase in GI bleeding risk)
Smoking
Older age
Significant alcohol use
Oral steroid medications
Other anticoagulants being administered
High dose or long duration of NSAID therapy
Poor general health

Data from 2005 US Food and Drug Administration labeling template for class of drug.

Table 11 Risks of NSAID therapy	
Risk	Comments
Renal toxicity	Especially preexisting renal dysfunction, or hypovolemia
Surgical bleeding	Nonspecific COX inhibitors only
Asthma	With preexisting disease, nasal polyps
GI bleeding	See Table 10
Impaired bone healing	Controversial; consider in high nonunion rate surgery
Fluid retention	Especially elderly

An additional clinical controversy involves impaired bone healing. There is some evidence that orthopedic surgery patients treated with NSAIDs may have an increased risk of a fracture nonunion or failed spinal fusion surgery [80]. Although the literature is not complete, one group reported that the rate of nonunion in spinal fusion surgery is higher with nonselective COX inhibitors than with COX-2 inhibitors [81].

Individual NSAIDs (Table 12) do not seem to have significant differences in analgesic efficacy; all seem to be effective at arthritic and musculoskeletal pain, and less effective for neuropathic pain [82–84]. Following surgery, patients treated with preoperative NSAIDs typically consume 25% to 33% fewer opioids and report lower pain scores [85].

Gabapentinoids

Gabapentin and pregabalin are 2 newer additions to the perioperative analgesic armamentarium. These medications were originally approved as anticonvulsants. Although named for their original intent of binding g-aminobutyric acid (GABA) receptors, in fact they do not act as either agonists or antagonists at GABA receptors, and their metabolites are likewise not active at GABA receptors. There are several proposed mechanisms that attempt to explain the analgesia observed with gabapentin and pregabalin. Gabapentinoids bind spinal cord and primary afferent nerve voltage-gated calcium channels, which

Table 12 Individual NSAIDs
Selective COX-2 agents
Celecoxib
Nonselective COX inhibitors
Aspirin
Ibuprofen
Naproxen
Indomethacin
Sulindac
Piroxicam
Ketoprofen
Ketrorolac (PO or IV)

seems to inhibit firing of wide dynamic range neurons involved in central pain sensitization [86]. Gabapentinoids are efficacious in neuropathic pain, and recent animal evidence points to a separate supraspinal mechanism of action in this particular pain state: gabapentin acts as an agonist on noradrenergic receptors, which stimulates descending pain inhibition pathways in neuropathic pain hypersensitivity states [87].

Gabapentinoids have been studied in a range of pain states (Table 13), and have well-established efficacy in neuropathic pain states, including diabetic neuropathy, post-herpetic neuralgia, postamputation pain, Guillain-Barré syndrome, spinal cord injury, and compressive neuropathies in cancer states [88–94]. In chronic neuropathic pain, low-dose gabapentin plus low-dose narcotic was more effective compared with high-dose opioids. In addition, gabapentinoids provide significant acute and subacute (7–10 days) postoperative analgesia [95]. Pregabalin also improves sleep disturbances associated with pain, without the side effects seen with benzodiazepines [96]. It is not known if gabapentin shares this efficacy. Finally, perioperative gabapentinoids decrease opioid-related side effects, such as sedation and nausea/vomiting.

Side effects of gabapentinoids include sedation and dizziness, which is dose dependent, and typically decreases over several days. Gabapentin is renally excreted, and does need significant dosage adjustment with renal impairment. Pregabalin does need dosage adjustment with renal insufficiency, but can be continued on dosages of up to 150 mg/d unless creatinine clearance is less than 15 mL/min [97]. The authors typically use gabapentin 1200 mg by mouth before major surgery, and continue gabapentin 300 mg by mouth three times a day after surgery (if patients are taking oral medications). If a patient has mild to moderate renal insufficiency, the authors will use pregabalin 150 mg preoperatively, and 50 mg by mouth twice a day in the postoperative phase.

Antidepressants

Tricyclic antidepressants (TCAs) have a long history of use in chronic pain states, particularly neuropathic pain conditions. In addition to analgesic efficacy, many patients with chronic pain conditions have concomitant depression and sleep disturbances. Tricyclic antidepressants have the potential to simultaneously treat all 3 conditions. Imipramine is a commonly chosen TCA, and is

Table 13
Gabapentinoids are effective in multiple painful conditions

Diabetic neuropathy
Phantom limb pain
Guillain-Barré syndrome
Post-herpetic neuralgia
Spinal cord injury
Cancer-related nerve compression pain
Postsurgical analgesia
Prevention of chronic pain following thoracotomy, mastectomy

believed to effect pain relief by enhancing descending inhibition of pain modulation in the CNS [98]. The authors commonly begin with 25 to 50 mg, by mouth at bedtime. Urinary retention is a risk with TCA medications, particularly with opioid therapy or neuraxial analgesia.

In addition to selective serotonin reuptake inhibitor (SSRI) class antidepressants, newer antidepressants combine the mechanisms of SSRI drugs with the adrenergic reuptake inhibition of TCAs. Duloxetine (trade name: Cymbalta) is such a medication, and has been approved by the United States FDA for use in patients with diabetic neuropathy or fibromyalgia. It is not currently known if duloxetine is more or less efficacious compared with the significantly less expensive imipramine.

NMDA receptor antagonists

NMDA receptor antagonists have become a mainstay in treating opioid-tolerant patients. The NMDA receptor is pivotal in pain transmission, serving as the predominant receptor for relaying pain signals from primary afferent neurons to second-order neurons in the dorsal horn of the spinal cord. Blockade of the NMDA receptor prevents glutamate from binding the receptor, and thereby precludes calcium entry into, and depolarization of, the second-order neuron. There are 3 NMDA receptor antagonists in clinical practice: ketamine, dextromethorphan, and memantine.

In Europe and much of Asia, dextromethorphan is available in parenteral administration formulations. In the United States, it is available only for oral administration, and is often used in cough suppressant combinations with other agents. A recent systematic review concluded that parenteral preoperative dextromethorphan was effective in producing sustained postsurgical analgesia [99]. Dextromethorphan likely does not have analgesic superiority compared with parenteral ketamine, but may have a lower incidence of psychological disturbances.

Memantine is an oral NMDA receptor antagonist that is used primarily in the treatment of Alzheimer disease. During the clinical trials process, it was evaluated in patients with long-standing neuropathic pain (10–15 years), and did not have significant analgesic efficacy. However, several recent reports highlight its efficacy in acute severe pain with a neuropathic component [100]. Memantine provides superior analgesia (compared with placebo) for up to 1 year after limb amputation, and has very effectively served as a rescue analgesic following traumatic amputations in Iraq War casualties [101]. Finally, memantine has shown promise in opioid-tolerant patients with acute severe pain [102]. In their practice, the authors often use systemic ketamine pre- and intraoperatively, and then switch to oral memantine if significant postsurgical acute neuropathic pain is anticipated or develops. The typical adult starting dose is 5 mg, by mouth twice a day, and can be titrated up to 20 mg, by mouth twice a day.

Ketamine remains the prototypical NMDA receptor antagonist, and has undergone a dramatic renaissance in clinical use as the number of opioid-tolerant and hyperalgesic patients has increased. Low-dose intravenous ketamine given just before surgical incision seems to diminish pain for several days following minor (knee arthroscopy) and major (total knee arthroplasty) orthopedic surgery [103,104]. Doses that are very unlikely to cause emergence delirium (10–15 mg in an adult) are effective in this application.

Ketamine is frequently coadministered with propofol for painful procedures performed under monitored anesthesia care. In this combination, respiratory depression seems significantly less common compared with propofol-opioid combinations.

Several recent reports also have defined the utility of combined opioid-ketamine intravenous patient-controlled analgesia (IV PCA) for postsurgical analgesia [105,106]. Dramatic reductions of opioid consumption are seen with this combination. One group determined the optimal combination to be a 1:1 mixture of ketamine and morphine (on a milligram to milligram basis) with a lockout of 8 mg [106]. Depending on the study, 0% to 10% of patients have unpleasant dreams when receiving morphine-ketamine IV PCA.

Local anesthetics

Local anesthetics have a wide variety of applications in perioperative analgesia. Nearly all health care providers are familiar with local anesthetic wound infiltration for short-term analgesia following minor surgery. Although there was some initial enthusiasm that protracted analgesia would result from "preemptive" surgical site local anesthetic infiltration, the preponderance of evidence does not support this concept. A long-established delivery route for local anesthetics in patients undergoing major surgery is continuous epidural analgesia. More recent applications of local anesthetics have included large-volume periarticular infiltration with total joint arthroplasty, deep wound catheters with laparotomy surgery, continuous nerve plexus catheters, and perioperative intravenous lidocaine. Several of these methods deserve more detailed discussion. Epidural analgesia is perhaps the gold standard for continuous postsurgical analgesia following major thoracic, abdominal, or lower extremity surgery, as well as providing analgesia following nonoperative trauma (eg, flail chest). Several recent systematic reviews suggest that epidural analgesia lowers major complications following thoracic or abdominal surgery [107].

In comparison with intravenous opiates, epidural analgesia is associated with a shorter duration of intestinal ileus following colorectal surgery [108]. Epidural anesthesia for total hip and total knee arthroplasty is associated with a significantly lower rate of postsurgical deep venous thrombosis compared with general anesthesia. In patients with opioid tolerance, the authors are more aggressive in using epidural analgesia. Epidural analgesia dampens the surgical inflammatory response and diminishes opioid consumption. Although the authors typically use opioid-local anesthetic combinations for postsurgical epidural infusates, in opioid-tolerant patients they use local anesthetic alone (usually 0.1% bupivacaine) in the epidural infusion and give intravenous opioids as needed. Great care must be taken not to unintentionally switch epidural and intravenous delivery devices in these patients. In addition, the widespread and increasing use of anticoagulant drugs for prophylaxis against deep venous thrombosis has complicated the placement and removal of epidural catheters (see www.ASRA.com for guidelines).

Although not commonplace, some centers are now using deep wound catheters to deliver local anesthetics. Following major abdominal surgery, preperitoneal infusion of ropivacaine via a preperitoneal catheter results in improved analgesia, less opioid need, and more rapid paralytic ileus recovery [109]. Although not specifically studied, this method might be especially useful in patients with opioid tolerance, particularly if epidural analgesia is contraindicated or refused.

Local anesthetics are increasingly being delivered via indwelling nerve plexus catheters [110]. This application is obviously an extension of traditional single-injection plexus blocks. Many different approaches have been used, including: interscalene, infraclavicular, and axillary brachial plexus catheters; lumbar plexus and femoral catheters for the lumar plexus; and parasacral, gluteal, infragluteal, and politeal approaches for the lumbosacral plexus. Nearly all studies show reduction in pain and improved patient satisfaction. Many of the studies report sending patients home with disposable local anesthetic delivery pumps. Dilute bupivacaine or ropivacaine (0.1%) typically is used, at 4 to 10 mL/h. Adding clonidine to the infusate may be beneficial, particularly with ropivacaine.

Local anesthetics in combination with other analgesics (see Table 8) are often used in infiltration techniques surrounding total joint arthroplasty procedures [111]. The combination of medications may dampen the inflammatory response following total joint arthroplasty, as the analgesic effects seem to outlast the expected local effects of the drugs. The authors routinely use this technique during total knee and total hip arthroplasty surgeries.

Perioperative intravenous lidocaine infusions are also rapidly gaining popularity for enhancing recovery following major abdominal surgery. Lidocaine has profound anti-inflammatory properties [112], manifested by suppressed release of surgical inflammatory mediators, diminished pain, and faster paralytic ileus recovery [113].

Many institutions are now employing multimodal analgesic techniques, including intravenous lidocaine infusions as part of "fast-track" colorectal surgery. Patients typically receive a loading dose of lidocaine (1.5 mg/kg) followed by a lidocaine infusion of 1 to 3 mg/kg/h, continued until several hours after surgery. Although epidural lidocaine is even more effective than intravenous lidocaine [114], intravenous lidocaine is both time- and cost-efficient.

CONVERTING ORAL AND PARENTERAL OPIOIDS

A frequent clinical challenge is the hospital admission of an opioid-tolerant patient for urgent or elective surgery. In the elective surgery patient, good communication between surgeons and an acute pain management service should allow a planned transition of opioids. There are several steps necessary to plan for opioid management in these patients (see Table 9):

1. Obtain an accurate history of opioid consumption. Sometimes it is also necessary to discuss this with the prescribing physician. There is frequently a difference between what the patient says he or she consumes, what a spouse states the patient consumes, and what the prescribing physician believes the patient is consuming.

2. If the patient will be nil per os for a period of time following surgery, then preoperative opioid prescriptions need to be converted to an intravenous opioid at equipotent doses. Although many conversion tables exist, Internet opioid converters are readily available and are much more time efficient. The authors use the opioid converter from the Kimmel Cancer Center at Johns Hopkins University, which is available either on the Web site (www.hopweb.org) or as a free PDA download. These converters allow simultaneous conversion of multiple opioids. As an example, a patient using transdermal fentanyl, oral morphine, and sustained-release oxycodone can have the equipotent dose of intravenous morphine rapidly estimated.

3. Convert all of the presurgical opioids to a 24-hour parenteral opioid dose. Divide this dose by 24 to obtain the hourly opioid dosage equivalent. This hourly dosage can be used as the basal rate of the intravenous opioid PCA.

4. Determine what amount of opioid to administer with demand doses of the PCA. Opioid-tolerant patients who undergo major surgery typically will have a 200% to 500% increase in their opioid requirements in the acute postoperative period. Thus, the PCA demand dosing should allow at least a 200% increase in the opioid consumption of the patient.

5. As has been emphasized previously, opioid-tolerant patients have a decreased analgesic response to opioids, yet remain at risk for opioid-induced respiratory depression. The goal of the treating physician should be to use nonopioid analgesics to the greatest extent that is prudent and reasonable, to educate the patient that excellent pain control will be difficult to safely achieve, and to safeguard the patient against opioid overdose.

6. It is essential to not overemphasize the "pain score" in opioid prescribing. The pain score number is only one data point, and the validity of the scoring system is widely debated. Many opioid-tolerant patients will have obvious sedation, slurred speech, decreased respiratory rate, and oxygen supplementation needs, yet will note a high pain score. Further opioid doses will place the patient at extreme risk of respiratory arrest and hypoxic injury. Explicit in nursing orders and opioid dosing policies should be to cease further opioid therapy if signs of opioid-induced respiratory depression are occurring.

7. Compounding this problem are issues of other coexisting diseases and organ dysfunctions. As an example, the opioid-tolerant patient that has (or is suspected of having) sleep apnea is at especially high risk of postsurgical apnea and hypoxia. These patients may warrant special monitoring, intensive care, and urgent evaluation for application of continuous positive airway pressure or other ventilatory support. Sleep apnea evaluation optimally occurs before elective surgery and appropriate therapy is instituted.

An interesting pharmacokinetic-pharmacodynamic approach to determining postsurgical PCA settings in opioid-tolerant patients has been the University of Utah fentanyl challenge test (Fig. 3) [115]. In brief, patients do not take their morning opioids; they are brought into a quiet operating room and attached to American Society of Anesthesiologists standard monitors. In addition, a tight-fitting anesthesia circle breathing system is attached. A fentanyl infusion is begun at 2 μg/kg/min, and continued until a respiratory rate of 5 is noted. Using established pharmacokinetic data, the appropriate settings of the fentanyl PCA are established that will allow the patient to approximate 30% of the serum level of fentanyl that caused respiratory depression. Patients report that this technique has met with high patient satisfaction and minimal need to adjust PCA settings.

CONVERTING PARENTERAL OPIOIDS TO ORAL OPIOIDS AND DISCHARGE PLANNING

This clinical challenge is a frequent source of acute pain management consultation requests. The methodology has many overlaps in converting the opioid-tolerant patient from oral to parenteral opioids. The essential elements include (see Table 9):

1. Review all analgesic medications the patient is receiving.
2. Contact the physician who will be prescribing opioids to the patient after discharge. Communication with this person is fundamental to ensuring an accurate exchange of information, particularly the expected duration of increased opioid needs, and that only one person is writing opioid prescriptions.
3. If adjuvant nonopioid analgesics are not being given and are appropriate, initiate therapy with these medications (gabapentinoid, TCA, acetaminophen, NSAID, memantine [in acute neuropathic pain]).
4. Determine 24-hour average consumption of parenteral opioids.
5. The goal is to prescribe approximately 60% to 75% of the opioids as sustained-release formulation, and 25% to 40% as breakthrough analgesics. Examples of sustained-release opioids are extended-release morphine, methadone, extended-release oxycodone, and transdermal fentanyl patch.
6. Use an opioid converter (www.hopweb.org) to establish equipotency between systemic and oral dosing. As an example, if a patient is receiving a total of 15 mg/24 hours of intravenous hydromorphone, this converts to 300 mg/24 hours of oral morphine. A reasonable starting place would be to order 60 mg of extended-release oral morphine every 8 hours (total 24-hour dose of 180 mg, which is 60% of 300 mg), and immediate-release oral morphine 20 to 30 mg every 6 hours as needed for pain (maximal 24-hour dose is 120 mg, which is the remaining 40% of the daily predicted opioid dose).
7. Allow the patient to have access to rescue parenteral opioids on the first day of opioid transition, as long-acting oral opioids slowly attain steady-state serum levels.

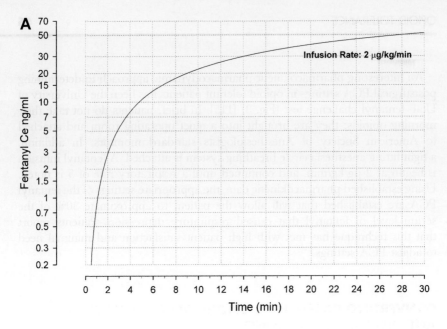

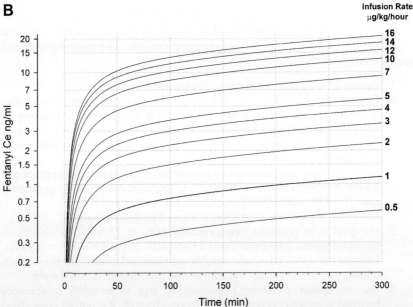

Fig. 3. The University of Utah fentanyl challenge test. (A) Fentanyl is infused in an awake opioid-tolerant patient at 2 μg/kg/min until a respiratory rate of less than 5 is obtained. Using established pharmacokinetic data, the effect site concentration of fentanyl can be estimated. As an example, if the patient took 11 minutes of fentanyl infusion before the respiratory rate was less than 5, the estimated effect site concentration was 21 ng/mL. Analgesia is usually obtained at 30% of the effect site concentration that induces significant respiratory depression. Thirty percent of 21 ng/mL is approximately 6 ng/mL: this is the analgesic target fentanyl effect site concentration. (B) With a target fentanyl effect site concentration of 6 ng/mL, the predicted hourly fentanyl need is approximately 6 μg/kg/h. Half this dosage is given as the basal rate of the PCA (3 μg/kg/h) and the second half is available via demand doses with the PCA device (for example, 1 μg/kg fentanyl dose available every 20 minutes).

8. Exercise extreme caution with rapidly escalating doses of methadone. Because steady-state levels of methadone are not achieved for several days after a change in methadone dose, it is important not to evaluate the efficacy of a new dose of methadone until at least several days have elapsed since a dosage adjustment. Also, it seems that the equipotent dose of methadone is not linear across a range of alternative opioids [116–120]. Thus, the use of methadone should be undertaken with significant caution and only by practitioners knowledgeable in the use of this opioid.

9. A plan should be established to taper the patient back to baseline opioid consumption in an interval appropriate for the surgery. For example, if patients that have anterior cruciate ligament reconstruction are typically off opioids by 1 month after surgery, then plan on tapering an opioid-tolerant patient back to baseline opioids over 1 month. Again, only one physician should be writing opioid prescriptions for these patients.

CLINICAL CHALLENGES: CASE PRESENTATIONS ILLUSTRATING APPLICATION OF PAIN MANAGEMENT PRINCIPLES IN OPIOID-TOLERANT PATIENTS

Clinical challenge #1: The patient on oral buprenorphine or Buprenorphine-naloxone combination therapy

There are several strategies to treat long-term opiate addiction. A popular current therapy is the use of the mixed agonist-antagonist opioid buprenorphine. Buprenorphine has a considerable affinity to the mu opiate receptor, and can be displaced only with high levels of other mu receptor agonists or antagonists.

There is a risk of illicit diversion of buprenorphine, principally involving crushing the buprenorphine capsules and injecting the drug intravenously. To discourage this practice, the combination prescription Suboxone (buprenorphine-naloxone) has been developed, approved, and marketed. Naloxone has minimal bioavailability when orally ingested. However, if Suboxone is injected intravenously, the naloxone is highly effective and will prevent a euphoric experience, and may cause immediate opioid withdrawal. This protocol may prevent criminal and recreational diversion of the buprenorphine and lowers the "street value" of this drug combination.

Individuals that are maintained on buprenorphine or Suboxone may need acute pain management for surgical procedures, childbirth, or trauma. Because of opioid tolerance and the high affinity of buprenorphine for the mu opioid receptor, pain is typically difficult to manage, particularly if standard doses of opioids are used. There are essentially 4 approaches to managing the buprenorphine population needing acute pain management: [121]

- Continue usual once or twice daily dose of buprenorphine, titrate a short-acting opioid analgesic, and monitor pain response, level of consciousness, and respiration.
- Divide the daily dose of buprenorphine and administer it every 6 to 8 hours (to maximize its analgesic effectiveness), and use additional short-acting opioid analgesia as needed.

- Discontinue buprenorphine and give full opioid analgesia. Resume buprenorphine maintenance with an induction period when pain is resolved.
- For hospitalized patients, discontinue buprenorphine and *give methadone*, 20 to 40 mg daily, with a short-acting opioid analgesic to treat pain. Keep naloxone available at the bedside. When pain is resolved, discontinue methadone and resume buprenorphine with an induction period. Be aware that methadone takes several days to achieve steady-state serum levels, and "overshoot" of methadone doses is common.

At the University of Vermont, the authors manage these patients individually, particularly depending on whether short- or long-term hospitalization is likely. As an example of short-term hospitalization, patients presenting in labor who are receiving buprenorphine continue that therapy, and receive higher doses of opioids and multimodal analgesia. If vaginal delivery occurs, very little post-hospitalization pain is likely, and resumption of the buprenorphine maintenance continues immediately on discharge.

This approach is modified if a longer hospital admission is anticipated, particularly when increased pain is likely. An example would be a buprenorphine-maintained patient presenting for elective colectomy. This patient would have buprenorphine discontinued the day before surgery, multimodal analgesia beginning before surgery, higher-dose opioids and ketamine during surgery, and postsurgical epidural analgesia. Rescue parenteral opioids are permitted, and the epidural is not removed until bowel function has returned. Patients are ultimately discharged on a tapering dose of opioids, and have buprenorphine resumed as an outpatient.

Clinical challenge #2: Opioid-tolerant patient requiring total knee arthroplasty

These patients are managed using the authors' total joint arthroplasty clinical pathway, with several modifications. Instead of a single-injection femoral nerve block, a continuous femoral nerve catheter is placed, low-dose bupivacaine or ropivacaine infused for 2 days. The authors continue their outpatient opioids at their usual dose, and allow approximately a 100% to 200% increase in their daily opioids for supplemental analgesia. Because these patients are able to consume oral medications, their opioids do not need to be converted to parenteral opioid equivalents.

Clinical challenge #3: Opioid-tolerant patient with traumatic lower extremity amputation

These patients represent a tremendous challenge. Trauma patients often have multiple concomitant injuries, and also typically receive anticoagulants to prevent deep venous thrombosis. Moreover, severe neuropathic pain accompanies amputation and frequently develops into chronic pain.

Depending on the nature and severity of other injuries, several approaches can be undertaken. Nearly all patients will benefit from multimodal analgesia. Depending on the location of the amputation, femoral or sciatic perineural catheters can be placed. Also, depending on anticoagulation therapy and presence or absence of spine trauma, epidural analgesia can be employed.

Another relatively new modality is using combined opioid-ketamine IV PCA [105,106]. Parenteral low-dose ketamine has a significant opioid-sparing effect, and seems to limit opioid-induced hyperalgesia [61]. Ketamine and other NMDA receptor antagonists are also highly effective at attenuating acute neuropathic pain, even in patients already consuming high-dose opioids [101]. The optimal dose ratio of morphine to ketamine in IV PCA applications seems to be 1 mg:1 mg, and the dosing lockout interval should be 8 minutes. In planning for discharge, an oral NMDA receptor blocker can be started, such as memantine at a dose of 5 to 10 mg twice a day.

SUMMARY

Perioperative management of the opioid-tolerant patient represents a new and major challenge of contemporary medical practice. Narcotic tolerance and opioid-induced hyperalgesia result in inadequacy of traditional pain management approaches. However, armed with multimodal techniques and judicious use of regional anesthesia, these patients can be successfully managed.

Acknowledgments

The authors wish to acknowledge Ms. Kellie Dutra's assistance with manuscript formatting, and Dr. Jennifer Davis' (Director of Acute Pain Service, University of Utah) contribution of figures and legend related to the fentanyl challenge test.

References

[1] Booth M. Opium: a history. New York: St. Martin's Press; 1986.

[2] Walid MS, Donahue SN, Darmohray DM, et al. The fifth vital sign—what does it mean? Pain Pract 2008;8(6):417–22.

[3] Kalb C. Taking a new look at pain. Newsweek 2003;141:44–6.

[4] Harstall C, Ospina M. How prevalent is chronic pain? Pain 2003;XI(2):1–4.

[5] Bennet M. The congressional briefing: the epidemic of pain in America. The Pain Practitioner 2006;16(3):76–8.

[6] Aronoff GM. Chronic pain and the disability epidemic. Clin J Pain 1991;7(4):330–8.

[7] Quality improvement guidelines for the treatment of acute pain and cancer pain. American Pain Society Quality of Care Committee. JAMA 1995;274(23):1881–2.

[8] Campbell J. Pain: the fifth vital sign. Paper presented at: Presidential Address, American Pain Society. Los Angeles, November 13, 1995.

[9] VHA. Pain as the fifth vital sign toolkit. Available at: http://www1.va.gov/pain_management/docs/TOOLKIT.pdf; 2000; Accessed January 25, 2009.

[10] Berry P, Dahl J. The new JCAHO pain standards: implications for pain management nurses. Pain Manag Nurs 2000;1(1):3–12.

[11] Kuehn BM. Opioid prescriptions soar: increase in legitimate use as well as abuse. JAMA 2007;297(3):249–51.

[12] Rowbotham M, Lindsey C. How effective is long-term opioid therapy for chronic noncancer pain? Clin J Pain 2007;23:300–2.

[13] Kelly J, Cook S, Kaufman D, et al. Prevalence and characteristics of opioid use in the US adult population. Pain Pract 2008;138:507–13.

[14] Taylor S, Voytovich AE, Kozol RA. Has the pendulum swung too far in postoperative pain control? Am J Surg 2003;186(5):472–5.

[15] Lucas CE, Vlahos AL, Ledgerwood AM. Kindness kills: the negative impact of pain as the fifth vital sign. J Am Coll Surg 2007;205(1):101–7.

[16] Koppert W, Schmelz M. The impact of opioid-induced hyperalgesia for postoperative pain. Best Pract Res Clin Anaesthesiol 2007;21(1):65–83.

[17] Simonnet G, Rivat C. Opioid-induced hyperalgesia: abnormal or normal pain? Neuroreport 2003;14(1):1–7.

[18] Carroll IR, Angst MS, Clark JD. Management of perioperative pain in patients chronically consuming opioids. Reg Anesth Pain Med 2004;29(6):576–91.

[19] Angst M, Clark J. Opioid-induced hyperalgesia. Anesthesiology 2006;104(3):570–87.

[20] Mao J. Opioid-induced abnormal pain sensitivity: implications in clinical opioid therapy. Pain 2002;100(3):213–7.

[21] Mao J. Opioid-induced abnormal pain sensitivity. Curr Pain Headache Rep 2006;10(1): 67–70.

[22] Celerier E, Rivat C, Jun Y, et al. Long-lasting hyperalgesia induced by fentanyl in rats: preventive effect of ketamine. Anesthesiology 2000;92(2):465–72.

[23] Rivat C, Laulin JP, Corcuff JB, et al. Fentanyl enhancement of carrageenan-induced long-lasting hyperalgesia in rats: prevention by the N-methyl-D-aspartate receptor antagonist ketamine. Anesthesiology 2002;96(2):381–91.

[24] Li X, Angst MS, Clark JD. Opioid-induced hyperalgesia and incisional pain. Anesth Analg 2001;93(1):204–9.

[25] Ibuki T, Dunbar SA, Yaksh TL. Effect of transient naloxone antagonism on tolerance development in rats receiving continuous spinal morphine infusion. Pain 1997;70(2-3): 125–32.

[26] Li X, Angst MS, Clark JD. A murine model of opioid-induced hyperalgesia. Brain Res Mol Brain Res 2001;86(1–2):56–62.

[27] Zissen MH, Zhang G, McKelvy A, et al. Tolerance, opioid-induced allodynia and withdrawal associated allodynia in infant and young rats. Neuroscience 2007;144(1): 247–62.

[28] Celerier E, Laulin JP, Corcuff JB, et al. Progressive enhancement of delayed hyperalgesia induced by repeated heroin administration: a sensitization process. J Neurosci 2001;21(11):4074–80.

[29] Aley KO, Green PG, Levine JD. Opioid and adenosine peripheral antinociception are subject to tolerance and withdrawal. J Neurosci 1995;15(12):8031–8.

[30] Aley KO, Levine JD. Different mechanisms mediate development and expression of tolerance and dependence for peripheral mu-opioid antinociception in rat. J Neurosci 1997;17(20):8018–23.

[31] Khasar SG, Wang JF, Taiwo YO, et al. Mu-opioid agonist enhancement of prostaglandin-induced hyperalgesia in the rat: a G-protein beta gamma subunit-mediated effect? Neuroscience 1995;67(1):189–95.

[32] Liang D, Shi X, Qiao Y, et al. Chronic morphine administration enhances nociceptive sensitivity and local cytokine production after incision. Mol Pain 2008;4:4–7.

[33] Vardanyan A, Wang R, Vanderah TW, et al. TRPV1 receptor in expression of opioid-induced hyperalgesia. J Pain 2009;10:243–52.

[34] Khasar SG, McCarter G, Levine JD. Epinephrine produces a beta-adrenergic receptor-mediated mechanical hyperalgesia and in vitro sensitization of rat nociceptors. J Neurophysiol 1999;81(3):1104–12.

[35] Liang DY, Liao G, Wang J, et al. A genetic analysis of opioid-induced hyperalgesia in mice. Anesthesiology 2006;104(5):1054–62.

[36] Liang DY, Liao G, Lighthall GK, et al. Genetic variants of the P-glycoprotein gene Abcb1b modulate opioid-induced hyperalgesia, tolerance and dependence. Pharmacogenet Genomics 2006;16(11).825 35.

[37] Mao J, Price DD, Mayer DJ. Thermal hyperalgesia in association with the development of morphine tolerance in rats: roles of excitatory amino acid receptors and protein kinase C. J Neurosci 1994;14(4):2301–12.

[38] Zhao M, Joo DT. Enhancement of spinal N-methyl-D-aspartate receptor function by remifentanil action at delta-opioid receptors as a mechanism for acute opioid-induced hyperalgesia or tolerance. Anesthesiology 2008;109(2):308–17.

[39] Haugan F, Rygh LJ, Tjolsen A. Ketamine blocks enhancement of spinal long-term potentiation in chronic opioid treated rats. Acta Anaesthesiol Scand 2008;52(5):681–7.

[40] Esmaeili-Mahani S, Shimokawa N, Javan M, et al. Low-dose morphine induces hyperalgesia through activation of G alphas, protein kinase C, and L-type Ca 2+ channels in rats. J Neurosci Res 2008;86(2):471–9.

[41] Celerier E, Simonnet G, Maldonado R. Prevention of fentanyl-induced delayed pronociceptive effects in mice lacking the protein kinase C gamma gene. Neuropharmacology 2004;46(2):264–72.

[42] Johnston IN, Milligan ED, Wieseler-Frank J, et al. A role for proinflammatory cytokines and fractalkine in analgesia, tolerance, and subsequent pain facilitation induced by chronic intrathecal morphine. J Neurosci 2004;24(33):7353–65.

[43] Vera-Portocarrero LP, Zhang ET, King T, et al. Spinal NK-1 receptor expressing neurons mediate opioid-induced hyperalgesia and antinociceptive tolerance via activation of descending pathways. Pain 2007;129(1–2):35–45.

[44] Van Elstraete AC, Sitbon P, Mazoit JX, et al. Gabapentin prevents delayed and long-lasting hyperalgesia induced by fentanyl in rats. Anesthesiology 2008;108(3): 484–94.

[45] Zhao M, Wang JY, Jia H, et al. Roles of different subtypes of opioid receptors in mediating the ventrolateral orbital cortex opioid-induced inhibition of mirror-neuropathic pain in the rat. Neuroscience 2007;144(4):1486–94.

[46] Wang JY, Zhao M, Huang FS, et al. Mu-opioid receptor in the nucleus submedius: involvement in opioid-induced inhibition of mirror-image allodynia in a rat model of neuropathic pain. Neurochem Res 2008;33(10):2134–41.

[47] Hamlin AS, McNally GP, Osborne PB. Induction of c-Fos and zif268 in the nociceptive amygdala parallel abstinence hyperalgesia in rats briefly exposed to morphine. Neuropharmacology 2007;53(2):330–43.

[48] Ram KC, Eisenberg E, Haddad M, et al. Oral opioid use alters DNIC but not cold pain perception in patients with chronic pain—new perspective of opioid-induced hyperalgesia. Pain 2008;139(2):431–8.

[49] Angst M, Chu L, Clark D. Opioid tolerance and hyperalgesia in chronic pain patients after one month of oral morphine therapy: a preliminary prospective study. J Pain 2006;7(1): 43–8.

[50] Hay JL, White JM, Bochner F, et al. Hyperalgesia in opioid-managed chronic pain and opioid-dependent patients. J Pain 2009;10:316–22.

[51] Axelrod D, Reville B. Using methadone to treat opioid-induced hyperalgesia and refractory pain. J Opioid Manag 2007;3(2):113–4.

[52] Vorobeychik Y, Chen L, Bush M, et al. Improved opioid analgesic effect following opioid dose reduction. Pain Med 2008;9(6):724–7.

[53] Doverty M, White J, Somogyi A, et al. Hyperalgesic responses in methadone maintenance patients. Pain 2001;90:91–6.

[54] Schall U, Katta T, Pries E, et al. Pain perception of intravenous heroin users on maintenance therapy with levomethadone. Pharmacopsychiatry 1996;29:176–9.

[55] Compton P, Charuvastra V, Ling W. Pain intolerance in opioid-maintained former opiate addicts: effect of long-acting maintenance agent. Drug Alcohol Depend 2001;63: 139–46.

[56] Chu L, Angst M, Clark D. Opioid-induced hyperalgesia in humans. Clin J Pain 2008;24(6): 479–96.

[57] Pud D, Cohen D, Lawental E. Opioids and abnormal pain perception: new evidence from a study of chronic opioid addicts and healthy subjects. Drug Alcohol Depend 2006;82: 218–23.

[58] Cohen S, Christo P, Wang S, et al. The effect of opioid does and treatment duration on the perception of a painful standardized clinical stimulus. Reg Anesth Pain Med 2008;33(3): 199–206.

[59] Ho AM, Tang NL, Cheung BK, et al. Dopamine receptor D4 gene -521C/T polymorphism is associated with opioid dependence through cold-pain responses. Ann N Y Acad Sci 2008;1139:20–6.

[60] Cooper D, Lindsay S, Rydall D. Does intrathecal fentanyl produce acute cross-tolerance to I.V. morphine? Br J Anaesth 1997;78:311–3.

[61] Xuerong Y, Yuguang H, Xia J, et al. Ketamine and lornoxicam for preventing a fentanyl-induce increase in postoperative morphine requirement. Anesth Analg 2008;107:2032–7.

[62] Guignard B, Bossard A, Coste C. Acute opioid tolerance: intraoperative remifentanil increases postoperative pain and morphine requirement. Anesthesiology 2000;93:409–17.

[63] Joly V, Richebe P, Guignard B. Remifentanil-induced postoperative hyperalgesia and its prevention with small-dose ketamine. Anesthesiology 2005;103:147–55.

[64] Cortinez L, Brandes V, Munoz H. No clinical evidence of acute opioid tolerance after remifentanil-based anaesthesia. Br J Anaesth 2001;87:866–9.

[65] Lee L, Irwin M, Lui S. Intraoperative remifentanil infusion does not increase postoperative opioid consumption compared with 70% nitrous oxide. Anesthesiology 2005;102: 398–402.

[66] Angst M, Koppert W, Pahl I. Short-term in fusion of the mu-opioid agonist remifentanil in humans causes hyperalgesia during withdrawal. Pain 2003;106:49–57.

[67] Koppert W, Sittl R, Scheuber K. Differential modulation of remifentanil-induced analgesia and postinfusion hyperalgesia by S-ketamine and clonidine in humans. Anesthesiology 2003;99:152–9.

[68] Koppert W, Dern S, Sittl R. A new model of electrically evoked pain and hyperalgesia in human skin: the effects of intravenous alfentanil, S(+)-ketamine, and lidocaine. Anesthesiology 2001;95:395–402.

[69] Hood DD, Curry R, Eisenach JC. Intravenous remifentanil produces withdrawal hyperalgesia in volunteers with capsaicin-induced hyperalgesia. Anesth Analg 2003;97(3):810–5.

[70] Compton P, Athanasos P, Elashoff D. Withdrawal hyperalgesia after acute opioid physical dependence in nonaddicted humans: a preliminary study. J Pain 2003;4:511–9.

[71] Angst MS, Chu LF, Tingle MS, et al. No evidence for the development of acute tolerance to analgesic, respiratory depressant and sedative opioid effects in humans. Pain 2009;142(1–2):17–26.

[72] Kehlet H, Wilmore DW. Multimodal strategies to improve surgical outcome. Am J Surg 2002;183(6):630–41.

[73] Oscier C, Milner O. Peri-operative use of paracetamol. Anaesthesia 2009;64:65–72.

[74] Bertolini A, Ferrari A, Ottani A, et al. Paracetamol: new vistas of an old drug. CNS Drug Rev 2006;12(3–4):250–75.

[75] Bonnefont J, Daulhac L, Etienne M, et al. Acetaminophen recruits spinal p42/p44 MAPKs and GH/IGF-1 receptors to produce analgesia via the serotonergic system. Mol Pharmacol 2007;71(2):407–15.

[76] McQuay H, Moore A, Justins D. Treating acute pain in hospital. BMJ 1997;314(7093): 1531–5.

[77] Tannenbaum H, Bombardier C, Davis P, et al. An evidence-based approach to prescribing nonsteroidal antiinflammatory drugs. Third Canadian Consensus Conference. J Rheumatol 2006;33(1):140–57.

[78] Moore RA, Derry S, Makinson GT, et al. Tolerability and adverse events in clinical trials of celecoxib in osteoarthritis and rheumatoid arthritis: systematic review and meta-analysis of information from company clinical trial reports. Arthritis Res Ther 2005;7(3):R644–65.

[79] Fored CM, Ejerblad E, Lindblad P, et al. Acetaminophen, aspirin, and chronic renal failure. N Engl J Med 2001;345(25):1801–8.

[80] Glassman SD, Rose SM, Dimar JR, et al. The effect of postoperative nonsteroidal anti-inflammatory drug administration on spinal fusion. Spine 1998;23(7):834–8.

[81] Reuben SS, Ablett D, Kaye R. High dose nonsteroidal anti-inflammatory drugs compromise spinal fusion. Can J Anaesth 2005;52(5):506–12.

[82] van Tulder MW, Scholten RJ, Koes BW, et al. Non-steroidal anti-inflammatory drugs for low back pain. Cochrane Database Syst Rev 2000;(2):CD000396.

[83] Vroomen PC, de Krom MC, Slofstra PD, et al. Conservative treatment of sciatica: a systematic review. J Spinal Disord 2000;13(6):463–9.

[84] McNicol E, Strassels SA, Goudas L, et al. NSAIDs or paracetamol, alone or combined with opioids, for cancer pain. Cochrane Database Syst Rev 2005;(1):CD005180.

[85] Jirarattanaphochai K, Jung S. Nonsteroidal antiinflammatory drugs for postoperative pain management after lumbar spine surgery: a meta-analysis of randomized controlled trials. J Neurosurg Spine 2008;9(1):22–31.

[86] Knotkova H, Pappagallo M. Adjuvant analgesics. Med Clin North Am 2007;91(1):113–24.

[87] Hayashida K, Obata H, Nakajima K, et al. Gabapentin acts within the locus coeruleus to alleviate neuropathic pain. Anesthesiology 2008;109(6):1077–84.

[88] Eckhardt K, Ammon S, Hofmann U, et al. Gabapentin enhances the analgesic effect of morphine in healthy volunteers. Anesth Analg 2000;91(1):185–91.

[89] Turan A, Karamanlioglu B, Memis D, et al. Analgesic effects of gabapentin after spinal surgery. Anesthesiology 2004;100(4):935–8.

[90] Rowbotham M, Harden N, Stacey B, et al. Gabapentin for the treatment of postherpetic neuralgia: a randomized controlled trial. JAMA 1998;280(21):1837–42.

[91] Rice AS, Maton S. Gabapentin in postherpetic neuralgia: a randomised, double blind, placebo controlled study. Pain 2001;94(2):215–24.

[92] Bone M, Critchley P, Buggy DJ. Gabapentin in postamputation phantom limb pain: a randomized, double-blind, placebo-controlled, cross-over study. Reg Anesth Pain Med 2002;27(5):481–6.

[93] Pandey CK, Bose N, Garg G, et al. Gabapentin for the treatment of pain in Guillain-Barré syndrome: a double-blinded, placebo-controlled, crossover study. Anesth Analg 2002;95(6):1719–23, table of contents.

[94] Tai Q, Kirshblum S, Chen B, et al. Gabapentin in the treatment of neuropathic pain after spinal cord injury: a prospective, randomized, double-blind, crossover trial. J Spinal Cord Med 2002;25(2):100–5.

[95] Tiippana EM, Hamunen K, Kontinen VK, et al. Do surgical patients benefit from perioperative gabapentin/pregabalin? A systematic review of efficacy and safety. Anesth Analg 2007;104(6):1545–56, table of contents.

[96] Crofford LJ, Rowbotham MC, Mease PJ, et al. Pregabalin for the treatment of fibromyalgia syndrome: results of a randomized, double-blind, placebo-controlled trial. Arthritis Rheum 2005;52(4):1264–73.

[97] Micromedex Healthcare Series. Available at: http://www.micromedex.com Accessed February 3, 2009.

[98] Pappagallo M, Werner M. Chronic pain, a primer for physicians. London: Remedica; 2008.

[99] McCartney CJ, Sinha A, Katz J. A qualitative systematic review of the role of N-methyl-D-aspartate receptor antagonists in preventive analgesia. Anesth Analg 2004;98(5):1385–400, table of contents.

[100] Buvanendran A, Kroin JS. Early use of memantine for neuropathic pain. Anesth Analg 2008;107(4):1093–4.

[101] Hackworth RJ, Tokarz KA, Fowler IM, et al. Profound pain reduction after induction of memantine treatment in two patients with severe phantom limb pain. Anesth Analg 2008;107(4):1377–9.

[102] Grande LA, O'Donnell BR, Fitzgibbon DR, et al. Ultra-low dose ketamine and memantine treatment for pain in an opioid-tolerant oncology patient. Anesth Analg 2008;107(4): 1380–3.

[103] Adam F, Chauvin M, Du Manoir B, et al. Small-dose ketamine infusion improves postoperative analgesia and rehabilitation after total knee arthroplasty. Anesth Analg 2005;100(2):475–80.

[104] Menigaux C, Guignard B, Fletcher D, et al. Intraoperative small-dose ketamine enhances analgesia after outpatient knee arthroscopy. Anesth Analg 2001;93(3):606–12.

[105] Sveticic G, Eichenberger U, Curatolo M. Safety of mixture of morphine with ketamine for postoperative patient-controlled analgesia: an audit with 1026 patients. Acta Anaesthesiol Scand 2005;49(6):870–5.

[106] Sveticic G, Gentilini A, Eichenberger U, et al. Combinations of morphine with ketamine for patient-controlled analgesia: a new optimization method. Anesthesiology 2003;98(5): 1195–205.

[107] Popping DM, Elia N, Marret E, et al. Protective effects of epidural analgesia on pulmonary complications after abdominal and thoracic surgery: a meta-analysis. Arch Surg 2008;143(10):990–9 [discussion: 1000].

[108] Kehlet H. Fast-track colorectal surgery. Lancet 2008;371(9615):791–3.

[109] Beaussier M, El'Ayoubi H, Schiffer E, et al. Continuous preperitoneal infusion of ropivacaine provides effective analgesia and accelerates recovery after colorectal surgery: a randomized, double-blind, placebo-controlled study. Anesthesiology 2007;107(3): 461–8.

[110] Ilfeld BM, Ball ST, Gearen PF, et al. Ambulatory continuous posterior lumbar plexus nerve blocks after hip arthroplasty: a dual-center, randomized, triple-masked, placebo-controlled trial. Anesthesiology 2008;109(3):491–501.

[111] Andersen LO, Husted H, Otte KS, et al. High-volume infiltration analgesia in total knee arthroplasty: a randomized, double-blind, placebo-controlled trial. Acta Anaesthesiol Scand 2008;52(10):1331–5.

[112] Omote K. Intravenous lidocaine to treat postoperative pain management: novel strategy with a long-established drug. Anesthesiology 2007;106(1):5–6.

[113] Marret E, Rolin M, Beaussier M, et al. Meta-analysis of intravenous lidocaine and postoperative recovery after abdominal surgery. Br J Surg 2008;95(11):1331–8.

[114] Kuo CP, Jao SW, Chen KM, et al. Comparison of the effects of thoracic epidural analgesia and i.v. infusion with lidocaine on cytokine response, postoperative pain and bowel function in patients undergoing colonic surgery. Br J Anaesth 2006;97(5):640–6.

[115] Davis JJ, Swenson JD, Hall RH, et al. Preoperative "fentanyl challenge" as a tool to estimate postoperative opioid dosing in chronic opioid-consuming patients. Anesth Analg 2005;101(2):389–95, table of contents.

[116] Ripamonti C, Groff L, Brunelli C, et al. Switching from morphine to oral methadone in treating cancer pain: what is the equianalgesic dose ratio? J Clin Oncol 1998;16(10): 3216–21.

[117] Lawlor PG, Turner KS, Hanson J, et al. Dose ratio between morphine and methadone in patients with cancer pain: a retrospective study. Cancer 1998;82(6):1167–73.

[118] Pereira J, Lawlor P, Vigano A, et al. Equianalgesic dose ratios for opioids. A critical review and proposals for long-term dosing. J Pain Symptom Manage 2001;22(2):672–87.

[119] Moryl N, Santiago-Palma J, Kornick C, et al. Pitfalls of opioid rotation: substituting another opioid for methadone in patients with cancer pain. Pain 2002;96(3):325–8.

[120] Bruera E, Sweeney C. Methadone use in cancer patients with pain: a review. J Palliat Med 2002;5(1):127–38.

[121] Alford DP, Compton P, Samet JH. Acute pain management for patients receiving maintenance methadone or buprenorphine therapy. Ann Intern Med 2006;144(2): 127–34.

Advances in Anesthesia 27 (2009) 55–71

ADVANCES IN ANESTHESIA

Preoperative Stress Syndromes and Their Evaluation, Consultation, and Management

Edward R. Norris, MD*, Muhamad Aly Rifai, MD,
Michael W. Kaufmann, MD

Department of Psychiatry, Lehigh Valley Health Network, 2545 Schoenersville Road, 5th Floor, Bethlehem, PA 18017, USA

Anxiety is a nonspecific symptom and everyone experiences this emotion. Sometimes anxiety is adaptive, such as in novel situations, as it helps to mobilize an individual for a quick response. Anxiety can heighten awareness and help to prepare a defense to a threatening situation. Anxiety can be experienced with emotional and physical symptoms. Emotional symptoms include excessive worry and fear, dread, feeling on edge, poor concentration, and irritability. Physical symptoms include increased heart rate, shortness of breath, upset stomach, sweating, tremors, fatigue, and muscle tension. Some aspects of these manifestations, considered the fear response, are adaptive in the sense that they may help to promote the survival of an individual and the species. It is no wonder why it is so highly conserved in vertebrates and essentially hardwired into our brains [1].

Many patients are justifiably anxious in reaction to the diagnosis or potential diagnosis of an illness and the performance of diagnostic tests and surgical procedures. Anxiety is often increased if uncertainty exists about the course and prognosis of their illness. Stressful treatment options can also create anxiety problems. Patients who have anxiety should be given periodic opportunities to express their questions, fears, and concerns with physicians who are attentive, empathetic, and supportive of patients'; concerns [2].

Anxiety and fear are two main issues that a physician must examine when evaluating patients who are emotionally aroused. Anxiety is the apprehensive anticipation of future danger. This anticipation is experienced as unpleasant and is often accompanied by somatic symptoms, such as muscle tension. Fear is a more appropriate term to use when a real threat or danger exists. Both emotions are regulated through the same fight-flight response. Often

*Corresponding author. Research and Education, Department of Psychiatry, Lehigh Valley Health Network, 1251 S. Cedar Crest Boulevard, Suite 202A, Allentown, PA 18103. E-mail address: edward.norris@lvh.com (E.R. Norris).

0737-6146/09/$ – see front matter
doi:10.1016/j.aan.2009.07.005

anxiety in patients can be subconsciously contagious and patients experiencing this emotion can evoke multiple responses in the evaluating physician [3].

PATHOPHYSIOLOGY

The normal fear response that occurs in the setting of a threat first includes a cognitive appraisal to recognize and remember the threat. A physiologic arousal then occurs to signal danger, enhance alertness, and prepare the body for action. This physiologic arousal is followed by one of many behaviors that include fighting, fleeing, or freezing [4].

Fear and anxiety are mediated through the same neurophysiologic systems located in the limbic system of the brain. The major neurotransmitters involved in the mediation of the symptoms of anxiety disorders appear to be norepinephrine and serotonin. Other neurotransmitters and peptides, such as cortico-trophin-releasing factor, may also be involved. Peripherally, the autonomic nervous system, especially the sympathetic nervous system, mediates many of the symptoms of anxiety. In the brain, the amygdala is responsible for the initiation of fear and anxiety. This initiation can involve a number of central neurotransmitters that create and modulate anxious symptoms. Noradrenergic systems in the brain originate from the locus coeruleus. Stimulation of the locus coeruleus can create panic attacks and its blockade by pharmaceutical agents can decrease these attacks [2].

Modulation of anxiety symptoms mainly occurs through gamma-aminobutyric acid (GABA) and serotonergic systems. GABA neurons in the limbic system mediate nonspecific anxiety and worry. The highly concentrated GABA neurons in the hippocampal areas also help to mediate vigilance. When GABA neurons bind to benzodiazepines in anxiety, this heightened sense of vigilance dissipates. Serotonergic neurons help to modulate the activity of noradrenergic neurons and GABA neurons. In some manner, serotonergic neurons are like a volume switch and help to fine tune the amount of activity needed by these different brain neurons to maintain homeostatsis [1].

Anxiety, when unchecked or untreated, results in an overactive noradrenergic system. Complications of anxiety include increased catecholamine secretion that leads to increased blood pressure, heart rate, myocardial contractility, and oxygen consumption. This catecholamine secretion also decreases the threshold for ventricular fibrillation. Patients who have increased anxiety will have changes in the cardiac output, heart rate, and total peripheral resistance, which can make anesthesia more complicated to administer and monitor [5,6].

EPIDEMIOLOGY

Anxiety disorders are very common and among the most prevalent psychiatric diseases in the general population. One fourth of the United States population will experience pathologic anxiety over the course of their lifetime [7,8]. Two major studies in the United States have estimated the prevalence rates for a variety of anxiety disorders; these studies are the Epidemiologic Catchment Area study [9] and the National Comorbidity Survey study [7,8]. Drawing on these studies and other data, Fig. 1 estimates lifetime prevalence rates for individual anxiety disorders.

Social phobia, the persistent fear of being exposed to public scrutiny, is the most common anxiety disorder with 2.6% to 13.3% lifetime prevalence [7,8]. Specific phobias with the persistent fear of circumscribed situations or objects, such as heights or flying, are also common with 10% lifetime prevalence. Generalized anxiety disorder has a lifetime prevalence of 4.1% to 6.6%, and panic disorder has a lifetime prevalence of 2.3% to 2.7%. The prevalence of posttraumatic stress disorder is approximately 1.9% to 3.0% in the general population [10]. These statistics point to the fact that almost 1 in 10 patients undergoing anesthesia may suffer from an anxiety disorder that may impact their preoperative care [9,11]. First-degree relatives of patients who have anxiety disorders demonstrate significantly increased risk for anxiety disorders themselves [7,8].

The unfortunate course of anxiety disorders is that they are often associated with significant impairments in physical and social functioning leading to an impaired quality of life. Often this impaired quality of life can be mediated with early detection and treatment, but patients who have anxiety disorders often go for many years undiagnosed or undertreated. Patients who have anxiety disorders have a lifelong pattern of being more psychophysiologically reactive. This reactivity often leads to increased health issues and premature disability, caused by chronic increased catecholamine exposure [4].

ANXIETY DURING THE PREANESTHESIA PERIOD

Normal anxiety in the setting of requiring surgery is a common reaction witnessed in the hospital setting. For example, the woman who is awaiting surgery for breast cancer may be anxious about death or may instead be concerned

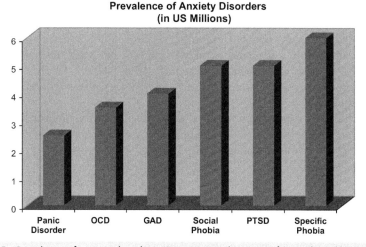

Fig. 1. Prevalence of anxiety disorders. (*From* National Institute of Mental Health.)

about disfigurement and recovery. It is important for the physician not to project their beliefs onto patients, and to acknowledge patients' anxiety while allowing them to express their anxious feelings. Acknowledging these emotions is often effective to decrease the anxiety of patients [2,12]. There are many reasons that are normal and expected for patients to experience anxiety in the preoperative setting. In the discussion and investigation of anxious symptoms, physicians can ask probing questions to better understand the source of the anxiety and to appropriately treat the symptoms [12,13].

Uncertainty of medical diagnosis often underlies anxiety when those with a personal or family history of illness undergo examinations. People may be afraid that they may have an undiscovered illness, and this anxiety is often heightened in the time period before the final diagnosis. This uncertainty can be prolonged as fears are left alone to go unchecked; however, with any diagnosis this uncertainty dissipates.

Everyone is afraid, at one point in their life, of dying. This fear is heightened immediately before surgery. Physicians should address this preoperative mortality fear in a calm and comfortable manner. This discussion can lead to specific reasons for the fear of death, understanding of specific irrationalities about death, surgery, and even existential thoughts regarding dying. Often this discussion can lead the physician to discover the underlying issue and solution to the short-term anxiety [13].

For many patients undergoing surgery there is an uncertainty of illness prognosis. Some patients have recurring illnesses, such as cancer and heart disease, which can activate anxiety leading up to the procedure. Unfavorable prognosis can increase anxiety, but anxiety can be present in benign cases. It is important to realize that patients' perspective can be different than the physician's, and even when an anticipated cure rate is 90%, patients may only be thinking about the 10% failure rate. Again it is important to explore these beliefs and fears with patients to allow for an open discussion.

Many will be less concerned with the current situation and much more concerned with how quickly they can recover. Anxiety about impact of illness can include concerns of lost income, ability to care for one's self, insurance costs, and the overall burden of illness that they place on their families. Inviting a social worker or financial counselor to speak with patients will often lessen their concerns.

As physicians, many are immersed in the hospital to the point that there is nothing inherently unique about going to the operating room every day, but for many not involved in health care, hospital visits are left only to the ill and dying. Fear of being in a hospital occurs often, and for many, it is difficult to trust a physician that they met only minutes before. In addition to being in a foreign location, they often feel alone, which heightens anxiety and dependency issues. Finally, patients may feel guilty about their personal habits that may have contributed to their need for surgery. This anxiety over guilt may lead some to not fully disclose personal information.

Primary anxiety disorders

Overview

Anxiety disorders are common psychiatric disorders but are often under recognized and undertreated. Anxiety disorders appear to be caused by an interaction of biopsychosocial factors, including genetic vulnerability, which interact with situations, stress, or trauma, to produce clinically significant syndromes. The presence of anxiety disorders is of particular interest in anesthesia and preoperative and postoperative care. Understanding the underlay of anxiety can help anesthesiologists better care for patients who have preexisting anxiety disorders.

Diagnosis

Symptoms of anxiety vary depending on the specific disorder. It is always important to rule out anxiety disorders secondary to general medical or substance abuse disorders. A detailed history and review of symptoms is essential and can help make this distinction. It is also essential to ask the patients' sleep partner about apneic episodes (sleep apnea) or myoclonic limb jerks. Concurrent depressive symptoms are common in all of the anxiety disorders. Patients who have anxiety disorders seldom receive appropriate treatment, most often because of under-recognition, misdiagnosis, and the complications of comorbidities. Severe anxiety disorders may produce agitation, suicidal ideation, and increased risk of completed suicide. While further inquiry into the symptoms of anxiety and depression is essential, it is always important to ask and inquire about suicidal ideation or suicidal intent in patients exhibiting symptoms of severe anxiety.

Diagnostic criteria of anxiety disorders

Panic disorder. Panic disorder is characterized by panic attacks that are recurrent and often unexpected; for example, panic attacks are periods of intense fear of abrupt onset peaking in intensity within 10 minutes. These symptoms are often coupled with anticipatory anxiety and phobic avoidance, which together impair the patient's professional, social, and familial functioning [4,14,15]. Panic attacks can also complicate the pre- and postoperative periods. Although not a diagnostic feature, suicidal ideation and completed suicide have been associated with panic disorder. Four of the following must be present to make a panic disorder diagnosis:

- Palpitations, pounding heart, or accelerated heart rate
- Sweating
- Trembling or shaking
- Shortness of breath or dyspnea
- Sensation of choking
- Chest pain or discomfort
- Nausea or abdominal distress
- Feeling dizzy, unsteady, lightheaded, or faint
- Derealization or depersonalization
- Fear of losing control or going crazy

- Fear of dying
- Paresthesias
- Chills or hot flashes

Generalized anxiety disorder. Generalized anxiety disorder (GAD) is characterized by persistent and uncontrollable worry, psychological anxiety, and somatic symptoms (eg, physical tension, difficulty concentrating) [16,17]. The symptoms of GAD are excessive and endure for most of the day, nearly every day, for a minimum of 6 months [16,18]. Although not a diagnostic feature, suicidal ideation and completed suicide have also been associated with generalized anxiety disorder. The anxiety and worry of GAD are associated with at least three of the following symptoms [17,19]:

- Restlessness or feeling on edge
- Easily fatigued
- Difficulty concentrating or mind going blank
- Irritability
- Muscle tension
- Sleep disturbance

Obsessive compulsive disorder. Obsessive Compulsive Disorder (OCD) is a disorder that is characterized by recurrent, intrusive thoughts and preoccupations, and rituals and behavioral compulsions [20]. The obsessions and compulsions are distressing, time consuming, and often lead to impairment in occupational, scholastic, or social functioning. Attempts are made to ignore or suppress thoughts, impulses, or images that are recognized by patients as being the product of the mind and not imposed from an outside force [20]. Obsessions include recurrent and persistent thoughts, impulses, or images that are intrusive, knowingly inappropriate, and cause anxiety or distress, and are not simply excessive worries about real-life problems. Compulsions include repetitive behaviors, such as hand washing, ordering, and checking, that people feel must be performed and occur to such an extreme that a person's ability to function is impaired.

Social anxiety disorder. Social Anxiety Disorder (SAD) is characterized by a persistent fear of negative evaluation or scrutiny by others in social situations [21] that results in excessive fear of humiliation or embarrassment, decrease in adaptive functioning, and clinical distress. Exposure to the feared social situation or anticipation of the situation can produce an intense and immediate anxiety reaction including physiologic symptoms, such as blushing and sweating [22]. These social anxiety concerns may involve circumscribed events or performances, such as public speaking, social interactions, or a pervasive fear encompassing a wide spectrum of generalized social situations [21–24]. These situations may also include the periods of pre- and postoperative care because of uncertainty and possible humiliation with the operative rituals (disrobing, manipulations, and loss of control) [21–24]. SAD is marked by at least two of the following [21–24]:

- Marked and persistent fear of social or performance situations to the extent that a person's ability to function at work or in school is impaired.
- Exposure to social or performance situation always produces anxiety.
- Fear/anxiety is recognized as excessive.
- Social or performance situations are avoided or endured with intense anxiety.

Posttraumatic stress disorder. Posttraumatic Stress Disorder (PTSD) develops when a severe trauma is experienced that includes actual or threatened death or serious injury, or threat to personal integrity of self or others, and includes responses that are characterized by intense fear, helplessness, or horror [25]. Life-threatening experiences and the attendant loss of control are key elements. Although not a diagnostic feature, suicidal and homicidal ideations have been associated with PTSD. PTSD symptoms include the following [10,25–30]:

Persistent re-experience of the event occurs by at least one of the following [10,25–30]:

- Recurrent and intrusive recollections
- Recurrent distressing dreams/nightmares
- Feelings of reliving traumatic event (ie, flashbacks)
- Intense psychological distress with internal or external cues to the trauma
- Physiologic reactivity on exposure to trauma cues

Persistent avoidance of stimuli of trauma and numbing/avoidance behavior demonstrated by at least three of the following:

- Avoidance of thoughts or conversation related to the trauma
- Avoidance of activities, places, or people related to the trauma
- Amnesia for important trauma-related events
- Decreased participation in significant activities
- Feeling detached or estranged from others
- Restricted affect
- Foreshortened sense of the future

Persistent symptoms of increased arousal demonstrated by two or more of the following:

- Difficulty staying or falling asleep
- Irritability or anger outbursts
- Difficulty concentrating
- Hypervigilance
- Exaggerated startle response

AWARENESS UNDER ANESTHESIA AND THE DEVELOPMENT OF POSTTRAUMATIC STRESS DISORDER

Anesthesia awareness (awareness with recall after surgery) occurs under general anesthesia when patients becomes cognizant and conscious of some or all events during surgery or a procedure, and has direct recall of those events after the surgery [26,31–33]. The frequency of anesthesia awareness has been found in multiple studies to range between 0.1 % and 0.2 % of all patients undergoing general anesthesia. Patients experiencing awareness report auditory recollections (48%), sensations of not being able to breathe (48%), and pain (28%) [26,31–33]. The occurrence of awareness is often thought to be the consequence of light-anesthetic techniques or smaller anesthetic doses. The awareness under anesthesia is an event of significant concern to patients and is associated with the development of prominent anxiety symptoms [26,31–33]. More than 50% of patients who experience awareness during anesthesia report experiencing mental distress following surgery, including the development of PTSD. For patients, awareness or recall while under general anesthesia is a frightening experience and may lead to debilitating anxiety. When concern about awareness under anesthesia is raised by patients, it is important for the physician to address this immediately, as early referral to psychiatric care can lead to a significant reduction in long-term psychological sequelae of this experience. Early intervention with psychotherapy and psychotropic medications has been show to reduce the risk of developing a debilitating anxiety disorder or PTSD [26,31–33].

DIFFERENTIAL DIAGNOSIS OF ANXIETY STATES

When patients who have medical illness become anxious, there is a large differential diagnosis including organic issues, substances, pain, delirium, and psychosis. In addition, anxious symptoms confer additional risk of morbidity in patients who have chronic medical illness. Therefore, patients who have chronic illness should undergo a thorough medical examination with neurologic examination, review of medication and substance use, and screening diagnostic studies. There are multiple medical conditions that cause anxiety (Table 1), but the most common include thyroid disease and pulmonary disease. Patients who have hyperthyroidism have symptoms that can mimic panic attacks and there is no routine method to determine the etiology by observation alone. A thyroid-stimulating hormone should be considered for all patients who have new anxiety [4].

Pulmonary disease and asthma can trigger anxiety attacks and some patients who have lung disease live with chronic anxiety about when their breathing may become difficult. Thus, this cycle can be triggered by either anxiety or respiratory illness in the preoperative setting [3].

Substances that are prescribed, over-the-counter, or illegal are important to consider when evaluating patients who have anxiety. Caffeine requires no prescription and is easily obtainable in many forms including caffeine-containing beverages (coffee, tea, soda), weight loss products (sympathomimetics), herbal medications, alertness medications, and headache preparations. For some, caffeine can induce anxiety, even in low doses. Fortunately, a reduction in caffeine can lead to a reduction in anxious symptoms [34]. Other common medications that cause anxiety are listed in Table 1.

Table 1	
Differential diagnosis of anxiety	
Medical conditions	Endocrine, vascular, cardiac, pulmonary, infectious disease, neurologic, metabolic
Substances	Caffeine, psychostimulants, theophylline, SSRI initiation, anticholinergic medications, dopaminergic medications
Substance withdrawal	Alcohol and benzodiazepine
Other	Pain, delirium (ICU psychosis)

The lack of some substances can cause significant and life-threatening anxiety. Chronic alcohol intake is common, particularly in victims of trauma. Patients are often hesitant, out of guilt or shame, to disclose their true intake of alcohol. The alcohol withdrawal syndrome can be life threatening if not detected and treated. Confusion, anxiety, agitation, and autonomic arousal are symptoms often seen in the withdrawal syndrome. Quick recognition and treatment with benzodiazepines can limit the severity of the symptoms. In addition, patients who misuse substances are more likely to have more chaotic home lives and increased anxiety while in the hospital [34].

Pain can also contribute to patients' discomfort and anxiety. While in the perioperative stages, pre- and postoperative pain is common. Patients who have their pain undertreated often become anxious about their current pain and the possibility that it will not be taken care of by staff. Regular scheduled pain medications can help to alleviate these concerns.

Finally, delirium or postoperative confusion can mimic anxiety states. However, waxing and waning of consciousness and confusion are the hallmarks of delirium. The medical causes of delirium are even more extensive than listed in Table 1, but in the postoperative setting, delirium is often related to the surgery and procedure.

MEDICAL CARE/PSYCHIATRIC CONSULTATION

The expectations for the treatment of anxiety disorder are manifold and demanding: fast response, disappearance of panic attacks, alleviation of general and anticipatory anxiety, decrease or disappearance of phobic avoidance, increased coping skills, improved quality of life, and decreased vulnerability to relapse. Patients who have an acute anxiety disorder frequently present to the emergency department with chest pain or dyspnea, fearing that they are dying of myocardial infarction. Anxiety symptoms often accompany, or can exacerbate, respiratory conditions, such as asthma and chronic obstructive pulmonary disease. If clinically indicated, further studies should be obtained to rule out myocardial infarction and pulmonary embolism (ECG, chest radiograph). Intravenous or oral acute sedation with benzodiazepines can be used, if the medical workup rules out any acute medical issues. Untreated panic attacks can subside spontaneously within 20 to 30 minutes, especially with reassurance and a calming environment. Long-term benzodiazepines for chronic anxiety disorders should be avoided and if this approach seems necessary, obtaining a confirming opinion from a consulting psychiatrist may be helpful.

Diet

Diet can contribute to the worsening of anxiety, and patients who have prominent anxiety should be advised to discontinue (or decrease to a low and reasonable level) caffeine-containing products, such as coffee, tea, and sodas. Over-the-counter preparations and herbal remedies should be reviewed with special caution because ephedrine and other herbal compounds may precipitate or exacerbate anxiety symptoms.

Medications for anxiety

Antidepressants, including tricyclic antidepressants (TCA), selective serotonin reuptake inhibitors (SSRI) and benzodiazepines were the first effective treatments for anxiety disorders and remain valuable tools in the management of panic and other anxiety disorders [4]. There are publications supporting the efficacy of all SSRI in the treatment of panic disorder, and the US Food and Drug Administration (FDA) has approved paroxetine and sertraline for panic treatment [14]. Meta-analyses suggest that high-potency benzodiazepines and antidepressants are effective in reducing panic attacks, achieving a panic-free state, and improving anxiety, agoraphobic avoidance, and overall functional impairment [14]. Antidepressants may hold a distinct advantage over benzodiazepines in their ability to reduce depressive symptoms, but drawbacks exist for each drug class. Benzodiazepines are associated with sedation, interdose anxiety, and rebound symptoms upon discontinuation. TCA provoke undesirable anticholinergic effects, which may be particularly troublesome for patients who have panic. SSRI have a slow therapeutic onset and may cause sexual side effects or hyperstimulation [35–37]. Maximizing the strengths and minimizing the weaknesses of these agents can result in a successful combination treatment.

Combined pharmacotherapy may accelerate response and improve tolerability. It is recommended to begin chronic treatment of anxiety disorders with a benzodiazepine plus an SSRI, to reduce early treatment somatic side effects (eg, jitteriness), then continuing to maintenance treatment with SSRI monotherapy [35–37]. A slow benzodiazepine taper reduces the potential for abuse or rebound symptoms. Patients who have panic tend to fear the physiologic sensations of fear and arousal (similar to those produced by many psychotropic agents), and these concerns may play a role in maintaining the disorder. It is therefore particularly important to minimize medication side effects early in treatment. Several studies offer evidence that a benzodiazepine plus an antidepressant has a faster onset of action than antidepressant monotherapy [35].

The management of individual anxiety disorders is dependent on the specific diagnosis. Antidepressant agents are the drugs of choice in the treatment of anxiety disorders, particularly the newer agents that have a safer adverse affect profile and higher ease of use than the older agents [38]; however, benzodiazepines, short-term (Table 2) and long-term, (Tables 3 and 4) can be used as

Table 2
Antidepressant medications in the treatment of anxiety disorders

Medication	Class	Dose	Indication	Special note
Fluoxetine (Prozac)	SSRI	10–60 mg	Major depression panic disorder OCD	May worsen anxiety initially
Paroxetine (Paxil)	SSRI	10–60 mg	Depression OCD, GAD panic disorder, social phobia PTSD	Significant withdrawal if dose reduced quickly
Sertraline (Zoloft)	SSRI	50–200 mg	Panic disorder PTSD GAD social phobia	Few drug-drug interactions
Citalopram (Celexa)	SSRI	10–60 mg	Depression	Few drug-drug interactions
Escitalopram (Lexapro)	SSRI	10–20 mg	Depression GAD	Few drug-drug interactions
Fluvoxamine (Luvox)	SSRI	50–300 mg	OCD	Significant cytochrome P-450 interactions
Venlafaxine (Effexor)	SNRI	37.5–300 mg	Panic disorder GAD social phobia	Risk of elevated blood pressure, worsening hypertension
Duloxetine (Cymbalta)	SNRI	30–60 mg	Depression GAD	Risk of elevated blood pressure, worsening hypertension
Mirtazapine (Remeron)	Special class	7.5–60 mg	Depression panic disorder GAD	Risk of bone marrow suppression
Buspirone (BuSpar)	Special class	15–60 mg	GAD	Few drug-drug interactions
Imipramine (Tofranil)	Tricyclic	75–300 mg	Depression panic disorder OCD	Risk of QTc prolongation

adjunctive treatment. SSRI and selective norepinephrine reuptake inhibitors (SNRI) are helpful in a variety of anxiety disorders, including generalized anxiety disorder, panic disorder, OCD, and social phobia [38]. Some anticonvulsant medications, such as divalproex and Gabitril, may have a role in the treatment of anxiety disorders, especially in patients who have high potential for abusing benzodiazepines. Atypical antipsychotics (eg, quetiapine) may

Table 3
Short acting benzodiazepines

Benzodiazepine	Equivalent dose/ class	Metabolism	Initial & maximum dose	Average half-life (hours)	Usual dose range
Alprazolam (Xanax)	0.5 mg Trazolo	Oxidation	0.25 mg 4–8 mg	6–12	0.25 mg po tid 1 mg po tid
Lorazepam (Ativan)	1 mg 3-Hydroxy	Conjugation	0.5 mg 10 mg	8–12	0.5 mg po tid 1 mg po tid 2 mg po tid
Oxazepam (Serax)	15 mg 3-Hydroxy	Conjugation	10 mg 120 mg	4–8	15 mg po hs 30 mg po hs 30 mg po tid
Temazepam (Restoril)	10 mg 3-Hydroxy	Conjugation	15 mg 60 mg	4–10	15 mg po hs 30 mg po hs
Triazolam (Halcion)	0.25 mg 3-Hydroxy	Oxidation	0.125 mg 0.5 mg	2–6	0.125 mg po hs 0.25 mg po hs

3-hydroxy Benzodiazepines are metabolized by oxidation.
More rebound anxiety effect and withdrawal reactions; better sedative/hypnotic; preferred over long acting in elderly (less accumulation) and in patients who have liver disorders (easier metabolized).

Table 4
Long acting benzodiazepines

Benzodiazepine	Equivalent dose/class	Metabolism	Initial & maximum dose	Average half-life (hours)	Usual dose range
Chlordiazepoxide (Librium)	25 mg 2-Keto	Oxidation	5 mg 200–400 mg	100	25 mg po tid 50 mg po tid
Clonazepam (Klonopin)	0.25 mg Nitro	Oxidation & Nitro reduction	0.25 mg 10–20 mg	32	0.5 mg po tid 1 mg po bid 2 mg po tid
Clorazepate (Tranxene)	10 mg 2-Keto	Oxidation	3.75 mg 60–90 mg	100	3.75 mg po bid 7.5 mg po bid 15 mg po bid
Diazepam (Valium)	5 mg 2-Keto	Oxidation	2 mg 40 mg	100	2 mg po tid 5 mg po tid 10 mg po tid
Flurazepam (Dalmane)	15 mg 2-Keto	Oxidation	15 mg 60 mg	100	15 mg po hs 30 mg po hs

2-Keto Benzodiazepines metabolized by conjugation and oxidation.
Less rebound symptoms; better choice when tapering off of benzodiazepines (eg, clonazepam/diazepam); withdrawal may be delayed 1 to 2 weeks for 2-Keto group; bedtime dose option for hypnotic and anxiolytic effect.

also be used in individuals where the long-term use of benzodiazepine may not be appropriate.

The FDA has granted specific indications to the following disorders and agents: generalized anxiety disorder (venlafaxine, buspirone, escitalopram, paroxetine, duloxetine) [39], social phobia (paroxetine, sertraline, venlafaxine), OCD (fluoxetine, sertraline, paroxetine, fluvoxamine), and PTSD (sertraline, paroxetine). All SSRI may be equal in the treatment of anxiety disorders; however, higher doses may be necessary in the treatment of OCD. Antidepressants that are not approved by the FDA for the treatment of a given anxiety disorder, such as nefazodone and mirtazapine, still may be beneficial. Mirtazapine, for example, may be used in patients who have prominent depression and anxiety in the context of cancer treatment and anxiety [40]. Patients who have panic disorder may be more sensitive to treatment with antidepressants and frequently need lower initial doses and slower titration to accomplish successful therapy.

Older antidepressants, such as tricyclic antidepressants and monoamine oxidase inhibitors (MAOI), also are effective in the treatment of anxiety disorders. Caution in their use is warranted because of their higher toxicity and potential lethality in overdose. Their use should be limited to cases where SSRI are not effective. MAOI may be especially indicated in treatment-refractory panic disorder. Clomipramine (Anafranil, a tricyclic agent) has an FDA indication in the treatment of OCD and is the only tricyclic agent effective in the treatment of this condition. Indeed, it can be effective in cases refractory to treatment with SSRI agents. MAOI agents also may have a role in the treatment of certain subtypes of OCD refractory to conventional treatment, such as patients who have symmetry obsessions or associated panic attacks.

TREATMENT OF ACUTE PREOPERATIVE ANXIETY

Benzodiazepines are especially useful in the management of acute situational anxiety disorder and adjustment disorder, where the duration of pharmacotherapy is anticipated to be 6 weeks or less, and for the rapid control of panic attacks. If long-term use of benzodiazepines seems necessary, obtaining a confirmatory opinion from a psychiatrist is helpful because chronic benzodiazepine use may be associated with tolerance, withdrawal, and treatment-emergent anxiety [35–37]. The risk of addiction potential with benzodiazepines should be carefully considered before use in the anxiety disorders. It is advisable to avoid use in patients who have a prior history of alcohol or other drug abuse. Closely monitor for evidence of unauthorized dose escalation or obtaining benzodiazepine prescriptions from multiple sources [35–37].

PSYCHOTHERAPY AND OTHER THERAPIES FOR ANXIETY

There is an emerging body of literature suggesting that long-term management of anxiety disorders can be best achieved with combinations of medications and psychotherapy [16,20,23,27]. Cognitive-behavioral therapy (CBT) is a specific form of psychotherapy that teaches patients about their thought processes and how to adopt newer, healthier ways of viewing their situations. It also uses behavior modification to help patients to react in healthier ways, improving the outcomes of anxiety-inducing circumstances. CBT differs from other forms of psychotherapy because it focuses on taking action rather than simply exploring the reasons behind anxiety. Patients are responsible for their own thoughts and behaviors, and eventually, they realize that changing their thoughts and behaviors changes their emotional reactions to life including their generalized anxiety. During the acute preoperative period, patients may be able to use CBT skills to better control anxiety around surgery and anesthesia [16,20,23,27].

COMPLEMENTARY AND ALTERNATIVE TREATMENT OF ANXIETY

Many patients seek out alternatives to conventional Western medicine in a search to relieve their symptoms, and it is important to remember to inquire about complimentary methods of treatment [41,42]. Although often thought of as innocuous, complimentary treatments involving herbal therapy and nutritional supplements can interfere with blood clotting, platelet aggregation, and augment central nervous system depression from typical anesthetics. It is estimated that 20% of the United States population uses herbal therapy and nutritional supplements [43] In a study of 16 hospitals representing different regions of the United States, 67% of all participants used complementary and alternative medicine and it was noted that there were potential anesthesia-herbal interactions in 34% of all participants [41,42]. Other treatments include physical interventions, such as acupuncture and aromatherapy, for preoperative anxiety and cognitive interventions, such as mindfulness-based stress reduction and meditation, that can help patients prepare and practice strategies to reduce anxiety during the preoperative time [43–45].

SUMMARY

Anxiety is a common symptom seen in all medical settings and can be heightened in the preoperative setting. Careful investigation into patients' symptoms and emotions can often elucidate the source of the anxiety and lead to simple solutions to alleviate it. However, when the anxiety is more intense investigation into the physiologic causes, including medical, pharmacologic, and psychiatric, will need to occur. Treatment with short-term agents (ie, benzodiazepines) in the preoperative setting is usually enough to bring relief to patients. In the setting of more chronic anxiety illness, patients are usually on long-term treatments that create stability when they encounter the increased stress of the preoperative setting.

References

[1] Weinberger DR. Anxiety at the frontier of molecular medicine. N Engl J Med 2001;344: 1247.

[2] Norris E, Raison C. Psychologic and emotional reactions to illness and surgery. In: Lubin M, Smith R, Dodson T, et al, editors. Medical management of the surgical patient. 4th edition. New York: Cambridge University Press; 2006. p. 490.

[3] Epstein S, Hicks D. Anxiety disorders. In: Levenson J, editor. Textbook of psychosomatic medicine. Washington (DC): American Psychiatric Publishing; 2005. p. 251.

[4] Walley EJ, Beebe DK, Clark JL. Management of common anxiety disorders. Am Fam Physician 1994;50:1745.

[5] Alpert J, Bernstein J, Rosenbaum J. Psychopharmacologic issues in the medical setting. In: Cassem N, Stern T, Rosenbaum J, et al, editors. The Massachusetts general hospital handbook of general hospital psychiatry. 4th edition. St. Louis (MO): Mosby; 1997. p. 249.

[6] Iosifescu D, Pollack M. Anxiety disorders. In: Stern T, Herman J, editors. Psychiatry update and board preparation. 2nd edition. New York: McGraw-Hill Publishers; 2004. p. 121.

[7] Kessler RC, Demler O, Frank RG, et al. Prevalence and treatment of mental disorders, 1990 to 2003. N Engl J Med 2005;352:2515.

[8] Kessler RC, McGonagle KA, Zhao S, et al. Lifetime and 12-month prevalence of DSM-III-R psychiatric disorders in the United States. Results from the National Comorbidity Survey. Arch Gen Psychiatry 1994;51:8.

[9] Regier DA, Narrow WE, Rae DS, et al. The de facto US mental and addictive disorders service system. Epidemiologic catchment area prospective 1-year prevalence rates of disorders and services. Arch Gen Psychiatry 1993;50:85.

[10] Grinage BD. Diagnosis and management of post-traumatic stress disorder. Am Fam Physician 2003;68:2401.

[11] Norquist GS, Regier DA. The epidemiology of psychiatric disorders and the de facto mental health care system. Annu Rev Med 1996;47:473.

[12] Norris E, Raison C. Anxiety and somatoform disorders. In: Lubin M, Smith R, Dodson T, et al, editors. Medical management of the surgical patient. 4th edition. New York: Cambridge University Press; 2006. p. 487.

[13] Norris E, Cassem N, Huffman J, et al. Cardiovascular and other side effects of psychotropic medications. In: Stern T, Herman J, editors. Psychiatry update and board preparation. 2nd edition. New York: McGraw-Hill Publishers; 2004. p. 385.

[14] Saeed SA, Bruce TJ. Panic disorder: effective treatment options. Am Fam Physician 1998;57:2405.

[15] Weinstein RS. Panic disorder. Am Fam Physician 1995;52:2055.

[16] Fricchione G. Clinical practice. Generalized anxiety disorder. N Engl J Med 2004;351:675.

[17] Gliatto MF. Generalized anxiety disorder. Am Fam Physician 2000;62:1591.

[18] Lavie CJ, Milani RV. Generalized anxiety disorder. N Engl J Med 2004;351:2239, author reply 2239.

[19] Magill MK, Gunning K. Generalized anxiety disorder in family practice patients. Am Fam Physician 2000;62:1497.

[20] Jenike MA. Clinical practice. Obsessive-compulsive disorder. N Engl J Med 2004;350:259.

[21] Bruce TJ, Saeed SA. Social anxiety disorder: a common, under-recognized mental disorder. Am Fam Physician 1999;60:2311.

[22] Woolf SH, Friedman CL. Social anxiety disorder. Am Fam Physician 2000;61:3245.

[23] Schneier FR. Clinical practice. Social anxiety disorder. N Engl J Med 2006;355:1029.

[24] Schwaber EA. Social anxiety disorder. N Engl J Med 2006;355:2702, author reply 2702.

[25] Davidson JR. Recognition and treatment of posttraumatic stress disorder. JAMA 2001;286:584.

[26] Osterman JE, Hopper J, Heran WJ, et al. Awareness under anesthesia and the development of posttraumatic stress disorder. Gen Hosp Psychiatry 2001;23:198.

[27] Schnurr PP, Friedman MJ, Engel CC, et al. Cognitive behavioral therapy for posttraumatic stress disorder in women. a randomized controlled trial. JAMA 2007;297:820.

[28] Spielmans GI, Gatlin ET. Posttraumatic stress disorder and cognitive behavioral therapy. JAMA 2007;297:2694.
[29] Stevens LM, Burke AE, Glass RM. JAMA patient page. Posttraumatic stress disorder. JAMA 2007;298:588.
[30] Stevens LM, Lynm C, Glass RM. JAMA patient page. Posttraumatic stress disorder. JAMA 2006;296:614.
[31] Ghoneim MM. Incidence of and risk factors for awareness during anesthesia. Best Pract Res Clin Anaesthesiol 2007;21:327.
[32] Ghoneim MM, Block RI, Haffarnan M, et al. Awareness during anesthesia: risk factors, causes and sequelae: a review of reported cases in the literature. Anesth Analg 2009;108:527.
[33] Sebel PS, Bowdle TA, Ghoneim MM, et al. The incidence of awareness during anesthesia: a multicenter United States study. Anesth Analg 2004;99:833.
[34] Cleary M, Hunt GE, Matheson S, et al. The association between substance use and the needs of patients with psychiatric disorder, levels of anxiety, and caregiving burden. Arch Psychiatr Nurs 2008;22:375.
[35] Gross HS. Use of benzodiazepines in anxiety disorders. N Engl J Med 1993;329:1501.
[36] Powell G. Use of benzodiazepines in anxiety disorders. N Engl J Med 1993;329:1500.
[37] Shader RI, Greenblatt DJ. Use of benzodiazepines in anxiety disorders. N Engl J Med 1993;328:1398.
[38] Stone KJ, Viera AJ, Parman CL. Off-label applications for SSRIs. Am Fam Physician 2003;68:498.
[39] Gelenberg AJ, Lydiard RB, Rudolph RL, et al. Efficacy of venlafaxine extended-release capsules in nondepressed outpatients with generalized anxiety disorder: a 6-month randomized controlled trial. JAMA 2000;283:3082.
[40] Hartmann PM. Mirtazapine: a newer antidepressant. Am Fam Physician 1999;59:159.
[41] Saeed SA, Bloch RM, Antonacci DJ. Herbal and dietary supplements for treatment of anxiety disorders. Am Fam Physician 2007;76:549.
[42] van der Watt G, Laugharne J, Janca A. Complementary and alternative medicine in the treatment of anxiety and depression. Curr Opin Psychiatry 2008;21:37.
[43] Norred CL. Complementary and alternative medicine use by surgical patients. AORN J 2002;76:1013.
[44] Grauer RP, Thomas RD, Tronson MD, et al. Preoperative use of herbal medicines and vitamin supplements. Anaesth Intensive Care 2004;32:173.
[45] Tsen LC, Segal S, Pothier M, et al. Alternative medicine use in presurgical patients. Anesthesiology 2000;93:148.

ADVANCES IN ANESTHESIA

ELSEVIER
MOSBY

Genomics: Implications for Anesthesia, Perioperative Care and Outcomes

Simon C. Body, MBChB, MPH

Department of Anesthesiology, Perioperative and Pain Medicine, Brigham and Women's Hospital, 75 Francis Street, Boston, MA 02115, USA

Advances in genetics as a result of the Human Genome Project and 100 years of prior human genetics have recently led to numerous studies associating genetic variation with common diseases such as coronary artery disease, type II diabetes, atrial fibrillation, autism and schizophrenia, amongst many others. Before 2005, the field was poorly represented by a small number of underpowered and unreplicated genetic association studies examining single genes, with only a few well-validated genetic risk factors for common disease. The fundamental advance in the field that enabled identification of important genetic associations with disease since 2005 was identification of most of the common variations in the human genome, and the technology to examine more than 500,000 of those variants in a single individual for a cost of less than US $600.

In contrast to common acquired diseases that make up most of the health care burden in the Western world, there are numerous genetic diseases that are rare in the overall population, but are profoundly debilitating or lethal in a much smaller number of individuals. These are often obvious earlier in life, are strongly inherited, and are little modified by other nongenetic influences. Because they are rare and inherited, they are often studied in small family kindreds. These are often called Mendelian disease because of the nature of their inheritance, and the first recognized example, alcaptonuia, was discovered more than 100 years ago. Other examples are sickle cell disease, malignant hyperthermia, and the pseudocholinesterase deficiencies.

This review outlines recent developments in human genetics that affect anesthesiologists in their clinical practice. The fundamental principles of genetic variation are discussed, and the technology used to identify genetic variation in studies of gene-disease associations is described with examples of its value, notably in common diseases such as coronary artery disease (CAD) and atrial

Sources of funding: this work was supported by a grant from the National Heart, Lung, and Blood Institute (K23HL068774).

E-mail address: body@zeus.bwh.harvard.edu

0737-6146/09/$ – see front matter
doi:10.1016/j.aan.2009.07.006

fibrillation. How identification of such relationships advances medicine in general and anesthesiology specifically is also discussed. In my experience, few anesthesiologists have a working knowledge of the fundamentals of genetics and genetic study methodology, especially those of us who graduated medical school before 1990. So a somewhat colloquial approach is used, emphasizing examples from my own experience.

FUNDAMENTAL PRINCIPLES OF GENETIC VARIATION AND IMPACT ON FUNCTION

The mechanisms of the effect of genetic variation on normal homeostasis and disease are multifactorial and are confounded by the tremendous interplay and redundancy in the human machine. An entire branch of biology, called systems biology, has been developed to try and make sense of these relationships, often with the goal of identifying key proteins and mechanisms in 1 or more pathways. For example, the currently known inter-relationships for the complement pathway are portrayed in Fig. 1. At the genetic level, the methodologies are somewhat simpler but still look pretty ugly. In principle and somewhat simplistically, genetic variation can be categorized into variations in chromatin folding, DNA coding, RNA expression, and RNA translation into functional protein. Of these 4 mechanisms, the variation in DNA code is most understood; however, the other 3 are likely to be just as important in human disease.

DNA is the fundamental template for protein coding, mediated through messenger RNA (mRNA) transcription. To create mRNA, the transcriptional machinery requires access to coding DNA; however, nuclear DNA exists in complex coils around protein units called histones that simplistically hide or expose a coding DNA sequence. Because the transcriptional machinery requires access to the coding DNA, the control of mRNA creation is under control of the way the histones and other proteins fold the DNA into the conglomerate known as chromatin. Overall, our knowledge of this important mechanism is rudimentary and is not discussed further in this review.

DNA transcription to mRNA is regulated by regulatory proteins, called transcription factors, which bind to specific DNA sequences close to the gene. Transcription factors bind to short (5–20 bp) promoter regions of DNA that are usually within a few hundred base pairs of the site where transcription starts (Fig. 2). Transcription factors alter the rate of transcription of DNA sequences into mRNA by binding to the DNA and increasing the ability of the transcriptional machinery responsible for formation of mRNA. This control mechanism for mRNA production may be the most important cause of variability in complex genetic disease. If a single base pair change alters the binding of a promoter to the DNA sequence, then more or less mRNA and subsequent protein may be created. In essence, the protein sequence is the same but the amount of protein being made is different.

Other mechanisms for increasing and decreasing mRNA production also exist. Enhancers are short regions of DNA similar to promoter sequences that bind to proteins, rather like the transcription factors to enhance

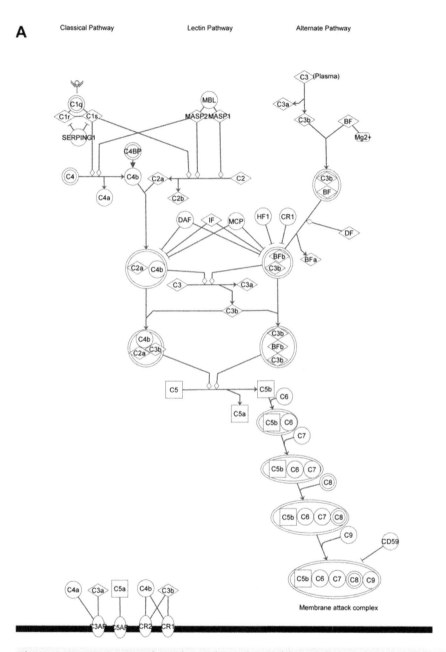

Fig. 1. Protein-protein inter-relationships within and around the complement pathway. (A) The relationships with linear sequential relationships between proteins in the complement pathway. (B) a single extension of the complement pathway into noncomplement proteins that interact with the pathway. The map was created using Ingenuity Pathway Analysis Software (http://www.ingenuity.com/; Redwood, CA) by J.D. Muehlschlegel.

B

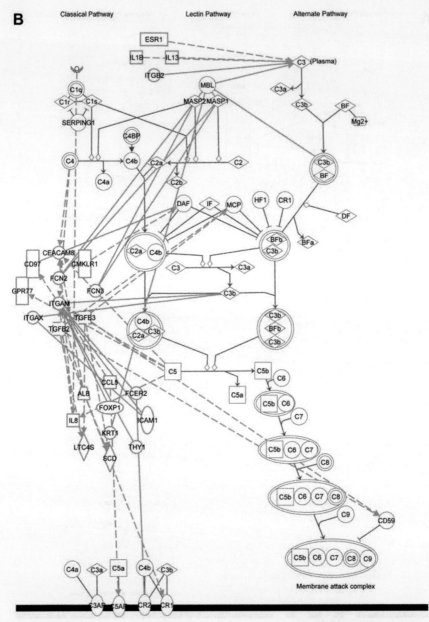

Fig. 1. (*continued*)

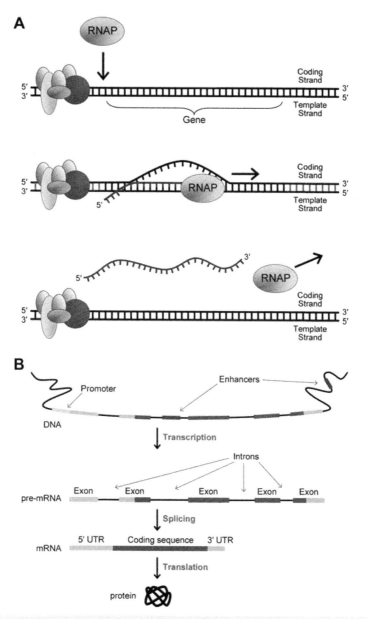

Fig. 2. Transcription of a DNA template into mRNA then into protein. (*A*) Transcription is the synthesis of mRNA from the DNA template by the enzyme RNA polymerase (RNAP). The regulatory sequence that lies before the coding sequence contains DNA sequences that bind proteins called transcription factors. Transcription factors control the transfer (or transcription) of genetic information from DNA to RNA. Transcription factors perform this function alone or with other proteins in a complex by promoting, or blocking, the recruitment of RNAP. (*B*) After transcription of mRNA, the intronic sections of mRNA are removed by the spliceosome. The processed mRNA is translated into a peptide sequence. The peptide may be further processed into a final protein. Figures are modified from http://en.wikipedia.org/wiki/File%3A Simple_transcription_initiation1.svg, http://en.wikipedia.org/wiki/File:Simple_transcription_ elongation1.svg, http://en.wikipedia.org/wiki/File:Simple_transcription_termination1.svg and http://en.wikipedia.org/wiki/File:Gene2-plain.svg.

transcription (Fig. 3). The fundamental difference between enhancers and promoters is that enhancers do not need to be close to the genes they act on. Although the enhancer sequencer may be far from the gene (as far as a million base pairs away), it is physically close to the gene when the DNA is folded around histones. Enhancers do not act on the promoter region itself, but are bound by activator proteins that enhance or repress transcription.

After transcription, the mRNA is further modified within the cell nucleus via splicing. Segments of the mRNA that do not code for a protein, called introns, are excised by enzymes called spliceosomes and the remaining exons (gene sequences that code for protein) are joined together. The final mature mRNA is then translocated to the cell cytoplasm, where the mRNA undergoes ribosomal translation into the corresponding amino acids of a protein. Another level of control exits at this point. Short sequences (~22 bp) of RNA that partially correspond to a complementary sequence of the mRNA may bind to the mRNA, thus preventing encoding of the protein. These microRNAs (miRNA) have only recently been identified and the role of the ~700 currently known human miRNAs is still poorly understood. Most miRNAs are transcribed in only 1 or a few tissues, and in only 1 or a few embryologic stages from conception to adulthood. miRNA levels are often profoundly altered in some diseases, but their role as initiators or perpetuators of disease are rarely

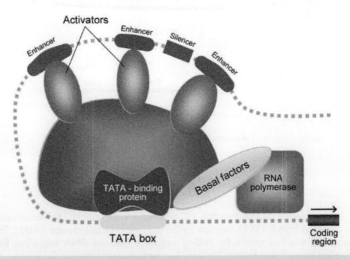

Fig. 3. The function of enhancers in transcription of DNA into mRNA. An enhancer is a short region of DNA that binds with activator proteins to enhance transcription of genes. An enhancer does not need to be particularly close to the genes it acts on, or near to the transcription initiation site, to affect the transcription of a gene. Enhancers do not act on the promoter region itself, but are bound by activator proteins that help recruit polymerase II and the general transcription factors, which then begin transcribing the genes. Genetic variation in an enhancer region may affect the binding of the enhancer to that region and the subsequent production of mRNA and protein.

known. DNA variation can alter the structure of a specific miRNA or the target of the miRNA. In addition, mRNA is degraded within the cell. The rate of degradation alters protein production.

As if we were not already overwhelmed with the options for altering the steps between DNA and protein, another vitally important step is possible. Although less than 2% of the human genome encodes the ~22,000 genes, these genes encode more than 100,000 different proteins. These different proteins result from different start, stop, and joining sites for mRNA production and splicing (Fig. 4). A single gene can encode hundreds of different proteins; there is even an example of a single fruit fly gene encoding more than 38,000 different proteins.

Although it may seem that there is an overwhelming number of ways to create variation in the human machine from its underlying complexity, the principles are relatively straightforward. Overall, the mechanism of variation can be thought of as occurring as a change in the protein structure, or a change in the amount of protein being produced.

VARIATION IN DNA AS A CAUSE OF HUMAN DISEASE

The most common type of human genetic variation is the single nucleotide polymorphism (SNP), in which 2 different bases are observed at the same position in the population and sometimes on the 2 homologous chromosomes in a single individual (Fig. 5A). Genetic variation also takes the forms of insertion or deletion of 1 or more base pairs; sometimes entire chromosomes (see Fig. 5B). When the number of inserted/deleted base pairs is large, an entire gene may be deleted or copied on the same chromosome, making a 50% decrease or 50% increase in the amount of mRNA being produced. These whole-gene insertions or deletions are called copy number variants, and are increasingly being recognized as causes of human disease. Large segments on

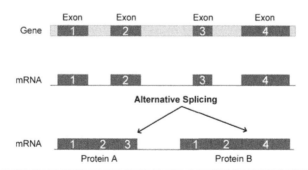

Fig. 4. Alternative splicing of messenger RNA into 2 different final proteins. Alternative splicing is a process by which the exons of the RNA produced by transcription of a gene are joined in more than 1 way during RNA splicing. The resulting different mRNAs are translated into different protein isoforms; thus, a single gene may code for multiple proteins. In humans, more than 80% of genes are alternatively spliced.

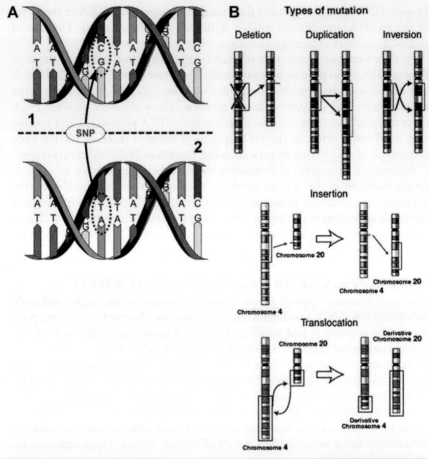

Fig. 5. DNA variation. Variation can occur at the single base level called a single nucleotide polymorphism (SNP) (A) or at a multiple base level (B). (*Figures from* http://en.wikipedia.org/wiki/File:Dna-SNP.svg, http://en.wikipedia.org/wiki/File:Types-of-mutation.png.)

the chromosomal scale can be swapped between chromosomes or inverted on the same chromosome.

The replication of DNA that is required for meiosis/mitosis and passage of DNA through generations has extremely high fidelity, with less than 1 error per million base pairs because of the extensive proof-reading capabilities of DNA replication. Even if an error occurs, the likelihood of it having functional importance is low. Redundancy exists in the amino acid code; 64 (4^3) possible combinations of base pair triplets exist to code for 21 possible amino acids, helping to limit the functional impact of errors. If the variant lies in a promoter or enhancer region, most of these variants have little effect on binding of transcription factors; yet some do.

On the simplest scale, an SNP can be seen 0, 1, or 2 times on the 2 of the 22 homologous nonsex chromosomes we each possess. The SNP may change the code for a protein if it lies within the coding sequence of the gene; many coding SNPs do not change the protein because of redundancy in the amino acid code. Even if the amino acid code is changed, most proteins have no alteration in function. The single base pair change that changes the β-hemoglobin sequence in sickle cell disease is a rare example of a functional protein change. Alternatively, the SNP may change binding of a transcription factor to a promoter or enhancer sequence, thus altering the quantity of protein being made, without changing the protein's structure. Finally, the SNP may occur at the boundary of an intron and an exon and cause the splicing machinery to code a very different and often truncated protein.

There is 1 more concept that we need to discuss. It is well known that variants close together on the same chromosome tend to be inherited together because it is rare for recombination to occur between adjacent chromosomal loci during meiosis. This is the phenomenon of linkage disequilibrium (LD). In simple terms, LD is the statistical correlation between 2 variants within a population. In general, the closer 2 variants are to each other on the chromosome, the more likely they are to be inherited together through future generations. However, there seem to be "hotspots" of recombination in the human genome that create a patchwork of "blocks" of variants that are almost always inherited together. These blocks average about 20 kbp in length, but vary widely. Within each block there is a lot of LD. Across the block boundary created by the hotspot there is much less LD. However, this block structure can vary from being well portrayed in part of the genome, to almost nonexistent in another region (Fig. 6).

When well delineated (see the F5/SELP example uppermost in Fig. 6), the limited diversity of polymorphisms within a block creates groups of alleles that are almost always inherited together, known as haplotypes. There are usually only a few haplotypes within a block that describe all of the genetic variation seen with tens to hundreds of variants. The block structure of the genome allows finer mapping of disease genes and alleles to the level of the individual haplotype block. Yet use of haplotype blocks for mapping genetic polymorphisms that contribute to disease complicates determination of a "responsible" variant below the level of the haplotype block, as there is strong LD between polymorphisms within the haplotype block. Often the investigator can say only that a group of highly related alleles are associated with a disease, without being able to pinpoint the variant specifically responsible. To find the actual causal variant requires molecular biology rather than genetics. The importance of this haplotype block structure is discussed later in this review.

TECHNOLOGY TO IDENTIFY GENETIC VARIATION
Measurement of DNA variation

The last 20 years have seen an exponential increase in the quality and quantity of genotyping. Five years ago, I paid US$0.50 for a single SNP measurement in

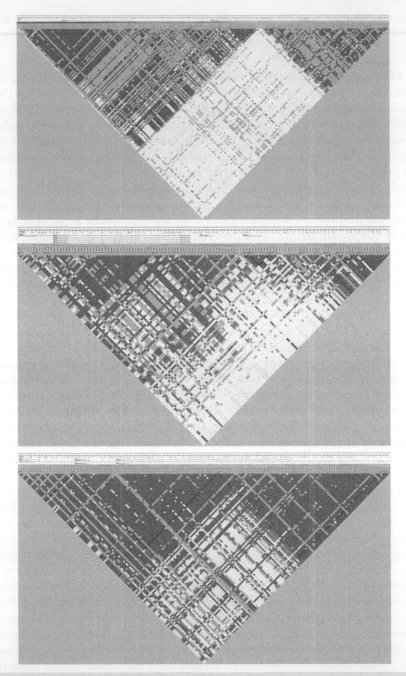

Fig. 6. LD structure of the genome. Each panel shows the correlation between variants within a genomic region. Each variant is plotted on the map and the more highly correlated a variant is with another variant, the redder the intersecting square is. The top panel shows the strong correlation between variants in the Factor V/P-selectin (*F5/SELP*) region, with a well-demarcated recombination point that breaks the region in 2. The middle panel shows mixed and low correlation in the A-natriuretic and B-natriuretic peptides (*NPPA/NPPB*) genomic region. The lower panel shows mixed and high correlation in the platelet adenosine diphosphate receptor (*P2RY12*) genomic region.

a single patient. On each plate of genotyping there were 368 patients in separate wells and in each well I could concurrently genotype 5 or 6 SNPs at a time. That scale and cost was considered miraculous at the time. Last year, we paid about US$0.0006 per SNP to genotype about 900,000 SNPs in a single patient (total cost per patient of about US$550). In 1 month in 2008, we doubled the total amount of genotyping we had performed in the previous 5 years.

How was this possible and how was it done? There are numerous genotyping technologies available, most of which fundamentally use the polymerase chain reaction (PCR) to amplify limited amounts of a specific sequence into larger quantities for analysis. Measurement of individual SNPs usually involves identifying the 2 different alleles using the molecular weight of the alleles, the length of different sequences depending on the allele, or making complementary sequences that bind to one or other of the alleles, which can then be identified by florescence or some other physicochemical property. These days, the methods are so accurate (>99.9%) and have such high success (>98%), that the choice of technique is usually dependent on price, the number of patients and SNPs being measured, and local expertise. However, 1 technique deserves closer review.

Whole-genome scanning (WGS) measures about 1 million SNPs and copy number variants, to cover the genome with high precision. For the 3 billion base pairs in the human genome, genotyping 1 million variants means that a genotype is measuring about every 3000 base pairs on average. Detailed analysis using real data shows that about 80% of all variations in a human is measured using about 1 million variants. This fidelity means that 1 or more SNPs are usually genotyped within each haplotype block. If an association is found, further genotyping of the SNPs in that region will likely identify 1 or more SNPs or haplotypes with the greatest association. Commercial WGS uses 2 technologies with similar accuracy and completeness. The chips are made by Affymetrix and Illumina, and the decision to use 1 or the other usually depends on local preference rather than on hard science. The physical characteristics of these chips are shown in Fig. 7.

Measurement of RNA variation

In general, the amount of mRNA produced within a cell determines the amount of protein made by the cell. There are several caveats to that statement but the general concept is correct. If a noncoding variant is found to be related to a disease, the proof of the relationship can be found by demonstrating increased or decreased mRNA production. Unfortunately, mRNA is a relatively unstable molecule made in small amounts, and complex techniques are required to accurately measure the amount of mRNA. Currently, the most common methods of measuring mRNA involve either: (1) measuring the amount of mRNA made through many cycles of PCR to quantify the original amount of mRNA present (slow and expensive, unsuitable for large-scale work), and (2) comparing the amount of mRNA present in 2 paired samples,

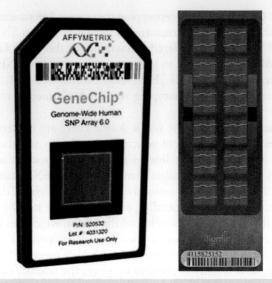

Fig. 7. Physical characteristics of "chips" used for whole-genome scans. Each of these chips is used for genotyping approximately 1 million SNPs and other variations in a single individual. The overall cost for genotyping a single individual at these ~1,000,000 variants is less than $1000.

often comparing before and after an event on chips, rather like the chips used for genotyping. This second technique is fast, can operate on industrial scales, and can compare signals for most proteins produced by the genome. However, interpretation of the signals is difficult as the comparison of different amounts of red and green light produced from fluorescent markers is inaccurate. In addition, the chips require detailed sequence knowledge of the mRNA being produced and cannot reliably measure splicing variants in many situations. The latest and greatest technology for mRNA measurement is a quantal improvement because of its ability to measure even a single mRNA molecule in a cell, measure mRNA sequences that we do not even know about, and give precise numeric estimates of the amount of every single mRNA in the cell. It does this by sequencing every mRNA present in a sample. However, its cost is high and its speed is slow. Both will improve with time.

PRINCIPLES OF STUDY OF GENE-DISEASE RELATIONSHIPS

Human gene-disease studies fall into 2 general classes; linkage studies and association studies, based on the nature of the inheritance pattern. Linkage studies are used in Mendelian disease, often in families with a high prevalence of a single disease that is observed early in life, in whom multigenerational trees of inheritance of disease can be traced. The basis of linkage studies is an observed principle in genetics that homologous chromosomes (ie, both copies of say chromosome 2) in a dividing germ cell exchange large common portions of the chromosome between each other, via a molecular process called recombination (Fig. 8). Those 2 chromosomes will have come from the individual's parents, and by comparing a large number (>1000) of genetic markers in multigenerational families the point of chromosomal swapping in the genome that is most significantly related to the disease can be established. This point is close to the gene responsible for the disease, but the fidelity of this technique is limited, often giving results that cover large portions (many millions of base pairs) of a chromosome. Narrowing the region down to 1 or more genes involves follow-up genotyping of progressively smaller regions with greater fidelity. A good example has been the use of linkage analysis in families with a high incidence of breast cancer at a young age to identify the *BRCA1* gene on chromosome 17. In general, linkage studies are only valuable when the disease is present at a young age and not significantly modified by environmental influences.

The contrast between Mendelian disease and complex disease is many-fold and can be simplistically thought of as a comparison of a predetermined genetic fate compared with a smaller risk that is often modified by nongenetic factors

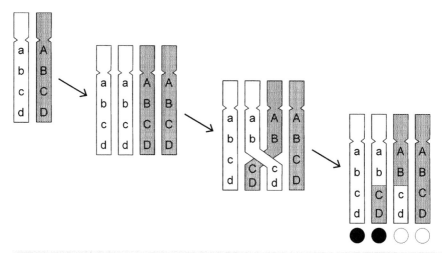

Fig. 8. Recombination and its use in linkage studies. In this example, the authors genotyped 4 markers (A, B, C, D) in a single individual. On the individuals maternal chromosome, the markers are variants called a, b, c, and d. On the individuals paternal chromosome, the equivalent markers are "normal" and called A, B, C, and D. Let us assume that the marker b causes a disease and so this person is a heterozygote, having 1 abnormal copy b and 1 normal copy B. During production of the 4 eggs or sperm resulting from a single germ cell, 2 adjacent chromosomes swap equal portions of the chromosome, an event called recombination or "crossing-over." Two of the 4 resulting gametes will pass the abnormal marker onto the next generation (marked with a black dot) and 2 will not (marked with a white dot). If 2 or more generations are genotyped in a single family, it can be seen that the disease occurs only in those with the a or b variants and not those with the c or d variants. If the genotyping is repeated in many families, the causative variant can be localized to a region around the marker b.

(Table 1). Despite the importance of individual Mendelian disease to those affected by it, the larger genetic burden on human health comes from complex diseases that often manifest only later in life. Simple examples are CAD, obesity, and hypertension. It is obvious that occurrence of these, and other complex diseases, is highly influenced by human behaviors and circumstances. For example, obesity and CAD are rarer outside the Western world. Other complex diseases have few environmental components, such as autism and schizophrenia. Their complexity seems to come from a likelihood that many variants, rather than 1 single variant, cause the disease either occurring together in a single individual or occurring rarely in many individuals.

Because diseases of old age can rarely be examined in large mutigenerational families (the parents and grandparents have often died by the time the children get the disease in their 60s or 70s), association studies are used to test whether a polymorphism occurs more or less frequently in many unrelated cases compared with many unrelated controls. Association studies have only become a common discovery tool now that much of the variation in the human genome is known. About 13 million SNPs in the human genome are known, about half of which are common (>1% frequency). This number far exceeds the density of markers used in linkage studies, so our ability to narrowly identify the polymorphism or region associated with disease is greatly improved. Another advantage is that association studies use conventional case-control methodology and do not require families to be studied. Consequently, association studies can allow us to examine genetic causes of diseases associated with surgery, drugs, or other interventions, where few individuals in the family have undergone the same surgery or taken the same drug. However, design, analysis, and interpretation of association studies require statistical rigor and expertise (see Table 1)[1].

Table 1
Comparison of single gene, strongly inherited disorders (often known as Mendelian diseases) with complex genetic disorders

Parameters	Mendelian disease	Complex disease
Number of diseases	4361 on 9 May 2009[a]	Most human disease
Frequency in population	Very rare	Common
Frequency of genetic variation	Very rare	Rare or common
Inheritance within a family	Strong	Weak
Risk ratio	>10–20	1–3
Genetic cause	Single gene	Often many genes
Nongenetic influence on frequency or severity of disease	Generally weak	Strong
Age at first recognition of disease	Often young	Often old
Method used for study of disease	Linkage study	Association study

[a]Online Mendelian Inheritance in Man (http://www.ncbi.nlm.nih.gov/Omim/mimstats.html).

An important concept in our understanding of complex human disease has been the role of many small-effect genes on common diseases. The so-called common disease/common variant hypothesis suggests that there are many common variants, each having a combined and incremental effect on the risk of a disease. Restated, several commonly occurring SNPs in several genes, each individually contribute a small increased or decreased risk to the overall risk of a disease in a single individual. We currently believe that this mechanism of complex disease is the most prevalent and accounts for many diseases of old age, such as diabetes and CAD. A simple and understandable example is height. There are several genes that have some role in determining height, but neonatal and childhood circumstances also play a strong role. Alternatively, the multiple rare variant hypothesis states that in any single individual, a few relatively rare variants, each with a relatively large effect, contribute to the disease, but because they are rare in the overall population, the effect appears to be complex. This mechanism is likely true for many genes of drug metabolism and obvious examples from the anesthesia realm are malignant hyperthermia and succinylcholine metabolism.

In 2005, the first genome-wide association studies (GWAS) emerged from the combination of the HapMap project (http://www.hapmap.org) with new technologies for testing hundreds of thousands of SNPs on a single chip. The studies are undertaken by measuring say 1 million known SNPs in say 10,000 individuals (5000 with the disease of interest and 5000 without). The SNPs are roughly spaced about 1 SNP every 3000 base pairs of the 3×10^9 base pair human genome, thus allowing almost complete coverage of all the variation in the genome. The coverage is not perfect; there are gaps, but we generally believe that we are able to observe about 80% of all common variations. The words common variation are important; it is likely that our ability to find associations of disease to variation that conforms to the multiple rare variant hypothesis is probably less than associations to variation that conforms to the common disease/common variant hypothesis.

These GWAS studies have successfully identified more than 30 genes associated with obesity, more than 30 genes associated with type II diabetes, more than 20 genes associated with CAD or myocardial infarction, more than 10 genes associated with breast or endometrial cancer, more than 5 genes associated with each of prostate cancer, schizophrenia, autism, and psoriasis, and 3 genes associated with atrial fibrillation (AF). In all, more than 400 genes have been associated with more than 75 complex diseases (mid-2009).

A SIMPLE EXAMPLE OF THE METHODS USED IN GENE-DISEASE ASSOCIATION STUDIES

A simple example of gene-disease association studies illustrates the general principles and serves as a basis for understanding the studies found in the anesthesiology literature. The methods used depend on the outcome being examined, the number and density of variants being examined, and the clinical factors that may alter the relationship between gene and disease.

The outcome of interest may be a continuous (such as duration of hospitalization), ordinal (such as American Society of Anesthesiologists [ASA] class), or dichotomous (such as postoperative myocardial infarction, or not) variable. Analysis methods exist for all these types of outcomes. The simplest example to illustrate is a dichotomous variable. The advantage of this type of analysis in unrelated individuals is its simplicity. It looks and behaves like the rudimentary 2×2 tables of epidemiology and χ^2 statistics. Let us say we have a population of 2000 patients who underwent coronary artery bypass graft (CABG) surgery at a single center and that 10% of them had a myocardial infarction (MI). Our hypothesis is that a single SNP in the chromosome 9p21 region is associated with MI. However, we could know that several pre- and perioperative factors affect the frequency of MI, such as age, race, current smoking, prior MI, severity of coronary disease, duration of cardiopulmonary bypass, and surgeon. We know this for our population because before we embarked on the genetic analysis, we examined many variables that may or may not predict MI and created a robust logistic regression model of the clinical variables that are associated with MI. We made this model for 2 reasons: (1) reducing other causes of variability in the relationship between SNP and MI may allow a stronger identification of the relationship, and (2) there may be situations where the signal is only present when a particular clinical covariate is also present. A theoretic example is that the SNP may only have an effect when the patient is a smoker. Although construction of a logistic regression model is essential in genetic studies of clinical outcomes, the overall principles can be demonstrated using a 2×2 table.

Looking at the 2×2 table in Table 2A, we have made a few assumptions: the minor (less frequent) allele occurs 1 or more times in 40% of the population, MI occurs at a rate of 10%, and there is a dominant genetic model. The null hypothesis of no relationship between SNP and MI would result in the distribution of individuals in the 2000 patient cohort illustrated in the upper panel. There is no difference in the frequency of MI between those with and without the SNP. However, let us say we actually observed the numbers in Table 2B. The chance of having an MI if you carried the SNP was observed to be 15%, but if you did not carry the SNP the chance of having an MI was 6.67%. The relative risk was increased 2.25-fold by carrying the SNP. The confidence interval of the relative risk of 2.25 is 1.72 to 2.94 and the result is statistically significant ($P<.0001$). This example is unrealistically simple. There are several factors that may confound this relationship between SNP and MI. One possible example is race. Let us say that the study population included 1000 white people and 1000 African Americans. The frequency of carrying 1 or more copies of the SNP is 50% in whites and 30% in African Americans and the MI frequency is 12.5% in whites and 7.5% in African Americans. In whites (see Table 2C), the relative risk from carrying the allele is 1.27 (0.91–1.77) and is not significant ($P=.15$) in this study. In African Americans (see Table 2D), the relative risk from carrying the allele is 4.67 (2.94–7.40) and is very significant ($P<.0001$). The effect of the SNP is only present in African

Table 2			
Example of a simple gene association study			
	SNP		
	Present	Absent	N
A: Null hypothesis: no relationship between SNP and MI			
MI Yes	80	120	200
No	720	1080	1800
	800	1200	2000
B: Observed relationship between SNP and MI in the whole population			
MI Yes	120	80	200
No	680	1120	1800
	800	1200	2000
C: Observed relationship between SNP and MI in white people			
MI Yes	70	55	100
No	430	445	875
	500	500	1000
D: Observed relationship between SNP and MI in African Americans			
MI Yes	50	25	75
No	250	675	925
	300	700	1000

Americans, an example of the relationship being stratified by population structure. We can opine on the biology that may cause such a difference, but the actual cause cannot be derived within this experiment. This probably unrealistic example shows the importance of including demographic and clinical variables in defining the relationship between an SNP and an outcome or disease.

WHAT ARE THE USES OF GENETIC STUDIES?

There are several potential uses of the results of genetic studies. We can think of them as being potentially valuable for a group of individuals, say white men with prostatic symptoms or white women with a family history of breast cancer. Alternatively, the benefit may only accrue to a single individual (Table 3). It is important to appreciate that most examples are still theoretic. We are at the early stages of applying genomics to medicine and there are many limitations to our knowledge and its applicability.

For a group of individuals, identification of a gene or region that is associated with a disease provides information on which genes or pathways are integral to disease. With extensive work, the molecular biology of the association may be established, a biomarker or drug target defined and perhaps a drug developed. These examples are currently few and far between. It is likely they will become more common; however, the greatest value of identifying a drug target or some other therapy may only be present for genetic factors with high relative risks. Illustrating the example, there are newly found regions that increase the risk of coronary disease by 15%. Many individuals and companies are working on identifying drug targets and drugs for this genetic risk factor. But, will I take

Table 3
Potential uses of a genetic test at a population and individual level

On a population level
  Identification of a disease-causing gene or region
  Identification of a biologic pathway associated with disease
  Identification of a biomarker of disease
  Identification of a drug target
On a personal level
  Identification of a risk prediction variable
  Identification of a pharmacogenomic risk or effect

a drug to prevent coronary disease if I am reducing my risk by only 15%? Probably not and especially if, on a population basis, everyone has to take the drug. In contrast, not starting, or stopping, smoking reduces risk by 50%. However, if I have severe coronary disease and a new drug will reduce my risk of MI by 50%, that reduction will likely be important to society and to me.

Another illustrative scenario is warfarin dosing. The *CYP2C9* and *VKORC1* genes are implicated in warfarin and vitamin K metabolism, and variants in these genes are strongly and consistently associated with bleeding while taking warfarin. Variation in these 2 genes outweighs all other clinical predictors including age, gender, and body weight. My father takes 1 to 2 mg of warfarin a day, most likely because he has 1 or both of these variants. There is a good chance my warfarin requirements will be similar, if I ever need warfarin. If I did not have that prior knowledge my warfarin dosing would likely be based on a population average until my internationalized normalized ratio (INR) has been measured several times. That may incur a risk of bleeding. Someone else may need much more warfarin than the population average and be at risk of thrombosis in those first few weeks of drug treatment. Several companies have developed rapid turnaround genotyping tests with high accuracy that cost about $400; however, the cost of saving a life using these tests is about $170,000 per quality-adjusted life-year [2]. Payment for the test was rejected by the Centers for Medicare and Medicaid Services earlier this year [3].

Another example may be illustrative. If a woman has a history of breast cancer in her family, there may be value in testing for the several variants that are associated with breast cancer (*BRCA1* and *BRCA2*). The lifetime risk of breast cancer for a woman is approximately 12%; but is increased to 60% for carriers of 1 of the *BRCA1* or *BRCA2* variants. At least 9 other genes have been associated with hereditary breast or ovarian cancers, but most hereditary breast cancers can be accounted for by inherited mutations in *BRCA1* and *BRCA2*. However, at a societal level there is no value in testing every woman for these variants. The reason is the low efficacy of determining the risk of breast cancer from these tests. Overall, *BRCA1* and *BRCA2* variants account for only 5% to 10% of breast cancers and 10% to 15% of ovarian cancers among white women, but 1 or more of these variants are carried by only

2.2% of white women. By contrast, the variant is present in 8.5% of Ashkenazi Jewish women (a population with a high rate of inherited breast cancer) and only 0.5% in Asian women (a population with a low rate of inherited breast cancer)[4]. The guidelines for testing for these mutations should reflect the relative frequency of the variants and family history [5]. Another example is Crohn disease, which has at least 32 genetic variants strongly associated with it. Because the average prevalence of the disease in the general population is less than 0.2%, people with several high-risk genes may have an approximately 20-fold increased risk, but still have a small probability (<4%) that they will get Crohn disease.

HOW DOES GENETIC INFORMATION ALTER RISK CLASSIFICATION

We are all familiar with classification of patients into risk classes. Daily examples are Mallampati classification for intubation difficulty, ASA class, and the many indices of cardiac risk. We are also aware of how these indices are not perfect predictors. Would having more information make them better predictors? The remainder of this discussion is predicated on several statements with varying degrees of truth:

(i) The value of risk classification only comes from what therapies and changes in therapies are driven by the risk

(ii) The value of a risk classifier is dependent on its positive and negative predictive value.

(iii) The value of the additional information to the patient is determined by the effectiveness of the therapy(ies).

The value of any additional information to a risk classification index is measured and determined by how many patients are correctly switched from 1 risk class to another and that a different and presumably better therapy is provided as a result of that information. Let us look at an example. The 9p21 chromosomal region has been strongly associated with CAD and MI. Papers that describe the association have P values better than 10^{-12} and have risk ratios of ~1.25 (ie, risk is increased by about 25% more than the general population). You can go to the web and order a kit to swab buccal cells, mail it back, and have your 9p21 status returned to you in a couple of weeks. You will be about $200 poorer; will you be wiser? By contrast, knowing several nongenetic facts may provide just as much, or likely more, predictive value. Using identified predictors from the Third Report of the National Cholesterol Education Program Expert Panel on Detection, Evaluation, and Treatment of High Blood Cholesterol in Adults (ATPIII) risk score, well-conducted studies have strongly predicted subsequent risk of cardiovascular events. As a perfect example of the relative value of genetic information, the study by Paynter and colleagues [6], using 22,129 white participants in the Women's Genome Health Study showed the ATPIII index (age, systolic blood pressure, cholesterol, high density lipoprotein cholesterol, smoking, antihypertensive use and diabetes) was strongly predictive of subsequent cardiovascular events. A measure of this prediction is the c-index which in this case was 0.803 ± 0.019, which is very strong. However, adding genetic information from the strongest genetic variant associated with CAD in the 9p21 region (rs10757274) only trivially improved the index to 0.805 ± 0.019. It is not statistically significant, and tells us little about the value of the genetic marker as a risk classifier for individual patients.

There is a better method. In the same study, they divided the ATPIII-predicted risk of cardiovascular events into 4 risk classes (<5%, 5% to <10%, 10% to <20%, and ≥20% risk of a cardiovascular event in the next 10 years). These classes are commonly used to tell patients about their risk. They then compared the assigned ATPIII risk categories for each participant without including any genetic information with the risk categories for the same participant with additional genetic information from the rs10757274 genotype included (Table 4). The proportion of participants who were reclassified into a different risk group by the ATIII index plus genetic information, versus the ATIII index only, can be estimated. Some of these reclassifications will be correct (ie, they correctly predict an event), and some will not be correct. If we added a variable to the model that had no effect on developing a cardiovascular event (eg, left vs right handedness), then the number of participants who correctly changed risk class would roughly equal the number who incorrectly changed risk class. By contrast, if the additional information was highly informative then the number correctly changed would far outweigh the number incorrectly changed. In this study, 606 of 22,129 participants were reclassified (see Table 4). Overall, 526 (87% of those reclassified) were reclassified correctly. This was a modest but significant ($P = .02$) improvement. But does it help us? This depends on what clinical value we assigned to each of the classes. If an effective therapy is only provided to patients with ≥5% risk,

Table 4
The effect of adding genotype to the ATPIII index on reclassification of participants

ATPIII risk class	ATPIII risk class and rs10757274 genotype				Reclassified correctly (%)/ reclassified (%)
	<5% risk	5% to <10% risk	10% to <20% risk	≥20% risk	
<5% risk, N (% reclassified)	18,609	205 (1.1)	–	–	1.1/1.1
5% to <10% risk, N (% reclassified)	181 (8.2)	1933	83 (3.8)	–	12.0/12.0
10% to <20% risk, N (% reclassified)	–	80 (9.9)	697	31 (3.8)	3.8/13.7
≥20% risk, N (% reclassified)	–	–	26 (8.4)	284	8.4/8.4

Modified from Paynter NP, Chasman DI, Buring JE, et al. Cardiovascular disease risk prediction with and without knowledge of genetic variation at chromosome 9p21.3. Ann Intern Med 2009;150(2):65–2.

then 205 additional patients will correctly receive the therapy and 181 will correctly not receive the therapy. No one will be incorrectly denied therapy. By contrast, if the effective therapy is only given to those with ≥20% risk, 31 additional patients will correctly get the therapy and 26 will correctly not get it. Although it may seem that these examples are pretty robust, they are actually trivial in numeric terms. Overall, few patients in this large cohort had a significant advantage conveyed by the additional genetic information. Why is that? The additional risk of having the rs10757274 genotype is small (about 25% more) and is outweighed by risks from smoking and other factors.

By contrast, the risk of atrial fibrillation during an individual's lifetime is approximately doubled by possessing a variant of a chromosome 4q25 SNP called rs2200733 [7]. Similarly, we have recently demonstrated that the risk of AF after cardiac surgery is approximately doubled by carrying minor alleles of rs2200733 [8]. This effect is independent of other well-known risk factors such as older age, a past history of AF, and the type of operation being performed. In a population of 959 patients undergoing CABG with or without concurrent valve surgery, we used a statistical model that included these variables, amongst others, to derive a predicted risk for each patient. We then classified individuals into 2 classes of risk of developing AF (Table 5) based on whether or not the risk was greater than or less than the population average AF rate of 30%. After adding the patients rs2200733 genotype status to the model, 53 patients in the low-risk group (<30% risk) were reclassified into the high-risk group (≥30% risk). Of these 53 patients, 21 (40%) developed postoperative AF and so can be construed as being correctly reclassified. After adding the patients rs2200733 genotype status to the model, 69 patients in the high-risk group (≥30% risk) were reclassified into the low-risk group (<30% risk). Of these 69 patients, 49 (71%) did not develop postoperative AF and so can be construed as being correctly reclassified. So, in this example, we have correctly reclassified 70 patients to a different risk group, but have incorrectly

Table 5
The effect of adding rs2200733 genotype to the risk of AF on reclassification of patients' risk

AF risk class without genotype status known	AF risk class with rs2200733 genotype		Reclassified correctly (%)/ reclassified (%)
	<30% risk	≥30% risk	
<30% risk, N (% reclassified)	532	53 (10.0)	4.0/10.0
≥30% risk, N (% reclassified)	69 (16.2)	427	11.5/16.2

The clinical risk model for AF included institution, age, gender, a prior history of AF, cardiopulmonary bypass duration, preoperative statin use and whether or not concurrent valve surgery was performed. Risk classes were created based on estimated risk of <30% risk and ≥30% risk from the clinical risk model.
Data from: Body S, Collard C, Shernan S, et al. Variation in the 4q25 chromosomal locus predicts new-onset atrial fibrillation after cardiac surgery. Circulation 2008;118:S882.

reclassified 52 patients, for a net gain of 18 patients. If we had put the patient on a drug, or not, based on the revised classification, we may have done some good or the effect may have been minimal. That would principally depend on the efficacy and side effects of the drug.

SUMMARY

There is considerable scope in genetic studies for identification of pathways of disease and determining therapies for individual patients. We should make ourselves aware of the unbiased evidence that supports a genetic test, its overall value to the population and to the individual, and its implications in determining clinical decision-making. However, much work needs to be done and most of what you will hear in the next 10 to 20 years will be hype rather than reality.

Acknowledgments

The authors thank all study the patients who participated in the CABG Genomics Program and the surgeons who collaborated by identifying their patients.

References

[1] Tabor HK, Risch NJ, Myers RM. Opinion: Candidate-gene approaches for studying complex genetic traits: practical considerations. Nat Rev Genet 2002;3(5):391–7.

[2] Eckman MH, Rosand J, Greenberg SM, et al. Cost-effectiveness of using pharmacogenetic information in warfarin dosing for patients with nonvalvular atrial fibrillation. Ann Intern Med 2009;150(2):73–83.

[3] Center for Medicare and Medicaid Services. Proposed decision memo for pharmacogenomic testing for warfarin response (CAG-00400N). Available at: https://www.cms.hhs.gove/mcd/viewdraftdecisionmemo.asp?id=224. Accessed August 10, 2009.

[4] John EM, Miron A, Gong G, et al. Prevalence of pathogenic BRCA1 mutation carriers in 5 US racial/ethnic groups. JAMA 2007;298(24):2869–76.

[5] National Cancer Institute. BRCA1 and BRCA2: cancer risk and genetic testing. Available at: http://www.cancer.gov/cancertopics/factsheet/risk.brca. Accessed August 10, 2009.

[6] Paynter NP, Chasman DI, Buring JE, et al. Cardiovascular disease risk prediction with and without knowledge of genetic variation at chromosome 9p21.3. Ann Intern Med 2009;150(2):65–72.

[7] Gudbjartsson DF, Arnar DO, Helgadottir A, et al. Variants conferring risk of atrial fibrillation on chromosome 4q25. Nature 2007;448(7151):353–7.

[8] Body S, Collard C, Shernan S, et al. Variation in the 4q25 chromosomal locus predicts new-onset atrial fibrillation after cardiac surgery [abstract]. Circulation 2008;118:S882.

Advances in Anesthesia 27 (2009) 95–110

ELSEVIER
MOSBY

ADVANCES IN ANESTHESIA

Retirement Planning for Physicians

J. Bruce Levis, Jr., MBA, CFP*, David S. Markle, CPA/PFS, CFP

McQueen, Ball & Associates, Inc., 561 Main Street, Suite 100, Bethlehem, PA 18018, USA

M ost physicians taking full advantage of their employer-sponsored retirement plans probably think that they are well on their way to a comfortable retirement. However, they may be quite surprised to find out that this savings strategy alone may not result in enough capital to support their lifestyle in retirement. Retirement planning deals with determining the amount of capital needed and the current action steps that should be taken to achieve this objective.

Traditionally, retirement income has come from three sources. The first source was your employer-sponsored defined benefit plan (pension), the second was Social Security, and the third was personal savings and investments.

"Pension Cuts Rise; So Do Concerns"
The New York Times, March 22, 2009

The employer-sponsored plan as a source of retirement income has been under pressure for several years. As legacy costs, which include medical and pension payments to retirees, place additional strain on the balance sheets and cash flows of many companies, the defined benefit plan has been jettisoned in favor of defined contribution plans. From 1975 to 2006, the number of defined benefit plans decreased by approximately 53%, according to the Department of Labor's *February, 2009 Private Pension Plan Bulletin* [1]. Over the same period, defined contribution plans have increased by 211%. Defined contribution plans usually permit employees to defer a portion of their current compensation, and may include an employer match into a tax-deferred account. This has proven to be a much cheaper solution for employers. If employees are fortunate enough to have a defined benefit plan that is well funded, they are in the minority.

"How to Prepare for the End of Social Security"
U.S. News & World Report, June 16, 2009

The second source of retirement income is Social Security. Regardless of whose numbers you look at or want to believe, the system faces the same actuarial challenges that the defined benefit plan faces: longer life expectancies and

*Corresponding author. *E-mail address*: blevis@mcqueenball.com (J.B. Levis, Jr.).

0737-6146/09/$ – see front matter
doi:10.1016/j.aan.2009.07.007

fewer workers supporting a larger number of retirees. Also, baby boomers are reaching retirement age and will surely place additional stress on the system. While it is impossible to say what will happen to the Social Security system as we know it, it is fair to say that this source of retirement income will be on less-stable footing.

"Consumers Are Saving More and Spending Less"
The New York Times, February 3, 2009

The third source is personal savings and investments, which include deferrals into 401(k) and 403 (b) defined contribution plans. According to the *April, 2009 Personal Income and Outlays* from the U.S. Department of Commerce, Bureau of Economic Analysis, the personal savings rate for the month was 5.7%, which is the highest number recorded since February of 1995 [2]. Personal savings is the focus of this article and the only source of retirement income over which the physician can exercise significant control.

One of the variables that affects retirement planning is life expectancy. The longer life expectancies that we enjoy in the United States place added strain on retirement budgets. According to the *32nd Report of Health, United States, 2008* by the Centers for Disease Control and Prevention, the life expectancy for a child born today is 78.1 years [3]. This same study shows that if you are turning age 65 today you are likely to live another 18.7 years and, if you are fortunate enough to have attained the age 75, you can expect on average another 12.0 years of life. It is not unrealistic for some young retirees to spend more time in their retirement years than they did in their working years.

Another variable specific to retirement planning for a physician deals with the delayed entry into the workforce due to lengthy educational requirements. The long educational commitment delays the start of a physician's professional career until sometime beyond age 30. The actual cost (usually in the form of student loans) can run into hundreds of thousands of dollars. The good news about choosing anesthesiology as a career is that, according to the occupational employment and wage estimates from the United States government, the average annual pay is $197,570 [4]. This above-average physician income helps both to compensate for the delayed career start and to pay down student loans.

The decline in the equity markets seen in 2008 and early 2009 has caused a number of individuals to delay their retirement altogether or consider working part-time to avoid drawing down their depleted portfolios. A recent article in the *AARP Bulletin Today* shows that the average retirement age has moved up since the mid-1980s, when individuals would typically retire at 62 or 63 [5], to an average retirement age in 2008 of 65.

During your professional career, you will likely face a number of financial commitments and obligations that may include living expenses, taxes, and housing costs, as well as your own educational debts and the costs of educating your children. Another responsibility that needs to be added to this list is that is building up enough capital to live comfortably during your retirement phase.

There are two major phases to the retirement planning process. The first is the accumulation phase. This is defined as the period at the beginning of your professional career when you are saving and building up your net worth to support the next phase of the process. The second phase of retirement planning is the distribution phase. This is the period when your professional career ends and you start to live off the capital you have accumulated. Regardless of which phase you are in, one common goal remains: to maximize your capital base from an investment and income tax standpoint.

TAX AND INVESTMENT STRATEGIES

Capitalizing on opportunities to grow or extend the life of your capital base is critical. To do so, it is important to note that rates of return are not earned in a vacuum and one of the main outflows from your capital base will be income taxes. Income tax planning has two primary objectives: (1) minimizing overall income tax liability and (2) fulfilling overall financial planning goals with minimal tax consequences.

These objectives are addressed through three broad strategies [6]:

1. Reducing the income tax consequences of a transaction or arrangement
2. Shifting the timing of a taxable event
3. Shifting income to another taxpayer

Each of the following six specific income tax and investment strategies may be incorporated into one or more of the broad strategies listed above.

Maximize contributions

The first strategy is to maximize your retirement plan contributions. This has the effect of both reducing current income and shifting the timing of the event to a future period. For example, the maximum salary deferral to a qualified plan for 2009 is $16,500. Taxpayers age 50 and above are eligible for an additional "catch-up" contribution of $5500 (Table 1). A contribution of $16,500 will reduce your taxable income, dollar for dollar. This contribution, assuming the taxpayer is subject to the Alternative Minimum Tax (AMT) at 28%, would save about $4,620 in current income tax liability. This tax saving opportunity also has the effect of helping to fulfill another important goal: saving for retirement. AMT is a separate tax calculation from the regular income tax and uses different rules. Some deductions taken for regular tax purposes are not allowed under AMT rules. Also, income and expenses are calculated differently under the AMT.

One opportunity available to many physicians (even physicians who are shareholders or partners in their own practices) is the opportunity to receive self-employment income for speaking engagements or other consulting services outside regular employment. In this situation, even if employees are covered under a qualified retirement plan, they may have the option to set up a simplified employee pension plan. The maximum contribution to a simplified employee pension plan for 2009 is 20% of self-employment compensation, or

Table 1
Retirement plan contribution limits

	2009	2010	2011
Traditional IRA and Roth IRA plans			
Limit	$5000	Indexed	Indexed
Catch-up	$1000	Indexed	Indexed
401(k), 403(b), and 457 plans			
Limit	$16,500	Indexed	Indexed
Catch-up	$5500	Indexed	Indexed
Simple IRA and simple 401(k) plans			
Limit	$11,500	Indexed	Indexed
Catch-up	$2500	Indexed	Indexed

Abbreviation: IRA, Individual Retirement Account.

$49,000. The maximum qualified compensation considered for the plan contribution is $245,000 for 2009.

Make tax-free investments

The second strategy involves investing in tax-free or tax-friendly investments. Municipal bonds provide interest income free from federal taxation. Municipal bonds currently yielding 3% have an after-tax effective yield of 4.17% for a taxpayer in the 28% bracket and 4.62% for someone in the 35% bracket. Physicians will probably want to avoid municipal bond interest from private activity bonds issued after August 7, 1986. The interest income from these bonds must be included in the tax calculation for AMT purposes. Arenas and sports stadiums are examples of private activity bonds.

Purchase stocks

A third strategy is the purchase of high-quality dividend-paying stocks. Qualified dividends are currently taxed at a maximum tax rate of 15%. This tax rate is scheduled to be in effect through 2010. Because of the current budget constraints of the federal government, it is probably not realistic to expect this rate to continue. However, some of the proposed legislation would limit the taxation of qualified dividends to 20%.

Investing in dividend-paying and growing stocks has another important potential benefit. One of the major challenges to a retiree's cash flow is inflation. Even small rates of inflation compounded over a 25- or 30-year retirement period can result in significant changes to your cash flow, buying power, and retirement lifestyle. An investment strategy focused on a diversified portfolio of dividend payers and growers can help supplement other sources of retirement income and provide a growing stream of cash. For example, take an initial investment of $500,000 in a diversified portfolio of equities that has an initial dividend yield of 3% and a history of raising these payments by 10% per year. Your starting dividend cash flow would be $15,000 per year; but your cash flow would quickly grow to over $24,000 in year 5 and to almost

$39,000 in year 10. This model for providing income growth can be a valuable component of an overall plan to protect purchasing power against inflation.

Investment assets purchased and held for over 1 year also receive discounted capital gains treatment of a maximum of 15% through 2010. In subsequent years, long-term capital gains tax rates are scheduled to increase to 20%. This is a good incentive to purchase high-quality assets that you plan to hold for at least 1 year.

Shift income

A fourth strategy is to shift income to another taxpayer, as in the case of parents giving assets to children under the annual gift-tax exclusion. The annual gift-tax exclusion amount for 2009 is $13,000 per recipient. A married couple can give a combined $26,000 to a single individual each year with no gift-tax consequences. The recipient can be any individual; there is no requirement that the gift be to a family member. For example, parents could give a combined gift of $26,000 to their daughter and an additional $26,000 to their son-in-law for a total of $52,000. However, one major pitfall of shifting income from parents to children is the "kiddie tax." The kiddie tax applies to unearned (investment) income a child earns over $1,800. This may be subject to tax based on their parents' income. The tax applies to all dependent children under age 18 and to full-time college students under the age of 24. Strategies to avoid the kiddie tax include moving income-generating securities into tax-free municipal bonds or growth stocks that do not generate dividends.

Fund education

The fifth strategy is education funding. A Qualified Tuition Program (QTP), or IRC Section 529 plan, effectively eliminates the income of the assets contributed from the grantor if used for qualified educational expenses. This allows a physician to save money for a child's education, removes the income tax burden, and allows flexibility to move money between siblings and other family members as needed. For example, if an older sibling earns a scholarship and does not need the full amount in the 529 plan, the residual can be transferred to a younger sibling or other close family member.

Because 529 plans are not included in the grantor's gross estate, they are also effective tools for reducing federal estate taxes. A Section 529 plan allows you to accelerate 5 years of giving ($65,000 for an individual or $130,000 joint gifts for husband and wife) in 1 year, without incurring gift taxes. If an accelerated gift is completed, no additional gifts can be made under the annual exclusion for the recipient for the next 5 years. Also, if the grantor passes away before the 5-year time line expires, the prorated amount of the gift would be pulled back into his or her gross estate.

Fund Roth individual retirement arrangement

The final strategy to consider during the accumulation phase is to fund a Roth Individual Retirement Account (IRA). A Roth IRA can be used to fund future retirement needs or accomplish estate-planning objectives. The Roth IRA is similar to a traditional IRA with one important difference: If you meet the 5-year holding requirement and are over age $59\frac{1}{2}$ upon distribution, there is no tax on the distributions (your nondeductible contributions are always available for tax-free withdrawal). To gain this tax benefit, you may not deduct the value of current contributions for federal income tax purposes, as you may (subject to income limits) with traditional IRAs.

The drawback to a Roth IRA is that it is subject to a modified adjusted gross income limit, but is not affected by qualified plan participation. The contribution limit for 2009 is $5000, plus a $1000 catch-up contribution allowed for taxpayers age 50 and over. The income phase-out range for 2009 for single individuals is $105,000 to $120,000 and $166,000 to $176,000 for married taxpayers who file a joint return. High-income individuals are precluded from making contributions to Roth IRAs. The strategy is to convert amounts in a regular IRA to a Roth IRA. Under current tax law, individuals may convert IRAs to Roth IRAs if their modified adjusted gross income is $100,000 or less. For tax years beginning after 2009, the modified adjusted gross income limit will be eliminated, allowing higher income taxpayers to convert traditional IRAs to Roth accounts [7]. This provides an opportunity for individuals to fund nondeductible IRAs in the years before 2010 and then convert the nondeductible IRAs into Roth IRAs. For example, if you contribute $5500 in 2009 and in 2010, and convert the nondeductible IRA to a Roth IRA in 2010, only the earnings the IRA has generated are taxable. The nondeductible contributions would not be taxable upon conversion. This strategy has the maximum benefit if your nondeductible IRA is your only IRA to date. If you have a rollover IRA or self-funded IRA, this strategy may not be advisable. This strategy can also be applied to a nonworking spouse. A nonworking spouse is still eligible to set up a nondeductible spousal IRA.

In 2010, when the traditional IRA is converted to a Roth IRA the taxable amount will be equally divided over the 2-year period of 2011 and 2012. With income tax rates scheduled to increase in 2011, this may not be the most effective tax strategy. It may be beneficial to elect to tax the full distribution in 2010 at a probable lower tax rate.

DISTRIBUTION PHASE

For some of you, the accumulation phase may have already happened, and you are now in, or about to enter, the distribution phase. There are some potentially unique planning opportunities during this period that warrant some consideration. What investment and tax strategies do most financial planners use to extend the life of accumulated capital?

In general, there are two schools of thought regarding the distribution phase. The first distribution method follows a rule of thumb sometimes used by financial advisors. This rule suggests that an annual withdrawal rate of 4% or 5% of your capital base can be used to support your personal budget. Given that each case is unique with a different set of circumstances and objectives (not to mention you may be one of the unfortunate individuals who decides to retire during a period when the stock market is performing poorly), picking a static drawdown rate can be dangerous. Clearly, an individual should be wary of overspending in the first few years of retirement, as it can be very difficult to recover from larger withdrawals made earlier in the process. In addition, the thought of being forced to sell equities in the middle of a 40% stock market decline for spending purposes can severely hurt your portfolio's ability to recover during a subsequent upturn.

The second distribution method is the bucket approach. The bucket approach divides your retirement capital into two pieces or buckets. The first bucket contains enough capital to provide for the first 10 years of predicted income need during your retirement. Investments in this bucket would include cash and high-quality fixed-income investments that mature over the 10-year time period. The second bucket contains longer-term assets, including long-term fixed-income and equity investments. This method gives the financial advisor some flexibility when it comes to the distribution phase. If the equity market performs well, some profits from the long-term bucket could be moved into the short-term bucket. At the same time, you would have a 10-year buffer in the short-term bucket if your retirement happens to coincide with a period of stock market decline.

Another strategy that you may want to consider in preparation for the distribution phase is to build up the first 2 years of your retirement capital in cash and other short-term liquid investments. By doing so, you remove the first couple of years of market risk from your portfolio and, if you are unfortunate enough to retire at the beginning of a stock market downturn, you could start to spend down the 2-year cash cushion. If you retire and the equity and fixed-income markets produce average or "excess" returns, you could draw down from this piece of the portfolio.

Regardless of which distribution method you use, having enough capital and flexibility to support a long retirement period is critical. The ideal situation is to have a personal budget supported by the cash flow from your capital base. This means that, if the interest and dividend income from your capital base is enough to support your personal budget needs, your situation becomes substantially easier to manage confidently for long-term security.

During the distribution phase, your income may decrease to the point where you find yourself in a lower tax bracket than during your working years. If this is the case, strategies can be employed to make use of the bottom tax rates. The strategies can include replacing municipal bonds with high-quality taxable bonds to seek higher after-tax rates of return. You may also want to consider taking distributions from your pretax retirement accounts in an effort to use up the bottom 10% to 15% tax brackets.

Required Minimum Distributions (RMDs) from your individual retirement account must begin by April 1 of the year following the year the account owner turns age $70\frac{1}{2}$. There is an exception to the RMD rules for defined contribution plans for nonowner employees who may delay the distribution until April 1 of the year following their retirement. For 2009, however, the RMD has been temporarily waived.

CASE STUDY

The case study section of this article works through and addresses the vital question of how much capital an individual or family will need.

Retirement planning follows a five-step process:

1. Estimate how much annual income you will need in retirement.
2. Determine the amount of capital needed to support your retirement budget.
3. Estimate how much capital you will have in the future.
4. Calculate the difference between what you need and what you are likely to have in the future.
5. Evaluate what can be done today and in years to come to address any deficit.

The test case attempts to take into consideration the important variables that have been discussed. Assumptions being used include:

- Married; both spouses are age 50
- Average annual compensation: $200,000
- Current savings total: $1,000,000
- Annual savings: maximum amount to 401(k) plan of $16,500, with an additional $5500 in the form of a catch-up contribution and a 4% employer match
- Retirement age: 65
- Death age: 90

The first step is to estimate how much annual income you will need in retirement. Two methods are routinely used to do this. The first is a rule of thumb: Most experts assume that you will need 60% to 90% of your current income to maintain your standard of living in retirement. You should be careful when using such rules of thumb, recognizing that every case is unique. However, this rule can be useful early in one's career as a goal when estimating how much to save. Under this method, you would need between $120,000 and $180,000 in annual retirement income, in today's dollars.

A second method requires more effort and thought, but is more precise. It requires you to actually track your spending and draw up a retirement budget. This tends to be an eye-opening exercise for most people, and forces thoughtful consideration about how they spend their time and money. Typical budget categories include housing, food, travel and entertainment, taxes, insurance, utilities, transportation, and health care costs not covered by insurance.

For purposes of this example, we will assume that 75% of your annual compensation is our target. This would amount to $150,000 per year in annual retirement income as your income-replacement goal.

The second step in the retirement planning process is determining the lump sum of capital that will be needed to support a $150,000 annual budget for the 25-year assumed term of your retirement.

At this point, it is appropriate to discuss inflation and rate of return. During some periods, our country has experienced very high inflation. For example, during the 1970s, inflation averaged about 8.5% per year. We have also experienced periods of very low inflation. During the 1990s, we had an average annual inflation rate of about 3%. It is likely that inflation will vary over a 25-year retirement period and will have a great deal of influence on your purchasing power. For purposes of the case study, we have assumed that inflation will average 4% over the period. Inflation is a volatile and important variable, and should be monitored closely in real-life applications of retirement planning.

The rate of return earned on the capital saved and invested is another variable that needs to be estimated. For the period of 1926 to 2008, rate of return for the equity market for the period of was about 9.6%. For the broad bond market, the rate of return was 5.5% over the same period. The equity markets have produced well below average rates of return over the last 10 years, which, for the record, as of this writing has been an average annual decline of 2.5%. The fixed-income markets have matched their long-term average of 5.5% over the last 10 years. The timing of your retirement relative to the timing of portfolio rates of return will also have a large impact on your capital base and quality of retirement. Let's assume that 40% of your capital is invested in fixed-income investments and earns 5.5%, and 60% is invested in equities and earns 8%. This would result in a blended portfolio rate of return of 7%.

With the estimated time variable of a 25-year retirement period, a $150,000 personal budget and an inflation rate of 4%, how much capital will need to be accumulated by age 65 to support the test case?

The first step in answering this question is to adjust the $150,000 personal budget for the 15 years from age 50 to the projected retirement date of age 65. This requires calculation of the future value of $150,000, by adjusting for 4% inflation compounded over 15 years. The answer to this question is $270,142 (see Appendix).

Table 2
Summary of first four steps of retirement planning in case study

Solve for:	Budget	Budget future value	Lump sum needed	Lump sum available	Projected shortfall
Step one	$150,000				
Step two		$270,142	$4,902,539		
Step three				$3,824,593	
Step four					$1,077,946

Table 3
Case study results if retirement age is 68 instead of 65

Solve for	Budget	Budget future value	Lump sum needed	Lump sum available	Projected shortfall
Step one	$150,000				
Step two		$303,873			
Step three			$5,040,580	$4,787,524	
Step four					$253,056

The next calculation to be made is to determine the sum of capital required to support a starting personal budget of $270,142 adjusted for a continuing 4% annual rate of inflation, the 7% portfolio rate of return, and the 25-year retirement period. The answer to this question is $4,902,539 (see Appendix).

Next, an estimation of how much capital should be available at age 65 is made, given in this case our starting capital base of $1,000,000, our annual savings rate (assumed to be $22,000 per year in addition to a 4% employer contribution), and our assumed 7% rate of return. Based on these assumptions, we should accumulate $3,824,593 (see Appendix).

Our retirement planning process then requires us to compare our estimated capital needs of $4,902,539 to our projected accumulation of $3,824,593. Bad news: We have a projected shortfall of $1,077,946!

Table 2 provides a summary for the first four steps in the retirement planning process for the case study.

Finally, what changes can be made today and in years to come to eliminate the projected $1,077,946 shortfall. Some of the important variables over which you can exercise degrees of control include working longer, spending less, and saving more.

Let's consider working longer. Table 3 shows the results if you move your retirement from age 65 to 68 and maintain the beginning budget amount of $150,000.

Now, let's consider spending less and saving more. The multiplier effect resulting from both a lower personal budget and a higher savings level produces dramatic results. Table 4 shows what happens if you are able to reduce your

Table 4
Case study results if personal budget reduced to $130,000 from $150,000 and difference added to savings

Solve for	Budget	Budget future value	Lump sum needed	Lump sum available	Projected surplus
Step one	$130,000				
Step two		$234,123			
Step three			$4,248,859	$4,382,354	
Step four					$133,495

personal budget from $150,000 to $130,000 and to apply this difference to increase your savings by the same amount.

SUMMARY

The progressive demise of traditional pension plans and the uncertainty of our Social Security system make the personal savings component of retirement planning more important than ever. Given the amount of capital needed to support the longer life expectancies, it is critical that the retirement planning process start early in one's career and be refined with new information frequently as one ages.

The average physician has some important advantages and disadvantages when it comes to retirement planning. The valuable services that a physician provides creates a level of job security, compensation, and predictable cash flow that is above the national average. However, physicians also must overcome the disadvantages of delayed entry into the workforce and, for many, substantial educational debt burdens. The key to successful retirement planning is recognizing these challenges and developing a plan. The plan should use the various strategies discussed in this article and incorporate issues related to income taxes, savings, investments, and anticipated needs.

Retirement planning can be overwhelming. For some, the enormity of the task can paradoxically lead to inaction. Physicians in this position should consider the assistance of a qualified financial planner. One starting point for locating this professional is to ask your accountant or attorney for a referral. You can also find a Certified Financial Planner by searching the following Web site: www.cfp.net.

References

[1] Private pension plan bulletin historical tables and graphs by U.S. Department of Labor, Employee Benefits Security Administration, February, 2009.
[2] Bureau of Economic Analysis. Personal income and outlays. 2009. Available at: http://www.bea.gov.
[3] Life expectancy data and mortality obtained from: the centers for disease control and prevention. Available at: www.cdc.gov.
[4] Wage estimates obtained from: Available at: http://finance.yahoo.com/career-work/article/107042/americas-best-and-worst-paying-jobs.
[5] AARP Bulletin Today. Available at: http://bulletin.aarp.org/states/hi/2009/13/articles/getting_older_but_working_longer_average.
[6] Available at: www.pfp.aicpa.org/resouces/Financial+Goals/Tax+Planning/Introduction+to+Personal+income+tax+planning.
[7] U.S. master tax guide. 92nd edition. Chicago: Wolters Kluwer; 2009.

Seletcted additional reading

Reference guide for financial planners, 2008 edition, Keir Educational Resources, Middletown (OH).
Schwab Charles R. 2001. You're fifty - now what? Crown Business, New York.
Tax planning for individuals quickfinder handbook, 2008 edition. Thomson Tax & Accounting.
Quickfinder handbook, 2008 edition. Thomson Reuters.

APPENDIX

Retirement Analysis

Retire at end of the year that you are age 65 on a $270,142 Retirement Budget

Rate Assumptions:
Inflation Rate   4.0%
Portfolio Return Rate   7.0%

Footnote #			(1)	(2)	(3)	(4)	(5)	(6)	(7)
Year End	Age H	Age W	Earned Income	Employer Cont.	Employee Savings	Retirement Budget	Invest Earnings	Retirement Savings	Lump-Sum Needed
2009								1,000,000	
2010	50	50	200,000	8,000	22,000	0	70,000	1,100,000	0
2011	51	51	208,000	8,320	22,000	0	77,000	1,207,320	0
2012	52	52	216,320	8,653	22,000	0	84,512	1,322,485	0
2013	53	53	224,973	8,999	22,000	0	92,574	1,446,058	0
2014	54	54	233,972	9,359	22,000	0	101,224	1,578,641	0
2015	55	55	243,331	9,733	22,000	0	110,505	1,720,879	0
2016	56	56	253,064	9,800	22,000	0	120,462	1,873,141	0
2017	57	57	263,186	9,800	22,000	0	131,120	2,036,060	0
2018	58	58	273,714	9,800	22,000	0	142,524	2,210,385	0
2019	59	59	284,662	9,800	22,000	0	154,727	2,396,912	0
2020	60	60	296,049	9,800	22,000	0	167,784	2,596,495	0
2021	61	61	307,891	9,800	22,000	0	181,755	2,810,050	0
2022	62	62	320,206	9,800	22,000	0	196,704	3,038,554	0
2023	63	63	333,015	9,800	22,000	0	212,699	3,283,052	0
2024	64	64	346,335	9,800	22,000	0	229,814	3,544,666	0
2025	65	65	360,189	9,800	22,000	0	248,127	3,824,593	4,902,539
2026	66	66	0		0	(270,142)	248,812	3,803,262	4,956,664
2027	67	67	0		0	(280,948)	246,562	3,768,877	5,003,016
2028	68	68	0		0	(292,186)	243,368	3,720,059	5,040,588
2029	69	69	0		0	(303,873)	239,133	3,655,319	5,068,284
2030	70	70	0		0	(316,028)	233,750	3,573,042	5,084,913
2031	71	71	0		0	(328,669)	227,106	3,471,479	5,089,180
2032	72	72	0		0	(341,816)	219,076	3,348,740	5,079,679
2033	73	73	0		0	(355,488)	209,528	3,202,779	5,054,884
2034	74	74	0		0	(369,708)	198,315	3,031,386	5,013,137
2035	75	75	0		0	(384,496)	185,282	2,832,172	4,952,645
2036	76	76	0		0	(399,876)	170,261	2,602,556	4,871,462
2037	77	77	0		0	(415,871)	153,068	2,339,753	4,767,481
2038	78	78	0		0	(432,506)	133,507	2,040,754	4,638,423
2039	79	79	0		0	(449,806)	111,366	1,702,314	4,481,819
2040	80	80	0		0	(467,799)	86,416	1,320,932	4,295,001
2041	81	81	0		0	(486,510)	58,409	892,831	4,075,085
2042	82	82	0		0	(505,971)	27,080	413,940	3,818,951
2043	83	83	0		0	(526,210)	0	0	3,523,233
2044	84	84	0		0	(547,258)	0	0	3,184,292
2045	85	85	0		0	(569,148)	0	0	2,798,204
2046	86	86	0		0	(591,914)	0	0	2,360,729
2047	87	87	0		0	(615,591)	0	0	1,867,298
2048	88	88	0		0	(640,215)	0	0	1,312,979
2049	89	89	0		0	(665,823)	0	0	692,456
2050	90	90	0		0	(692,456)	0	0	0

Retirement Analysis

Retire at end of the year that you are age 68 on a $303,873 Retirement Budget

Rate Assumptions:
Inflation Rate	4.0%
Portfolio Return Rate	7.0%

			(1)	(2)	(3)	(4)	(5)	(6)	(7)
Footnote #			Earned	Employer	Employee	Retirement	Invest	Lump-Sum	Lump-Sum
Year End	Age H	Age W	Income	Cont.	Savings	Budget	Earnings	Available	Needed
2009								1,000,000	
2010	50	50	200,000	8,000	22,000	0	70,000	1,100,000	0
2011	51	51	208,000	8,320	22,000	0	77,000	1,207,320	0
2012	52	52	216,320	8,653	22,000	0	84,512	1,322,485	0
2013	53	53	224,973	8,999	22,000	0	92,574	1,446,058	0
2014	54	54	233,972	9,359	22,000	0	101,224	1,578,641	0
2015	55	55	243,331	9,733	22,000	0	110,505	1,720,879	0
2016	56	56	253,064	9,800	22,000	0	120,462	1,873,141	0
2017	57	57	263,186	9,800	22,000	0	131,120	2,036,060	0
2018	58	58	273,714	9,800	22,000	0	142,524	2,210,385	0
2019	59	59	284,662	9,800	22,000	0	154,727	2,396,912	0
2020	60	60	296,049	9,800	22,000	0	167,784	2,596,495	0
2021	61	61	307,891	9,800	22,000	0	181,755	2,810,050	0
2022	62	62	320,206	9,800	22,000	0	196,704	3,038,554	0
2023	63	63	333,015	9,800	22,000	0	212,699	3,283,052	0
2024	64	64	346,335	9,800	22,000	0	229,814	3,544,666	0
2025	65	65	360,189	9,800	22,000	0	248,127	3,824,593	0
2026	66	66	374,596	9,800	22,000	0	267,721	4,124,114	0
2027	67	67	389,580	9,800	22,000	0	288,688	4,444,602	0
2028	68	68	405,163	9,800	22,000	0	311,122	4,787,524	5,040,588
2029	69	69	0		0	(303,873)	313,856	4,797,507	5,068,284
2030	70	70	0		0	(316,028)	313,704	4,795,183	5,084,913
2031	71	71	0		0	(328,669)	312,656	4,779,169	5,089,180
2032	72	72	0		0	(341,816)	310,615	4,747,968	5,079,679
2033	73	73	0		0	(355,488)	307,474	4,699,954	5,054,883
2034	74	74	0		0	(369,708)	303,117	4,633,363	5,013,137
2035	75	75	0		0	(384,496)	297,421	4,546,287	4,952,645
2036	76	76	0		0	(399,876)	290,249	4,436,660	4,871,462
2037	77	77	0		0	(415,871)	281,455	4,302,244	4,767,481
2038	78	78	0		0	(432,506)	270,882	4,140,619	4,638,423
2039	79	79	0		0	(449,806)	258,357	3,949,170	4,481,819
2040	80	80	0		0	(467,799)	243,696	3,725,068	4,295,001
2041	81	81	0		0	(486,510)	226,699	3,465,256	4,075,084
2042	82	82	0		0	(505,971)	207,150	3,166,435	3,818,951
2043	83	83	0		0	(526,210)	184,816	2,825,041	3,523,233
2044	84	84	0		0	(547,258)	159,445	2,437,228	3,184,292
2045	85	85	0		0	(569,148)	130,766	1,998,845	2,798,203
2046	86	86	0		0	(591,914)	98,485	1,505,416	2,360,729
2047	87	87	0		0	(615,591)	62,288	952,113	1,867,297
2048	88	88	0		0	(640,215)	21,833	333,731	1,312,978
2049	89	89	0		0	(665,823)	0	0	692,456
2050	90	90	0		0	(692,456)	0	0	0

Retirement Analysis

Footnotes:

1. Earned income is based on a starting salary of $200,000 and adjusted annually by the rate of inflation.

2. Employer contributions are assumed to be 4% of your annual salary up to the current federal maximum considered compensation of $245,000.

3. Employee contributions are the current maximum deferral of $16,500 plus the $5,500 catch-up contribution for those age 50 or older.

4. Retirement budget represents your desired spending level of $150,000 assumed to increase at the rate of inflation.

5. Investment earnings are based on the balance of your investment account earning 7.0%.

6. Your investment accounts along with annual savings are assumed to grow at 7%. Upon retirement this account is used to support your retirement budget.

7. The amount of capital needed to support the retirement budget until age 90.

Retirement Analysis

Retire at end of the year that you are age 65 on a $234,123 Retirement Budget

Rate Assumptions:
Inflation Rate	4.0%
Portfolio Return Rate	7.0%

Footnote #			(1)	(2)	(3)	(4)	(5)	(6)	(7)	(8)
Year End	Age H	Age W	Earned Income	Employer Cont.	Employee Savings	After Tax Savings	Retirement Budget	Invest Earnings	Retirement Savings	Lump-Sum Needed
2009									1,000,000	
2010	50	50	200,000	8,000	22,000	20,000	0	70,000	1,120,000	0
2011	51	51	208,000	8,320	22,000	20,000	0	78,400	1,248,720	0
2012	52	52	216,320	8,653	22,000	20,000	0	87,410	1,386,783	0
2013	53	53	224,973	8,999	22,000	20,000	0	97,075	1,534,857	0
2014	54	54	233,972	9,359	22,000	20,000	0	107,440	1,693,656	0
2015	55	55	243,331	9,733	22,000	20,000	0	118,556	1,863,945	0
2016	56	56	253,064	9,800	22,000	20,000	0	130,476	2,046,221	0
2017	57	57	263,186	9,800	22,000	20,000	0	143,235	2,241,257	0
2018	58	58	273,714	9,800	22,000	20,000	0	156,888	2,449,944	0
2019	59	59	284,662	9,800	22,000	20,000	0	171,496	2,673,241	0
2020	60	60	296,049	9,800	22,000	20,000	0	187,127	2,912,167	0
2021	61	61	307,891	9,800	22,000	20,000	0	203,852	3,167,819	0
2022	62	62	320,206	9,800	22,000	20,000	0	221,747	3,441,367	0
2023	63	63	333,015	9,800	22,000	20,000	0	240,896	3,734,062	0
2024	64	64	346,335	9,800	22,000	20,000	0	261,384	4,047,247	0
2025	65	65	360,189	9,800	22,000	20,000	0	283,307	4,382,354	4,248,860
2026	66	66	0	0	0	0	(234,123)	290,376	4,438,607	4,295,768
2027	67	67	0	0	0	0	(243,488)	293,658	4,488,778	4,335,940
2028	68	68	0	0	0	0	(253,227)	296,489	4,532,040	4,368,502
2029	69	69	0	0	0	0	(263,356)	298,808	4,567,491	4,392,505
2030	70	70	0	0	0	0	(273,890)	300,552	4,594,153	4,406,917
2031	71	71	0	0	0	0	(284,846)	301,651	4,610,958	4,410,615
2032	72	72	0	0	0	0	(296,240)	302,030	4,616,749	4,402,381
2033	73	73	0	0	0	0	(308,089)	301,606	4,610,266	4,380,891
2034	74	74	0	0	0	0	(320,413)	300,290	4,590,142	4,344,711
2035	75	75	0	0	0	0	(333,230)	297,984	4,554,897	4,292,285
2036	76	76	0	0	0	0	(346,559)	294,584	4,502,922	4,221,926
2037	77	77	0	0	0	0	(360,421)	289,975	4,432,476	4,131,810
2038	78	78	0	0	0	0	(374,838)	284,035	4,341,672	4,019,959
2039	79	79	0	0	0	0	(389,831)	276,629	4,228,470	3,884,236
2040	80	80	0	0	0	0	(405,425)	267,613	4,090,658	3,722,328
2041	81	81	0	0	0	0	(421,642)	256,831	3,925,848	3,531,734
2042	82	82	0	0	0	0	(438,507)	244,114	3,731,454	3,309,752
2043	83	83	0	0	0	0	(456,048)	229,278	3,504,685	3,053,463
2044	84	84	0	0	0	0	(474,290)	212,128	3,242,523	2,759,715
2045	85	85	0	0	0	0	(493,261)	192,448	2,941,710	2,425,106
2046	86	86	0	0	0	0	(512,992)	170,010	2,598,729	2,045,962
2047	87	87	0	0	0	0	(533,511)	144,565	2,209,783	1,618,322
2048	88	88	0	0	0	0	(554,852)	115,845	1,770,777	1,137,913
2049	89	89	0	0	0	0	(577,046)	83,561	1,277,292	600,128
2050	90	90	0	0	0	0	(600,128)	47,402	724,566	0

Retirement Analysis

Footnotes:

1. Earned income is based on a starting salary of $200,000 and adjusted annually by the rate of inflation.

2. Employer contributions are assumed to be 4% of your annual salary up to the current federal maximum considered compensation of $245,000.

3. Employee contributions are the current maximum deferral of $16,500 plus the $5,500 catch-up contribution for those age 50 or older.

4. The increased level of savings as a result of the reduced budget are assumed to be invested in after-tax assets.

5. Retirement budget represents your desired spending level of $130,000 assumed to increase at the rate of inflation.

6. Investment earnings are based on the balance of your investment account earning 7.0%.

7. Your investment accounts along with annual savings are assumed to grow at 7%. Upon retirement this account is used to support your retirement budget.

8. The amount of capital needed to support the retirement budget until age 90.

Advances in Anesthesia 27 (2009) 111–142

ADVANCES IN ANESTHESIA

ELSEVIER
MOSBY

Nonopioid Adjuvants in Multimodal Therapy for Acute Perioperative Pain

Bryan S. Williams, MD, MPH, Asokumar Buvanendran, MD*

Division of Pain Medicine, Department of Anesthesiology, Rush University Medical Center, Rush Medical College, 1653 W. Congress Parkway, #739, Chicago, IL 60612, USA

Advancements in surgical technique have led to increasingly more procedures being performed on an outpatient basis. In North America, the number of outpatient procedures has increased to nearly 70% of all surgical procedures [1–4]. Improvements in surgical techniques similarly have led to the performance of more invasive procedures. These procedures cause increased tissue disruption and associated pain. There are several inflammatory mediators released with the surgical trauma including histamine, bradykinin, and prostaglandins. Increased sensitivity to painful stimuli is mediated by repetitive, excitatory amino acids (glutamate and aspartate) with expression of c-fos, nitric oxide (NO) synthase, and the cyclooxygenase-2 (COX-2) gene, with ensuing sensitization. The amplification of painful stimuli increases the concentration of prostaglandins and NO, which may be the primary mediators of central sensitization (secondary hyperalgesia) [5]. Preventing or inhibiting this sensitization by addressing transmission by multimodal pathways may reduce acute postoperative pain and may prevent chronic postoperative pain from developing [6–8].

The literature indicates that up to 75% of postsurgical patients have reported pain, and 80% of these patients experienced severe acute pain during their hospital stay [9]. Postoperative pain is the most common reason for delayed discharge, and the main reason for unanticipated hospital admission [10]. Improvements in morbidity and mortality related to anesthesia have led to an emphasis on secondary outcome measures such as perioperative pain, because poor patient satisfaction resulting from inadequate perioperative pain control is associated with increased cytokine and acute-phase reactant release, elevated levels of stress hormones, activation of the renin-angiotensin-aldosterone cascade, impaired coagulability, and an altered immune response [11,12].

Opioid medications have been the mainstay of postoperative pain management, but these medications are not without adverse effects. Adverse events such as nausea and vomiting, constipation, ileus, confusion, sedation, urinary retention, delirium, pruritus, headache, respiratory depression, or other effects

*Corresponding author. E-mail address: asokumar@aol.com (A. Buvanendran).

0737-6146/09/$ – see front matter
doi:10.1016/j.aan.2009.07.008

such as muscle rigidity and hypotension secondary to histamine release are potentially more serious effects [13,14]. In addition, the paradoxic phenomenon of opioid-induced hyperalgesia (OIH) has been described in animal models, human volunteers, and surgical patients, indicating that even short-term use of high-dose opioids may lead to opioid-induced hyperalgesia or tolerance [15–17]. OIH is now recognized to reflect a sustained sensitization of the nervous system in which excitatory amino acid neurotransmitter systems play a critical role, especially via N-methyl-D-aspartate (NMDA) receptors. From a medical viewpoint, abnormal persistence of excitatory neuroplasticity is now considered to be a major, if largely unrecognized, candidate mechanism for the development of chronic pain [18]. A multimodal approach has been advocated as a method to best treat pain in the perioperative period. The addition of adjuvant medications permits the use of lower doses of opioids while addressing pain by alternative mechanisms (Fig. 1). Synergistically or additively, these adjuvants enhance analgesia provided by opioids and reduce potential adverse effects of opioids. In addition, acute opioid tolerance has

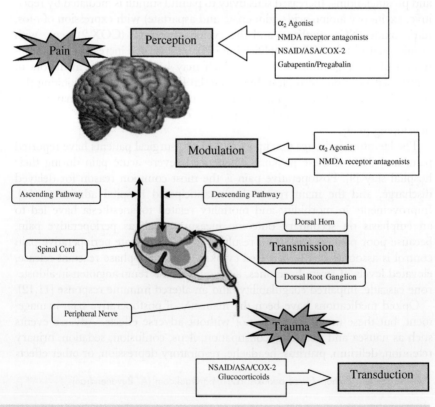

Fig. 1. Site of action of adjuvant medications.

been described, and a correlation between high-dose intraoperative opioid administration has necessitated that postoperative opioid requirements be increased [19,20].

Kehlet and Dahl [21] may have been the first to describe the term "multimodal analgesia," referring to balancing analgesic agents and techniques to address postoperative pain by different analgesic mechanisms. The goal of this mechanistic multimodal analgesia approach is to provide improved perioperative analgesia and minimize adverse effects. Multimodal techniques reduce the total dose of any one medication by attending to patient analgesic requirements through various receptor modulations. Multimodal analgesic techniques are becoming increasingly more prevalent as an approach for balanced analgesia and thus, a reduction in postoperative pain.

This review focuses on adjuvant medications (nonopioid) and the mechanism by which these medications improve postoperative analgesia and decrease the amount of opioid medications needed to achieve pain relief, thus decreasing the incidence of opioid-related adverse effects.

NONSTEROIDAL ANTI-INFLAMMATORY DRUGS, CYCLOOXYGENASE-2 INHIBITORS, AND ACETAMINOPHEN

Nonsteroidal anti-inflammatory drugs (NSAIDs) are among the most widely used analgesic medications in the world because of their ability to reduce pain and inflammation [22–24]. The NSAIDs are structurally diverse, but all have antipyretic, anti-inflammatory, and analgesic or antihyperalgesic properties. The salicylates (aspirinlike medications) have been used to treat pain conditions for thousands of years, with the Ebers Papyrus recommending the application of a decoction of the dried leaves of myrtle to the abdomen and back to expel rheumatic pains from the womb; and Hippocrates recommending the juices of the poplar tree to treat eye diseases, and those of willow bark to relieve the pain of childbirth and to reduce fever [25]. NSAIDs have both peripheral and central mechanisms of action [23,26,27]. The mechanism of action of the NSAIDs is inhibition of prostaglandin production by either reversible or irreversible acetylation of the COX enzyme. It is the COX-2 isoform that is induced by proinflammatory stimuli and cytokines, causing fever, inflammation, and pain, and thus forming the target for anti-inflammation by NSAIDs [25]. The COX-1 isoform is constitutive, causing hemostasis, platelet aggregation, and the production of prostacyclin, which is gastric mucosal protective. The inhibition of COX-1 isoform may be responsible for the adverse effects related to the nonselective NSAIDs [28]. NSAIDs are administered in the setting of minimal to moderate pain or as an adjuvant to other medications, such as opioids, for their opioid-sparing properties [23,29].

NSAID medications act synergistically with opioids to provide better analgesia than either medication alone, decreasing the required opioid dose [23,30–32]. Although nonselective NSAIDs have shown benefit in multimodal perioperative pain management, the routine use of NSAIDs raises concerns with respect to their adverse effects such as gastric irritation, impaired coagulation, wound healing, osteogenic activity and fracture healing, and renal dysfunction [33–35].

Nonselective nonsteroidal anti-Inflammatory drugs

Acetylsalicylic acid (aspirin; ASA) covalently modifies COX-1 and COX-2, irreversibly inhibiting cyclooxygenase activity. This modification is an important distinction among the NSAIDs because aspirin's duration of action is related to the turnover rate of cyclooxygenases in different target tissues. The duration of action of nonaspirin NSAIDs, which competitively inhibit the active sites of the COX enzymes, relates more directly to the time course of drug disposition [36]. Furthermore, NSAIDs traditionally referred to as nonselective now have been shown to be selective. For example, meloxicam, an enolic acid, shows dose-dependent COX selectivity whereby 7.5 mg is more selective for COX-2, whereas at 15 mg meloxicam becomes less selective [36].

Aspirin

Aspirin (ASA) is the most widely used drug in the world [37]. The analgesic effect is secondary to the inhibition of prostaglandin synthesis (Fig. 2). In a meta-analysis, Edwards and colleagues [38] reviewed the efficacy of single-dose ASA in postoperative pain. The number needed to treat (NNT) was used as an outcome measure. In the analysis, significant benefit of ASA over placebo was shown for ASA 600/650 mg, 1000 mg, and 1200 mg, with NNTs for at least 50% pain relief of 4.4 (4.0–4.9), 4.0 (3.2–5.4), and 2.4 (1.9–3.2), respectively [38]. Single-dose aspirin 500 mg did not prove to be effective in reducing postoperative pain. These results are also reflected in a study by Rees and colleagues [39]. In a study by Laska and colleagues [40], ASA was evaluated for its efficacy in 3 different pain states (postepisiotomy, uterine cramping, and postsurgical patients) with NNT as the outcome measure. The investigators concluded that at ASA 650 mg the NNT for uterine cramping was 3.55 and 3.15 for moderate and severe uterine pain, respectively. Moderate episiotomy pain yielded a NNT of 3.44 and 3.77 for severe episiotomy pain. The NNT for postsurgical pain was 3.58, and with these NNTs the investigators conclude that ASA was effective at treating postsurgical pain [40].

Most studies investigating ASA to treat acute pain or postoperative pain evaluate the effectiveness of ASA in dental patients. Pain after third molar extraction has become the model most frequently used in acute pain trials, because third molar extraction is a common procedure with pain frequently moderate or severe in intensity, and with sufficient numbers of patients to make studies relatively easy to perform [41]. Investigators assert that analgesic effectiveness may vary substantially between pain models [40,42], whereas others argue that there may be no differences in the analgesic efficacy between dental and other postoperative pain models [41]. As previously mentioned, Rees and colleagues [39] investigated the effectiveness of single-dose aspirin in the treatment of acute pain and postsurgical pain. The review comprised mostly dental pain

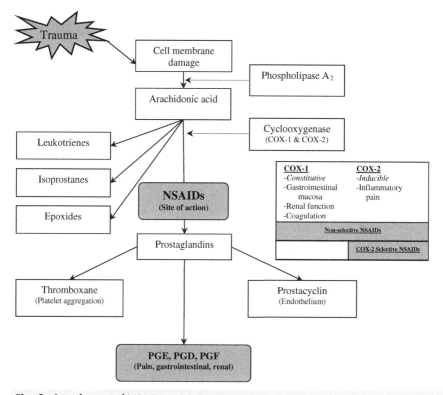

Fig. 2. Site of action of NSAIDs.

(68%) models but also included other pain models (episiotomy, mixed orthopedic surgery, urogenital surgery, gynecologic surgery, and other nonspecified surgeries). The investigators concluded that for doses greater than 600/650 mg, ASA was effective at reducing the number of patients with at least 50% pain relief in this mixed study population.

The trepidation in prescribing ASA still remains in its ability to irreversibly inhibit COX activity and possibly increase adverse effects such as gastric irritation and impaired coagulation. For aspirin in particular, the irreversible inhibition of COX-1 has limited its use in the postoperative period as compared with the nonselective NSAIDs that reversibly inhibit COX-1. Thus, the consequences of inhibition of platelet COX-1 last for the lifetime of the platelet. Inhibition of platelet COX-1-dependent thromboxane formation therefore is cumulative with repeated doses of aspirin (at least as low as 30 mg/d) and takes 8 to 12 days, and increased bleeding time or decreased platelet aggregation [36]. Unique to postsurgical patients is the risk of platelet dysfunction resulting from preoperative ASA administration, which increases the risk of perioperative bleeding and gastric irritation [39].

Diclofenac

Diclofenac is a phenylacetic acid derivative that is a nonsteroidal anti-inflammatory medication, and has been used to treat the pain and inflammation by inhibiting COX-1 and COX-2. Diclofenac is available in 2 enteral formulations, diclofenac sodium and diclofenac potassium. Diclofenac potassium is formulated to be released and absorbed in the stomach. Diclofenac sodium, usually distributed in enteric-coated tablets, resists dissolution in low pH gastric environments, being released instead into the duodenum [43]. Other formulations of diclofenac include topical gels and transdermal patches. In addition, diclofenac is available in a parenteral formulation for infusion (Voltarol ampoules), and more recently a formulation for intravenous bolus has been developed (diclofenac sodium injection [DIC075V; Dyloject]). In comparison with other analgesics a single 50-mg dose of diclofenac, NNT 2.3 (2.0–2.7), is equivalent to ibuprofen 400 mg, NNT 2.4 (2.3–2.6), and significantly more effective than a single dose of paracetamol 1000 mg, NNT 3.8 (3.4–4.4), and aspirin 600/650 mg, NNT 4.4 (4.0–4.9) [44]. A randomized double-blind, placebo-controlled trial investigated the opioid-sparing effect of diclofenac (suppository) after cesarean sections [45]. The investigators concluded that the diclofenac significantly reduced the cumulative administration of morphine. In a randomized, placebo-controlled trial, Hynes and colleagues [46] demonstrated equal analgesic efficacy of parenteral paracetamol (propacetamol) 2 g to diclofenac 75 mg intramuscularly (n = 40) in treating postoperative hip arthroplasty pain. In a Cochrane Collaborative meta-analysis, diclofenac was shown to be effective for treating acute postoperative pain [47]. The meta-analysis assessed 7 trials (n = 945) and provided an NNT for at least 50% relief over 4 to 6 hours for diclofenac of 2.8 (2.1–4.3), 2.3 (2.0–2.7), and 1.9 (1.6–2.2) for 25 mg, 50 mg, and 100 mg, respectively. These results indicate a dose-response relationship, with increasing doses providing better pain relief. The Cochrane group concluded that oral diclofenac is an effective single-dose treatment for moderate to severe postoperative pain. There was no significant difference between diclofenac and placebo in the incidence of adverse effects. The risk of adverse events with the administration of diclofenac is equal to that of other NSAIDs, but the COX selectivity may provide a theoretical advantage to less selective or COX-1 NSAIDs.

Ketorolac

Ketorolac tromethamine is an NSAID with activity at COX-1 and COX-2 enzymes, thus blocking prostaglandin production. Administration of ketorolac is available for enteral, ophthalmic, and parenteral delivery, and is the only parenteral NSAID currently available in the United States. Ketorolac has an onset of action of approximately 10 minutes, peak analgesic effect of 2 to 3 hours, and analgesic duration of 6 to 8 hours, making it attractive for postoperative analgesia [48]. Ketorolac has been used to treat mild to severe pain following major surgical procedures including general abdominal surgery, gynecologic surgery, orthopedic surgery, and dentistry. Multiple studies have investigated the analgesic potency of ketorolac, and in animal models the analgesic potency has be estimated to be between 180 and 800 times that of aspirin [49,50]. When compared with morphine, ketorolac 30 mg intramuscular (IM) has been shown to be equivalent to 12 mg morphine IM and 100 mg meperidine IM [51]. Ketorolac has shown usefulness in postoperative pain control and is has been advocated in ambulatory surgical procedures, because of the lack of respiratory or central nervous system depression and its ability to diminish postoperative nausea and vomiting associated with opioid medications. In a randomized, double-blind, placebo-controlled study involving patients undergoing total hip or knee replacement procedures, the analgesic efficacy of parenteral ketorolac (15 or 30 mg) was compared with propacetamol (2g) and placebo [52]. The primary efficacy measures were visual analog scale (VAS) and verbal rating scale (VRS) pain assessments. The investigators concluded that propacetamol 2 g had a shorter duration of analgesia than ketorolac 30 mg, but the analgesic response was not significantly different from ketorolac 15 mg or 30 mg. This conclusion is supported by a prior study showing consistent findings whereby enteral acetaminophen (1 g) was shown to be similar to ketorolac 10 to 20 mg orally for postoperative orthopedic pain [53]. A systemic review of the analgesic efficacy of ketorolac in moderate to severe postoperative pain calculated the relative benefit and NNT for one patient to achieve at least 50% pain relief to be 3.4 (2.5–4.9) for intramuscular ketorolac and 2.6 (2.3–3.1) for enteral ketorolac [54].

Opioid sparing is the purported advantage of adjuvant medication additions to postoperative analgesic regimens. In a double-blind, randomized controlled trial using the primary outcome variable of the proportion of subjects who reported a 50% decrease in pain intensity 30 minutes after the initiation of the intravenous infusion, Cepeda and colleagues [55] evaluated the effectiveness of ketorolac compared with morphine. Patients were also evaluated for the presence and severity of opioid requirements and opioid-related adverse effects. The morphine group required more morphine to achieve the desired pain intensity levels than did the ketorolac + morphine group, and with this increase in morphine dosing the risk of development of any side effects also increased. The calculated risk of developing adverse effects increased 1.3% (1.3–1.4) for every 1-mg increment of morphine consumed. Comparing ketorolac with morphine the calculated NNT is 5 [4–10], and the number needed to harm for morphine compared with the combination of ketorolac + morphine is 9 [6–20]. In addition, a prospective, double-blind, randomized trial evaluated the effectiveness of combination (NSAIDs + opioid) analgesics versus morphine alone and ketorolac alone in the management of postoperative pain after orthopedic surgery [56]. The investigators found that morphine + ketorolac provided significantly better analgesia versus ketorolac or morphine alone, and consumption of morphine in the morphine + ketorolac groups was significantly less than in the morphine alone groups at study end (24.2 mg vs 64.2 mg). The side effects observed in the study were not significantly different between the groups except that urinary retention was significantly higher in the morphine alone group (41.6%) compared with the morphine + ketorolac group (12.5%). The investigators concluded that the combination of morphine + ketorolac provided better analgesia in the postoperative period than morphine alone. In addition, the combination potentiated the effects of each medication and the reduction of morphine (opioids) decreased the risk and occurrence of adverse side effects associated with morphine. In a systematic review of randomized, controlled trials of ketorolac versus placebo with opioids given for breakthrough pain, ketorolac reduced opioid dose requirements by a mean of 36% (range 0%–73%) depending on the type of surgery, but this did not result in a concomitant reduction in all opioid side effects (eg, nausea and vomiting) [57].

Acetaminophen

Acetaminophen (paracetamol) produces its analgesic effect by inhibiting central prostaglandin synthesis with minimal inhibition of peripheral prostaglandin synthesis [48,58]. Often labeled as an NSAID, acetaminophen and NSAIDs have important differences, such as acetaminophen's weak anti-inflammatory effects and its generally poor ability to inhibit COX in the presence of high concentrations of peroxides, as are found at sites of inflammation; [48,58] nor does it have an adverse effect on platelet function [59] or the gastric mucosa [58]. Acetaminophen is absorbed rapidly, with peak plasma levels seen within 30 minutes to 1 hour, and is metabolized in the liver by conjugation and hydroxylation to inactive metabolites, with a duration of action of 4 to 6 hours [48,60]. Paracetamol is perhaps the safest and most cost-effective nonopioid analgesic when it is administered in analgesic doses [61]. Paracetamol is available in parenteral form as propacetamol, and 1 g of propacetamol provides 0.5 g paracetamol after hydrolysis [62]. The addition of acetaminophen to patient-controlled analgesia (PCA) morphine has been shown to improve the quality of pain relief and patient satisfaction after major orthopedic procedures [63]. A double-blind, randomized, placebo-controlled, parallel study investigated the effect of a combination of acetaminophen + morphine after open reduction and internal fixation of acute limb fractures. The investigators concluded that the mean pain scores in the acetaminophen group were significantly lower than those in the control group on day 1 (2.1 vs 3.3; $P = .03$), the average duration of PCA use was significantly reduced in the acetaminophen group (35.8 vs 45.4 h; $P = .03$) and the mean morphine consumption was 16% less in the acetaminophen group, but did not reach significance ($P = .27$). The nausea and sedation scores and the incidence of emesis were comparable between the 2 groups. In a qualitative systematic review, the analgesic and adverse effects of paracetamol and NSAIDs in the postoperative period found no significant difference between NSAIDs and paracetamol in major abdominal-gynecologic and orthopedic surgical procerdures [64]. Furthermore, in a double-blind, randomized, parallel group trial the analgesic efficacy and safety of propacetamol in combination with morphine administered by PCA were studied [65]. Primary efficacy measures included total dose of morphine over 24 hours

n the action of selective agonists:
pionic acid (AMPA), kainic acid
tor has a crucial role in excitatory
degeneration in the central nervous
modulate the excitatory effects of
particularly preincisionally [86,87],
d and increased responses at the
ral pain perception originating in
DA receptors, which are thought
and maintenance of chronic pain,
nistered to produce analgesia. Ket-
available NMDA antagonist [88],
e and chronic pain [89]. Ketamine
an NMDA receptor antagonist to
t in chronic pain syndromes [90].
or antagonists lies in the reduction
ration or hemodynamic parameters

been studied at subanesthetic doses.
onist at NMDA receptors but also
binds weakly to opioid receptors,
tors, facilitates $GABA_A$ signaling,
y neuroregenerative properties [92–
as been used to attenuate opioid
ociated undesirable psychomimetic
allucinations) observed with larger
nized study, Urban and colleagues
erative administration of ketamine
on. A numerical rating scale (NRS)
d as a primary measure of effective-
cantly ($P \le .05$) less pain during the
continued to have less pain during
h physical therapy, but differences
stoperative day 2. The cumulative
etween the 2 groups, but the inves-
administration of ketamine reduced
prospective, randomized, double-
the effectiveness of perioperative
nine) consumption with the primary
consumption 48 hours after major
mine was administered at induction
ntinued as an infusion into the post-
ne PCA. Group 2 received ketamine

(PCA bolus + PCA basal flow + titration) and the number of boluses requested. Other efficacy measures were pain intensity scores and global efficacy. Morphine consumption was significantly decreased in the propacetamol group at 24 hours (37% decrease, $P = .01$), and both the total 24-hour PCA morphine dose (24% decrease, $P = .03$) and the PCA dose + titration (20% decrease, $P = .02$) were significantly less. The conclusion was that propacetamol demonstrated a morphine-sparing effect but there was no significant difference in pain scores and adverse effects (respiratory depression, sedation, and hypotension) between the 2 groups. In a systematic review of the morphine-sparing effect of acetaminophen combined with PCA, Remy and colleagues [66] evaluated its efficacy and effects on opioid-related adverse effects in 7 prospective, randomized controlled trials (265 patients in the group with PCA morphine + acetaminophen and 226 patients in the group with PCA morphine alone). Outcome measures included morphine consumption over the first 24 hours after surgery, patient satisfaction, and the incidence of opioid-related adverse effects, including nausea and vomiting, sedation, urinary retention, pruritus, and respiratory depression. Acetaminophen combined with PCA morphine induced a significant morphine-sparing effect but did not change the incidence of morphine-related adverse effects in the postoperative period.

The comparative efficacy of different analgesics has also been shown to vary with the type and extent of surgical procedure [67]. This variation in efficacy has led to the coined term "procedure-specific postoperative pain management [68]." A qualitative systematic review comparing acetaminophen and NSAIDs in postoperative pain management found NSAIDs to be superior after dental surgery; acetaminophen had comparable efficacy in many of the studies, but no significant differences were found after orthopedic surgery [64]. Although no advantage was found, comparative tables provide useful information for the prescriber. The League Table provides a useful measure of the effectiveness of different analgesics [69]. The comparative effectiveness of the medications is compiled from information from systematic reviews of randomized, double-blind, single-dose studies in patients with moderate to severe pain. The efficacy measure for each review is reliable: at least 50% pain relief over 4 to 6 hours.

COX-2 inhibitors

Nonselective NSAIDs inhibit both COX-1 and COX-2, and with increased COX-1 selectivity increases the tendency toward gastrointestinal toxicity [70]. Celecoxib at supratherapeutic dosages of up to 1200 mg/d (600 mg twice daily) had no significant effect on collagen- and arachidonate-induced platelet aggregation or bleeding time in humans [71]. Furthermore, although overall incidence of renal adverse events was significantly higher among patients treated with celecoxib or comparator NSAIDs than in those receiving placebo, there were no reports of celecoxib-associated acute renal failure, nephrotic syndrome, interstitial nephritis, or renal papillary necrosis [71]. COX-2 inhibitors, which selectively target COX-2 while sparing COX-1, were developed in an attempt to obtain the therapeutic benefits of NSAIDs while overcoming their limitations, and highlight responsible medication administration [72].

COX-2 inhibitors (celecoxib, rofecoxib, and valdecoxib) were approved for use in the United States and Europe, but both rofecoxib and valdecoxib have now been withdrawn from the market due to their adverse event profile. Parecoxib and etoricoxib recently have been approved in Europe but still await approval in the United States. The newest drug in the class, lumiracoxib, is under consideration for approval in Europe and the United States. On administration most of the coxibs are distributed widely throughout the body, with celecoxib possessing an increased lipophilicity that enables transport into the central nervous system. Lumiracoxib is more acidic than the others, which may favor its accumulation at sites of inflammation. Despite these subtle differences, all of the coxibs achieve sufficient brain concentrations to have a central analgesic effect [73], and all reduce prostaglandin formation in inflamed joints. The estimated half-lives of these medications vary (2–6 hours for lumiracoxib, 6–12 hours for celecoxib and valdecoxib, and 20–26 hours for etoricoxib). Likewise, the relative degree of selectivity for COX-2 inhibition is lumiracoxib = etoricoxib > valdecoxib = rofecoxib >> celecoxib [48].

The efficacy of COX-2–specific inhibitors for the management of postoperative pain has been evaluated in numerous controlled clinical trials. For example, in a prospective randomized placebo-controlled trial, opioid-sparing effects and rehabilitative results after perioperative COX-2 administration for total knee arthroplasty (TKA) were investigated [74]. Primary efficacy measures were pain scores measured by VAS and range of motion (ROM) outcomes. The COX-2 group showed less postoperative VAS pain at rest than the control group. The COX-2 group showed significant improvement postoperatively in knee ROM. Both investigators concluded that perioperative administration of a selective COX-2 inhibitor reduced postoperative VAS pain scores at rest and decreased opioid usage while providing better ROM rehabilitation results. In a systematic review assessing the analgesic efficacy and adverse effects of a single oral dose of celecoxib for moderate to severe postoperative pain, 8 studies (1380 participants) were analyzed, providing an NNT of 4.2 (3.4–5.6) and 2.5 (2.2–2.9) compared with placebo for celecoxib 200 mg and 400 mg, respectively [75]. Furthermore, a 200-mg dose of celecoxib was at least as effective as aspirin 600/650 mg and acetaminophen 1000 mg for relieving postoperative pain, whereas a 400-mg dose was at least as effective as ibuprofen 400 mg. Adverse events occurred at a similar rate as celecoxib and placebo.

The preceding review of selective NSAIDs and acetaminophen highlights the effectiveness of nonsteroidal medications in the treatment of postoperative pain. Other NSAID medications have been administered to treat postoperative pain but are not discussed in detail. For example, the NSAIDs ibuprofen and diclofenac in single oral doses for moderate to severe postoperative pain have been compared with placebo in a recent Cochrane Review [76]. In postoperative pain the NNT (to achieve at least 50% pain relief) for ibuprofen

be further divided into 3 subtypes based α-amino-3-hydroxy-5-methylisoxazole-4-pr (KA), and *NMDA* [84]. The NMDA rece synaptic transmission, plasticity, and neuro system [85], and has become an avenue t glutamate. Inhibition of NMDA receptors, reduces the excitement of the spinal co dorsal horn (wind-up), thus reducing ce the periphery. Through inhibition of NM to play a crucial role in the generation NMDA receptor antagonists can be admi amine, currently the most potent clinicall has been studied in the treatment of acu has been used at subanesthetic doses as inhibit the processing of nociceptive inpu The clinical importance of NMDA recept of pain perception without depressing resp that are induced by opioids [91].

Ketamine

For postoperative analgesia, ketamine has Ketamine functions not only as an antag blocks non-NMDA glutamate receptors, antagonizes muscarinic cholinergic rece and possesses local anesthetic and possibl 94]. At subanesthetic doses, ketamine requirements while minimizing the ass side effects (confusion, dysphoria, and anesthetic doses. In a prospective rando [90] evaluated the effectiveness of posto in opioid-tolerant patients after spinal fus at rest and during physical therapy was u ness. The ketamine group exhibited signi first postoperative hour after surgery, an the first postoperative day at rest and w in NRS score were not significant at p opioid use was not significantly different tigators did conclude that postoperative pain scores in opioid-tolerant patients. blind, placebo-controlled study compare ketamine administration on opioid (morp outcome measure of cumulative morphi abdominal surgery [95]. In group 1, ket of anesthesia, intraoperatively, and was c operative period concurrently with morp

(PCA bolus + PCA basal flow + titration) and the number of boluses requested. Other efficacy measures were pain intensity scores and global efficacy. Morphine consumption was significantly decreased in the propacetamol group at 24 hours (37% decrease, $P = .01$), and both the total 24-hour PCA morphine dose (24% decrease, $P = .03$) and the PCA dose + titration (20% decrease, $P = .02$) were significantly less. The conclusion was that propacetamol demonstrated a morphine-sparing effect but there was no significant difference in pain scores and adverse effects (respiratory depression, sedation, and hypotension) between the 2 groups. In a systematic review of the morphine-sparing effect of acetaminophen combined with PCA, Remy and colleagues [66] evaluated its efficacy and effects on opioid-related adverse effects in 7 prospective, randomized controlled trials (265 patients in the group with PCA morphine + acetaminophen and 226 patients in the group with PCA morphine alone). Outcome measures included morphine consumption over the first 24 hours after surgery, patient satisfaction, and the incidence of opioid-related adverse effects, including nausea and vomiting, sedation, urinary retention, pruritus, and respiratory depression. Acetaminophen combined with PCA morphine induced a significant morphine-sparing effect but did not change the incidence of morphine-related adverse effects in the postoperative period.

The comparative efficacy of different analgesics has also been shown to vary with the type and extent of surgical procedure [67]. This variation in efficacy has led to the coined term "procedure-specific postoperative pain management [68]." A qualitative systematic review comparing acetaminophen and NSAIDs in postoperative pain management found NSAIDs to be superior after dental surgery; acetaminophen had comparable efficacy in many of the studies, but no significant differences were found after orthopedic surgery [64]. Although no advantage was found, comparative tables provide useful information for the prescriber. The League Table provides a useful measure of the effectiveness of different analgesics [69]. The comparative effectiveness of the medications is compiled from information from systematic reviews of randomized, double-blind, single-dose studies in patients with moderate to severe pain. The efficacy measure for each review is reliable: at least 50% pain relief over 4 to 6 hours.

COX-2 inhibitors

Nonselective NSAIDs inhibit both COX-1 and COX-2, and with increased COX-1 selectivity increases the tendency toward gastrointestinal toxicity [70]. Celecoxib at supratherapeutic dosages of up to 1200 mg/d (600 mg twice daily) had no significant effect on collagen- and arachidonate-induced platelet aggregation or bleeding time in humans [71]. Furthermore, although overall incidence of renal adverse events was significantly higher among patients treated with celecoxib or comparator NSAIDs than in those receiving placebo, there were no reports of celecoxib-associated acute renal failure, nephrotic syndrome, interstitial nephritis, or renal papillary necrosis [71]. COX-2 inhibitors, which selectively target COX-2 while sparing COX-1, were developed in an attempt to obtain the therapeutic benefits of NSAIDs while overcoming their limitations, and highlight responsible medication administration [72].

COX-2 inhibitors (celecoxib, rofecoxib, and valdecoxib) were approved for use in the United States and Europe, but both rofecoxib and valdecoxib have now been withdrawn from the market due to their adverse event profile. Parecoxib and etoricoxib recently have been approved in Europe but still await approval in the United States. The newest drug in the class, lumiracoxib, is under consideration for approval in Europe and the United States. On administration most of the coxibs are distributed widely throughout the body, with celecoxib possessing an increased lipophilicity that enables transport into the central nervous system. Lumiracoxib is more acidic than the others, which may favor its accumulation at sites of inflammation. Despite these subtle differences, all of the coxibs achieve sufficient brain concentrations to have a central analgesic effect [73], and all reduce prostaglandin formation in inflamed joints. The estimated half-lives of these medications vary (2–6 hours for lumiracoxib, 6–12 hours for celecoxib and valdecoxib, and 20–26 hours for etoricoxib). Likewise, the relative degree of selectivity for COX-2 inhibition is lumiracoxib = etoricoxib > valdecoxib = rofecoxib >> celecoxib [48].

The efficacy of COX-2–specific inhibitors for the management of postoperative pain has been evaluated in numerous controlled clinical trials. For example, in a prospective randomized placebo-controlled trial, opioid-sparing effects and rehabilitative results after perioperative COX-2 administration for total knee arthroplasty (TKA) were investigated [74]. Primary efficacy measures were pain scores measured by VAS and range of motion (ROM) outcomes. The COX-2 group showed less postoperative VAS pain at rest than the control group. The COX-2 group showed significant improvement postoperatively in knee ROM. Both investigators concluded that perioperative administration of a selective COX-2 inhibitor reduced postoperative VAS pain scores at rest and decreased opioid usage while providing better ROM rehabilitation results. In a systematic review assessing the analgesic efficacy and adverse effects of a single oral dose of celecoxib for moderate to severe postoperative pain, 8 studies (1380 participants) were analyzed, providing an NNT of 4.2 (3.4–5.6) and 2.5 (2.2–2.9) compared with placebo for celecoxib 200 mg and 400 mg, respectively [75]. Furthermore, a 200-mg dose of celecoxib was at least as effective as aspirin 600/650 mg and acetaminophen 1000 mg for relieving postoperative pain, whereas a 400-mg dose was at least as effective as ibuprofen 400 mg. Adverse events occurred at a similar rate as celecoxib and placebo.

The preceding review of selective NSAIDs and acetaminophen highlights the effectiveness of nonsteroidal medications in the treatment of postoperative pain. Other NSAID medications have been administered to treat postoperative pain but are not discussed in detail. For example, the NSAIDs ibuprofen and diclofenac in single oral doses for moderate to severe postoperative pain have been compared with placebo in a recent Cochrane Review [76]. In postoperative pain the NNT (to achieve at least 50% pain relief) for ibuprofen

400 mg was 2.7 (2.5–3.0), for ibuprofen 600 mg 2.4 (1.9–3.3), for diclofenac 50 mg 2.3 (2.0–2.7), and for diclofenac 100 mg 1.8 (1.5–2.1).

Regarding the choice of NSAIDs or acetaminophen, The Agency for Healthcare Research and Quality found no clear difference in efficacy between celecoxib and nonselective NSAIDs, based on results from published trials and meta-analyses of published and unpublished trials with respect to osteoarthritis [77]. The key question is which medication should be administered with the greatest efficacy and opioid-sparing effect, and fewest adverse effects. The addition of the medication in the perioperative period is dependent on the intent and the potential for adverse effects. For example, in the patients with high potential for postoperative bleeding it may be prudent to withhold medications such as aspirin or ketorolac because of the COX-1 effect and the risk of bleeding. The procedure may dictate the choice of medication, optimizing the medication choice and analgesia. Procedure-specific medication choices correspond to the magnitude of surgical trauma, the risk of adverse effects of the medication, and the underlying patient characteristics. Prudent medication administration dictates that inhibition of platelet aggregation and, therefore, risk of bleeding that is associated with NSAIDs will be more relevant in those operations in which there is greater potential for bleeding complications (eg, tonsillectomy, plastic surgery, major joint replacement) than in others (eg, cholecystectomy, herniorrhaphy, and so forth) [68]. In contrast, NSAIDs that do not inhibit platelet aggregation (COX-2) or have less selectivity toward COX-1 inhibition are better choices. The selective and nonselective medications have been administered concurrently, but the use of low-dose aspirin for primary or secondary prevention of cardiovascular disease may negate the gastroprotective effect of COX-2–selective NSAIDs. In contrast, the beneficial effect of aspirin may be attenuated by concomitant use of nonselective NSAIDs, such as ibuprofen or naproxen [78].

The recent retraction of several manuscripts published by Dr Scott Reuben has led to several editorials [79–83] questioning the validity of multimodal analgesia for perioperative pain management. Some of the retracted articles were themed on the use of COX-2 inhibitors for perioperative pain management. However, it is vital to realize that there are several other published studies on the use of COX-2 inhibitors demonstrating the reduction in opioid use in the postoperative period. Recognizing the implications of falsified data on COX-2 inhibition and spinal surgery, the retracted articles [80–82] authored by Dr Reuben on the use of COX-2 inhibitors for spinal fusion surgery necessitates reevaluation of the coxibs before these medications can be routinely used perioperatively in spine surgery patients.

N-METHYL-D-ASPARTATE RECEPTOR ANTAGONISTS

Glutamate is a major excitatory neurotransmitter in the brain and spinal cord, exerting its effects postsynaptically. This excitation is caused by the activation of both ionotropic and metabotropic receptors. The ionotropic receptors can be further divided into 3 subtypes based on the action of selective agonists: α-amino-3-hydroxy-5-methylisoxazole-4-propionic acid (AMPA), kainic acid (KA), and *NMDA* [84]. The NMDA receptor has a crucial role in excitatory synaptic transmission, plasticity, and neurodegeneration in the central nervous system [85], and has become an avenue to modulate the excitatory effects of glutamate. Inhibition of NMDA receptors, particularly preincisionally [86,87], reduces the excitement of the spinal cord and increased responses at the dorsal horn (wind-up), thus reducing central pain perception originating in the periphery. Through inhibition of NMDA receptors, which are thought to play a crucial role in the generation and maintenance of chronic pain, NMDA receptor antagonists can be administered to produce analgesia. Ketamine, currently the most potent clinically available NMDA antagonist [88], has been studied in the treatment of acute and chronic pain [89]. Ketamine has been used at subanesthetic doses as an NMDA receptor antagonist to inhibit the processing of nociceptive input in chronic pain syndromes [90]. The clinical importance of NMDA receptor antagonists lies in the reduction of pain perception without depressing respiration or hemodynamic parameters that are induced by opioids [91].

Ketamine

For postoperative analgesia, ketamine has been studied at subanesthetic doses. Ketamine functions not only as an antagonist at NMDA receptors but also blocks non-NMDA glutamate receptors, binds weakly to opioid receptors, antagonizes muscarinic cholinergic receptors, facilitates $GABA_A$ signaling, and possesses local anesthetic and possibly neuroregenerative properties [92–94]. At subanesthetic doses, ketamine has been used to attenuate opioid requirements while minimizing the associated undesirable psychomimetic side effects (confusion, dysphoria, and hallucinations) observed with larger anesthetic doses. In a prospective randomized study, Urban and colleagues [90] evaluated the effectiveness of postoperative administration of ketamine in opioid-tolerant patients after spinal fusion. A numerical rating scale (NRS) at rest and during physical therapy was used as a primary measure of effectiveness. The ketamine group exhibited significantly ($P \leq .05$) less pain during the first postoperative hour after surgery, and continued to have less pain during the first postoperative day at rest and with physical therapy, but differences in NRS score were not significant at postoperative day 2. The cumulative opioid use was not significantly different between the 2 groups, but the investigators did conclude that postoperative administration of ketamine reduced pain scores in opioid-tolerant patients. A prospective, randomized, double-blind, placebo-controlled study compared the effectiveness of perioperative ketamine administration on opioid (morphine) consumption with the primary outcome measure of cumulative morphine consumption 48 hours after major abdominal surgery [95]. In group 1, ketamine was administered at induction of anesthesia, intraoperatively, and was continued as an infusion into the postoperative period concurrently with morphine PCA. Group 2 received ketamine intraoperatively (induction and intraoperatively) with a morphine PCA postoperatively, and group 3 received morphine PCA alone. Ketamine administered perioperatively (group 1) significantly ($P = .008$) reduced the cumulative consumption of morphine compared with the other groups, but there was no difference in morphine consumption between groups 2 and 3. In addition, the VAS scores at 4, 24, and 48 hours postoperatively were significantly lower in groups 1 and 2 compared with group 3 ($P = .004$, $P = .0001$, $P = .001$, respectively). Group 1 experienced significantly less ($P = .005$) nausea or vomiting compared with group 3. There was no difference in sedation scores and adverse psychomimetic effects between the groups. The conclusion was that opioid (morphine) consumption and nausea or vomiting can be reduced in the postoperative period by administration of low-dose ketamine in the perioperative period. In a prospective, randomized, double-blind study, Kollender and colleagues [96] compared the efficacy of morphine alone and morphine (65% of control) plus subanesthetic ketamine for postoperative pain control in orthopedic oncology patients. The morphine + ketamine group used significantly less ($P<.05$) morphine and diclofenac than the morphine only group over the 96-hour study duration. Throughout the study duration the morphine only group consistently reported significantly ($P<.001$) higher VAS scores. The rate of nausea and vomiting was significantly higher ($P<.05$) in the morphine only group, and no ketamine-related specific side effects were reported in the morphine + ketamine group. The investigators concluded that subanesthetic ketamine provides a morphine-sparing effect, while consistently lowering pain scores without psychomimetic side effects. The use of subanesthetic ketamine has been studied in several other studies, with favorable results of low-dose ketamine in the perioperative period as an adjuvant for analgesia [97–99]. A Cochrane Review [100] evaluated the administration of ketamine in the perioperative period by analyzing 37 studies (n = 2240), and concluded that subanesthetic ketamine dosing is effective at reducing morphine requirements in the first 24 hours after surgery, reducing postoperative nausea and vomiting, and was not associated with significant adverse effects related to ketamine administration.

Dextromethorphan

Dextromethorphan (DM) is a noncompetitive antagonist of the NMDA-sensitive inotropic glutamate receptor [101,102]. The neurophysiologic activity of DM resembles that of ketamine, although it has a lower affinity to the receptor [103], which may contribute to its tolerability and improved side-effect profile compared with ketamine. DM possesses a weak affinity for the μ-opioid receptor and has a sedative effect [104], and has been used as an antitussive since its Food and Drug Administration approval in the mid twentieth century. Dextromethorphan has been reported to produce a reduction in postoperative pain and opioid consumption. A randomized, placebo-controlled, double-blind study investigated the analgesic effectiveness of dextromethorphan in orthopedic oncology patients [91]. The participants were randomly assigned to placebo, DM 60 mg, or DM 90 mg given 90 minutes before the operative procedure and on each of the 2 days after surgery. The DM groups reported significantly ($P<.01$) less pain compared with the placebo group both immediately and up to 3 days postoperatively. In addition, both DM groups consumed less morphine than the placebo group ($P<.01$), their demand for rescue drugs on the first postoperative day was significantly lower ($P<.01$), and sedation was significantly ($P<.01$) less in the DM groups. The investigators concluded that perioperative administration of DM reduced pain intensity, sedation, and analgesic requirements in patients that expectedly would need higher opioid requirements. Administration of preincisional or postincisional DM on postoperative analgesia was investigated in a randomized, placebo-controlled, double-blind study [105]. The administration of preincisional DM significantly ($P<.001$) reduced postoperative opioid (meperidine) consumption compared with both postincisional DM administration and placebo. A qualitative review of NMDA receptor antagonists (ketamine, memantine, amantadine, dextromethorphan, magnesium, and methadone) reported that ketamine and DM produced a significant preventive analgesic benefit in 58% and 67% of studies, respectively [106]. In a randomized, placebo-controlled, double-blind study, Wadhwa and colleagues [107] examined the effectiveness of a large dose (800 mg per 24 hours in divided doses) of DM, and whether DM could potentiate morphine analgesia while simultaneously causing a significant improvement in the management of the postoperative pain. The administration of a large dose of oral DM (200 mg every 8 hours) given postoperatively after knee surgery produced a significant but modest reduction in morphine requirements (29.3%; $P<.05$) but no reduction in postoperative pain levels. Dextromethorphan at the 200-mg dose was associated with a reduction in opioid requirements but doses greater than 200 mg were associated with DM-related side effects such as sedation and nausea. The investigators concluded that oral dextromethorphan is not clinically useful in the treatment of postoperative pain after knee surgery. In a qualitative systematic review of the analgesic efficacy of DM in postoperative patients, Duedahl and colleagues [108] reviewed 28 randomized, double-blind, clinical studies, and found inconsistent results for the use of DM in the perioperative period. Significant decreases in supplemental opioid consumption were observed in the majority of parenteral DM studies and in about one-half of the oral studies, but the inconsistencies led to a limited clinical application (not routine) of DM in perioperative pain management.

Magnesium

Similar to ketamine and dextromethorphan, the magnesium ion acts to block the NMDA receptor channel. Magnesium sulfate is available as a 500 mg/mL preservative-free solution for injection. Magnesium administered intravenously lacks efficacy in the cerebrospinal fluid at 4 g; however, 50 mg administered intrathecally has been demonstrated to be effective [109]. Perioperative intravenous magnesium sulfate at very high doses has been reported to reduce postoperative morphine consumption but not postoperative pain scores [110,111]. Both studies conclude that intravenous magnesium (3–3.5 g) can be a useful adjuvant in perioperative analgesia, but the exact dose needs to be determined. A recent dose-finding study for intravenous magnesium determined that administration of magnesium at 40 mg/kg before induction, followed by a 10 mg/kg/h infusion, resulted in a reduction in perioperative analgesic requirements without any major hemodynamic consequences [110]. Higher-infusion doses did not offer any advantage. However, because the magnesium ion crosses the blood-brain barrier poorly in humans [112], it is not clear whether the therapeutic effect is related to NMDA antagonism in the central nervous system.

GABAPENTINOIDS
The gabapentinoid group of drugs, gabapentin and pregabalin, have been shown to be effective in several chronic pain states [113–119]. This class of medications recently has gained favor in the treatment of acute postoperative pain.

Gabapentin
Gabapentin, 1-(aminomethyl)cyclohexane acetic acid, is a structural analogue of the neurotransmitter γ-aminobutyric acid (GABA), initially synthesized to mimic the chemical structure of the GABA, but is not believed to bind directly to GABA receptors or have any effect on the uptake or breakdown of GABA. The primary mechanism of action for gabapentin is via the modulation or binding to the $\alpha_2\delta$ subunit of presynaptic voltage-dependent calcium channels (VDCC) [120,121]. The upregulation of $\alpha_2\delta$ subunit of VDCC in the dorsal root ganglia and spinal cord has been demonstrated after experimental peripheral nerve injury [122] and surgical incision [123], and it is at these calcium channel subunits that gabapentin is purported to have its mechanism of action. Gabapentin may produce its antinociception effect by inhibiting calcium influx via these channels, and subsequently inhibiting the release of excitatory neurotransmitters such as substance P and calcitonin gene-related peptide from the spinal cord [121]. Gabapentin has a half-life of about 5 to 7 hours, and its bioavailability is inversely related to the dose administered. Multiple studies support the use of gabapentin for the treatment of postoperative pain. In a randomized, double-blind, placebo-controlled study, Dirks and colleagues [124] investigated the effect of gabapentin on morphine consumption and postoperative pain in patients undergoing radical mastectomy. A significant clinical response was found, with a total morphine consumption reduction compared with placebo ($P<.0001$). Multiple studies have replicated the positive response of gabapentin on postoperative analgesia and opioid sparing in various surgical procedures (abdominal hysterectomy, spinal surgery, laparoscopic cholecystectomy) [125–128]. In addition, 2 meta-analyses have demonstrated gabapentin to be an effective analgesic adjunct in the perioperative period [11,129]. Doses ranged from 300 to 1200 mg, and were generally given as a single dose 1 to 2 hours before surgery. Compared with placebo, the perioperative

administration of gabapentin produced significantly better postoperative analgesia. In a systematic review of 16 randomized trials, 1200 mg gabapentin was administered as an adjunct to opioids and led to decreased pain scores and 24-hour opioid consumption postoperatively. Decreased pain scores, but with less dramatic reduction in opioid use, were observed when the dose was less than 1200 mg. However, gabapentin was associated with an increased risk of sedation, but fewer opioid-related side effects such as vomiting and pruritus occurred [130]. Although the exact mechanism of action of gabapentin is not wholly elucidated, clinical trials support its use in the perioperative period as a clinically useful analgesic adjunct for postoperative pain management.

Pregabalin

Pregabalin is the active S-enantiomer of racemic 3-isobutyl GABA, modifying VDCC in a similar manner to gabapentin. Potent binding at this site reduces calcium influx at nerve terminals and therefore, reduces the release of several neurotransmitters including glutamate, norepinephrine, and substance P [113,131]. Compared with gabapentin, pregabalin has greater lipid solubility, thus improving diffusion across the blood-brain barrier, has better pharmacokinetic properties, and has fewer drug interactions, due to an absence of hepatic metabolism [132]. Pregabalin is more potent than gabapentin and achieves its efficacy at lower doses, and therefore may be associated with fewer side effects. Systemic pregabalin reduces hyperalgesia in an animal model of postoperative pain [133].

For both pregabalin and gabapentin, most studies have focused on the treatment of chronic pain conditions, but recently studies have emerged evaluating the use of pregabalin in the treatment of acute postoperative pain. In a randomized, double-blind, parallel, placebo-controlled trial, pregabalin was examined for its analgesic efficacy in an ambulatory day-surgery population experiencing acute visceral pain [134]. Patients undergoing minor gynecologic surgery received either 100 mg of pregabalin or placebo 1 hour before surgery, with the primary outcome measure being pain VAS scores. The study found no statistical difference between the pregabalin group and the placebo group. Jokela and colleagues [135] investigated the analgesic effectiveness of perioperative pregabalin administration in laparoscopic hysterectomy patients. Pregabalin was administered at doses of 150 mg and 300 mg preoperatively, and repeated 12 hours from the initial dose. An active placebo (diazepam) was used preoperatively and a placebo was used 12 hours after initial dose. The doses of oxycodone during hours 0 to 12 after surgery were similar in the 3 study groups, whereas the consumption of oxycodone during hours 12 to 24 after surgery was significantly reduced in the pregabalin 300 mg pre- and postoperative group compared with the pregabalin 150 mg pre- and postoperative group ($P = .025$). The VAS scores for pain at rest, pain in motion, and when coughing during the whole recovery period were similar in the 3 study groups. Satisfaction with anesthesia and pain medication was equal in all 3 study groups. The study did not significantly prove an opioid-sparing effect of pregabalin or a decrease in VAS scores. Similar results were reported in a prospective, randomized, double-blind, placebo-controlled clinical study investigating the efficacy of a single preoperative dose of pregabalin for attenuating postoperative pain and fentanyl consumption after laparoscopic cholecystectomy [136].

The results from the pregabalin studies are surprising, considering the results of the published studies on gabapentin. Tiippana and colleagues [121] reviewed the effectiveness of the perioperative administration of gabapentinoids for postoperative pain relief, and concluded that the class of medications was effective in reducing postoperative pain, opioid consumption, and opioid-related adverse effects after surgery, but only one study included pregabalin [137]. Multimodal postoperative analgesia including the gabapentinoids and other medications has shown promise in postoperative analgesia, possibly by synergistic mechanisms. In a randomized, double-blind, placebo-controlled trial, Mathiesen and colleagues [138] investigated the postoperative analgesic effect of preoperative pregabalin and dexamethasone in patients undergoing total hip arthroplasty. The study groups were (1) placebo + placebo; (2) pregabalin (300 mg) + placebo; and (3) pregabalin (300 mg) + dexamethasone (8 mg). The primary outcome measure was PCA morphine consumption from 0 to 4 and 0 to 24 hours after surgery, and secondary outcome measures were postoperative pain VAS score at rest and during mobilization, and side effects (nausea, vomiting, sedation, and dizziness). In the initial 4 hours after surgery, no significant differences between the groups in morphine consumption were found. At 24 hours the total morphine consumption was significantly reduced in groups 2 and 3 compared with group 1 ($P<.003$), and no significant difference was found between groups 2 and 3. VAS pain scores at rest, or during movement, showed no significant difference between the groups. Preoperative pregabalin resulted in a significant reduction in opioid requirements (opioid sparing) but was not associated with a reduction in the incidence of postoperative nausea and vomiting (PONV). The addition of dexamethasone reduced PONV but had no effect on opioid requirements or analgesia. In another study, pregabalin and dexamethasone in combination with paracetamol were evaluated for the synergistic analgesic effect in the postoperative period [139]. The study groups were (1) paracetamol (1000 mg) + placebo + placebo; (2) pregabalin (300 mg) + paracetamol (1000 mg) + placebo; and (3) paracetamol (1000 mg) + pregabalin (300 mg) + dexamethasone (8 mg). The investigators reported that the combination of pregabalin and para-cetamol did not improve 24-hour postoperative morphine consumption or pain scores for patients in abdominal hysterectomy, compared with paracetamol alone. In addition, the combination of paracetamol, pregabalin, and dexamethasone reduced nausea and vomiting compared with paracetamol alone, but did not exert any further effect on the pain treatment outcomes.

α_2-ADRENERGIC AGONISTS

The analgesic activity of α_2-agonists may be mediated by both supraspinal and spinal mechanisms. The central α_2-adrenoceptors in the locus ceruleus (a supraspinal site) and in the dorsal horn of the spinal cord is a primary site of action by which the antinociceptive effect occurs [140–145]. The α_2 receptors at the spinal cord level are thought to be responsible for the analgesic properties of α_2-adrenegic agonists, which inhibit the release of substance P [146]. The sedative effect is secondary to action on the locus ceruleus [146,147]. The α_2-adrenergic agonists, clonidine and dexmedetomidine (DEX), have been administered as adjuvant medications in the perioperative period to produce significant anesthetic and analgesic-sparing effects. Clonidine is a selective partial agonist for α_2-adrenoceptors, with a ratio of approximately 220:1 (α_2:α_1). Clonidine is rapidly and almost completely absorbed after oral administration, with a time to maximum plasma concentration of between 1.5 and 2 hours and elimination half-life of 8 to 12 hours [148,149]. DEX is more selective for the α_2 receptors (8 times more than clonidine), with an α_2:α_1 binding ratio of 1620:1. The half-life of DEX is shorter (2 hours) than that of clonidine (9–12 hours) [146,150,151].

Clonidine

Clonidine can be administered either orally or intravenously, but with systemic clonidine the dose is limited by centrally mediated side effects including hypotension, tachycardia, rebound hypertension, and sedation. In a randomized, double-blind study the analgesic and opioid-sparing properties of clonidine were evaluated [152]. The investigators randomized patients to morphine PCA or morphine PCA + clonidine. The outcome measures were pain, sedation, and PONV. Pain scores were significantly lower in the first 12 hours in the morphine + clonidine group compared with the morphine only group, but the difference was insignificant after 12 hours. Decreased morphine consumption only achieved statistical significance in the morphine + clonidine group compared with the morphine only group at 36 hours postoperatively. There were no differences in sedation scores between the groups. PONV was significantly ($P<.05$) less in the morphine + clonidine group compared with the morphine only group. The investigators concluded that perioperative use of clonidine in addition to morphine produced analgesic improvement only in the first 12 hours. In a prospective, double-blind, placebo-controlled trial, Park and colleagues [149] evaluated the effect of perioperative oral clonidine on postoperative analgesia and PCA morphine requirements in adult patients after major orthopedic knee surgery. Primary outcome measures included VAS pain scores and morphine consumption. The cumulative morphine consumption was significantly ($P = .031$) lower in the clonidine + morphine group compared with the morphine only group, although the VAS for pain was not significantly different between the 2 groups. The use of perioperative systemic clonidine has an opioid-sparing effect, but central neuraxial administration has shown the most promise in acute and chronic pain management compared with systemic administration [153,154].

Dexmedetomidine

DEX is an α_2 receptor agonist that has been available in the United States since 1999 as a short-term sedative for mechanically ventilated, critically ill patients.

DEX possesses potent and highly selective α_2-adrenoreceptor agonist attributes (analgesia, sedation, anxiolysis, and no respiratory depression), making it attractive for postoperative analgesia. The unique sedative properties of DEX are not mediated by the GABA-mimetic system, such as that of benzodiazepines, thus it does not depress the respiratory drive. The actions of DEX may be mediated through postsynaptic α_2-adrenoceptors [151]. DEX significantly reduced opioid requirements compared with placebo in postsurgical, critically ill patients requiring mechanical ventilation and sedation [151]. These patients required almost 50% less morphine for pain during each study period than did placebo recipients, and approximately 43% required no morphine compared with approximately 17% for placebo [151]. This initial outcome in intensive care patients has prompted evaluation of dexmedetomidine use in the treatment of perioperative pain. In a prospective, randomized, double-blind study, Gurbet and colleagues [142] compared the effectiveness of the intraoperative infusion of DEX versus placebo on postoperative analgesia in patients undergoing total abdominal hysterectomy. Morphine consumption, VAS pain scores, and sedation were outcome measures. The DEX group consumed significantly ($P<.05$) less PCA morphine during the postanesthesia care unit stay, and had significantly ($P<.01$) lower mean cumulative morphine consumption than placebo patients at study end (48 hours). In addition, nausea and vomiting requiring treatment was significantly ($P<.05$) lower in the patients randomized to DEX. The investigators concluded that continuous perioperative intravenous DEX during abdominal surgery provided effective postoperative analgesia and reduced postoperative morphine requirements without increasing the incidence of side effects. The analgesic benefits of the adjuvant DEX were demonstrated in a prospective, randomized, double-blind study comparing morphine PCA to morphine + DEX PCA [155]. One hundred patients undergoing total abdominal hysterectomies were allocated to receive morphine PCA or morphine + DEX PCA with cumulative PCA requirements, pain intensities, and PCA-related adverse events as the outcome measures. Patients in the morphine + DEX group required significantly less PCA morphine than those from the morphine only group at all times in the study period ($P<.01$), as well as the cumulative PCA morphine consumption at the conclusion (24 hours) of the study period ($P<.01$). The incidence of PONV was significantly ($P<.05$) lower in the morphine + DEX group only from 4 to 24 hours. These results indicate that morphine + DEX mixture significantly enhanced the analgesic effect of morphine, and reduced PCA morphine requirement and morphine-induced nausea, without clinically relevant bradycardia or hypotension, oversedation, or respiratory depression. The opioid-sparing effects of DEX have been replicated [156,157], whereas others have failed to replicate such findings [158].

GLUCOCORTICOIDS

The glucocorticoid receptor resides predominantly in the cytoplasm in an inactive form until it binds glucocorticoids. Steroid binding results in receptor activation and translocation to the nucleus, where it can bind to DNA sequences known as glucocorticoid-responsive elements. This complex can either directly inhibit or activate the expression of target genes (such as cytokines like interleukin-2), or can interact with certain transcription factors such as nuclear factor (NF)-κB, which in turn limit expression of these genes. Inhibition of inflammation can occur at various sites, especially within the prostaglandin synthesis pathway. Glucocorticoids can induce the activation of lipocortin-1 (annexin-1), which then acts to block production of the prostaglandin substrate arachidonic acid, by inhibition of cytosolic phospholipase A_2 (PLA_2). Downstream, glucocorticoids inhibit expression of COX-2, probably by blocking NF-κB. Side effects of glucocorticoids are due to their lack of selectivity, so that healthy metabolic processes are impaired [143,159].

Glucocorticoids act on diverse targets through multiple mechanisms to control inflammation. Inflammatory, metabolic, hormonal, and immune responses to surgery are activated immediately after the surgical incision, so preoperative administration of steroids may be important to obtain the full postoperative benefit [160–162]. Also, a direct inhibitory effect of locally administered steroids on signal transmission in nociceptive C-fibers has been demonstrated [163]. Prostaglandins are key inducers of inflammation after tissue injury, and one mechanism by which glucocorticoids reduce prostaglandin synthesis is by inhibiting the expression of COX-2 without affecting COX-1 [164]. Corticosteroids have been used as anti-inflammatory and anti-immunologic agents, and have been evaluated for their effectiveness postoperatively for analgesia. Several clinical investigations have evaluated the effectiveness of glucocorticoids in the perioperative period.

In a randomized, double-blind, parallel trial, Romundstad and colleagues [165] evaluated the time course and magnitude of the analgesic effect of methylprednisolone 125 mg compared with ketorolac 30 mg and placebo in orthopedic surgery patients. Both methylprednisolone ($P<.02$) and ketorolac ($P<.0005$) significantly reduced pain intensity compared with placebo; no significant difference was found between methylprednisolone and ketorolac. Pain relief was likewise significantly reduced in the methylprednisolone and ketorolac groups compared with placebo ($P<.05$). First perceptible pain relief was registered after a median of 3 minutes for ketorolac, 5 minutes for placebo, and 7 minutes for methylprednisolone. The ketorolac group had meaningful pain relief after a median of 5 minutes, whereas both the placebo and methylprednisolone groups had meaningful pain relief after a median of 9 minutes. Opioid consumption for the 72 hours after drug intake was significantly lower in the methylprednisolone group compared with both ketorolac ($P<.02$) and placebo ($P<.003$). The investigators concluded that methylprednisolone 125 mg 1 day after surgery gave a similar early reduction of pain to ketorolac 30 mg. In addition, less pain than placebo 24 hours after methylprednisolone, and lower opioid consumption for 72 hours compared with ketorolac and placebo, indicated sustained analgesic effects of methylprednisolone. Other studies report glucocorticoid benefit with respect to PONV but not in postoperative pain

Table 1
Nonopioid medications for perioperative analgesia

Medication	dose	side effects	comments
NSAIDs			
Aspirin	650–1000 mg by mouth every 4–6 h, as needed, not to exceed 4000 mg/d	Inhibits platelet aggregation, gastrointestinal irritation	Should be avoided in patients and procedures with high risk of bleeding; may produce hypoprothrombinemia; caution when used in combination with anticoagulants
Diclofenac	50 mg by mouth 3 times a day or 4 times a day, as needed, not to exceed 200 mg/d	Gastrointestinal irritation, abnormal renal function, edema	Available in combination with misoprostol
Ketorolac	20 mg by mouth once followed by 10 mg every 4–6 h as needed, not to exceed 40 mg/d 30 mg intravenous/intramuscular every 6 h, as needed, not to exceed 120 mg/d	Inhibits platelet aggregation, gastrointestinal irritation, abnormal renal function	Should not be used greater than 5 days. Contraindicated in patients with previously documented peptic ulcers or gastrointestinal bleeding
Celecoxib	200 mg by mouth 2 times a day, as needed, not to exceed 400 mg/d	Cardiac and cerebrovascular complications	Celecoxib is contraindicated for the treatment of perioperative pain in the setting of coronary artery bypass graft surgery; should be used with caution in patient with known cardiac or cerebrovascular disease
Acetaminophen	500–1000 mg by mouth every 4–6 h, as needed, not to exceed 4000 mg/d	Hepatotoxicity, nephrotoxicity, hypersensitivity reactions	May produce hypoprothrombinemia; caution when used in combination with anticoagulants, but has no antiplatelet or gastric effects

NMDA receptor antagonist

Drug	Dose	Side effects	Comments
Ketamine	0.25–0.50 µg/kg intravenous bolus preincisional followed by 250–500 µg/kg/h infusion intraoperatively; 120 mg/kg/h infusion postoperatively for 24 h, then 60 µg/kg/h as needed	Psychotomimetic, sedation, nausea, diplopia, sympathomimetic	Intraoperative infusion to be stopped 60 min before end of surgery; increased incidence of adverse effects with infusion greater than 10 mg/h
	0.25–0.50 mg/kg intravenous bolus preincision followed by 0.125–250 mg/kg bolus at 30-min intervals		
	intraoperatively; patient-controlled analgesia bolus of ketamine 1 mg + morphine 1 mg (or equivalent) 20 µg/kg/h infusion postoperatively for 24 h, then 60 µg/kg/h as needed		
Dextromethorphan	30–90 mg by mouth preincisional followed by 30–90 mg by mouth postoperative as needed	Sedation, dizziness, xerostomia	
Magnesium	Exact dose needs to be determined	Sedation, hemodynamic derangement, muscle weakness	

(continued on next page)

Table 1
(continued)

Medication	dose	side effects	comments
Antiepileptic medications			
Gabapentin	300–1200 mg by mouth as a single dose 1–2 h before surgery, followed by 300–1200 mg by mouth postoperatively	Somnolence, dizziness, ataxia, diplopia, xerostomia, nausea	
Pregabalin	150–300 mg by mouth as a single dose 1–2 h before surgery, followed by 75–300 mg by mouth postoperatively	Somnolence, dizziness, ataxia, diplopia, xerostomia, nausea	
Glucocorticoids			
Dexamethasone	8–10 mg intravenous as a single dose preincisional or intraoperative		Suppression of the hypothalamic-pituitary-adrenal axis
α-2 Agonist			
Dexmedetomidine	0.2–0.7 μg/kg/h infusion intraoperatively	Hypotension, hypertension, and bradycardia	Expense of medication may be prohibitive to use

scores and analgesic requirements [166]. Dexamethasone is a synthetic gluco-corticoid with high potency and long duration of action (half-life: 2 days), but with no mineralocorticoid activity. In a prospective, randomized, double-blind, placebo-controlled study, either a single dose of dexamethasone 40 mg or saline placebo was administered to 50 consecutive patients before under-going unilateral primary total hip arthroplasty [167]. Although there were no significant differences in NRS pain scores at rest or cumulative morphine consumption throughout the 48-hour study period, patients in the dexametha-sone group reported significantly lower dynamic NRS scores (2.7, 95% confi-dence interval 2.2–3.1 vs 6.8, 95% confidence interval 6.4–7.2; $P<.0001$) compared with placebo.

Although there is modest evidence for the analgesic actions of corticoste-roids, widespread clinical use of these glucocorticoids for the management of postoperative pain has not followed, perhaps because of the adverse effects of corticosteroids when given in repeated doses. Inflammatory pain continues after the immediate postoperative period, and the benefits of corticosteroids might be maximized by repeated dosing, but the fear of adverse side effects (adrenal suppression, wound healing, gastrointestinal ulceration) may limit glucocorticoid administration.

SUMMARY

The management of acute postoperative pain continues to pose a major chal-lenge for health care providers. Postoperative pain remains a major reason for delayed discharge, unplanned admission after ambulatory surgery, and patient dissatisfaction. Table 1 provides suggestions of useful nonopioid medi-cations for perioperative pain management. Advances in understanding the mechanisms of pain, including the receptors involved in the transmission of pain, have led to improvements in postoperative pain management. Pain and pain treatment is multifactorial and complex. The use of a multimodal approach for analgesia makes use of the analgesic properties of adjuvant medi-cations with the goal of limiting the adverse effects of any one medication. The integration of multimodal analgesic techniques will continue to advance, further facilitating patient satisfaction and improving patient outcomes.

References

[1] Deutsch N, Wu CL. Patient outcomes following ambulatory anesthesia. Anesthesiol Clin North America 2003;21(2):403–15.

[2] McGrath B, Chung F. Postoperative recovery and discharge. Anesthesiol Clin North Amer-ica 2003;21(2):367–86.

[3] Pregler JL, Kapur PA. The development of ambulatory anesthesia and future challenges. Anesthesiol Clin North America 2003;21(2):207–28.

[4] Apfelbaum JL, Chen C, Mehta SS, et al. Postoperative pain experience: results from a national survey suggest postoperative pain continues to be undermanaged. Anesth Analg 2003;97(2):534–40, table of contents.

[5] Fanelli G, Berti M, Baciarello M. Updating postoperative pain management: from multi-modal to context-sensitive treatment. Minerva Anestesiol 2008;74(9).409–500.

[6] White PF. The role of non-opioid analgesic techniques in the management of pain after ambulatory surgery. Anesth Analg 2002;94(3):577–85.

[7] Perkins FM, Kehlet H. Chronic pain as an outcome of surgery. A review of predictive factors. Anesthesiology 2000;93(4):1123–33.

[8] Obata H, Saito S, Fujita N, et al. Epidural block with mepivacaine before surgery reduces long-term post-thoracotomy pain. Can J Anaesth 1999;46(12):1127–32.

[9] Warfield CA, Kahn CH. Acute pain management. Programs in U.S. hospitals and experiences and attitudes among U.S. adults. Anesthesiology 1995;83(5):1090–4.

[10] McGrath B, Elgendy H, Chung F, et al. Thirty percent of patients have moderate to severe pain 24 hr after ambulatory surgery: a survey of 5,703 patients. Can J Anaesth 2004;51(9):886–91.

[11] Hurley RW, Cohen SP, Williams KA, et al. The analgesic effects of perioperative gabapentin on postoperative pain: a meta-analysis. Reg Anesth Pain Med 2006;31(3):237–47.

[12] Cohen SP, Christo PJ, Moroz L. Pain management in trauma patients. Am J Phys Med Rehabil 2004;83(2):142–61.

[13] Bowdle TA. Adverse effects of opioid agonists and agonist-antagonists in anaesthesia. Drug Saf 1998;19(3):173–89.

[14] Moote C. Efficacy of nonsteroidal anti-inflammatory drugs in the management of postoperative pain. Drugs 1992;44(suppl 5):14–29 [discussion: 29–30].

[15] Angst MS, Clark JD. Opioid-induced hyperalgesia: a qualitative systematic review. Anesthesiology 2006;104(3):570–87.

[16] Woolf CJ. Intrathecal high dose morphine produces hyperalgesia in the rat. Brain Res 1981;209(2):491–5.

[17] Mercadante S, Ferrera P, Villari P, et al. Hyperalgesia: an emerging iatrogenic syndrome. J Pain Symptom Manage 2003;26(2):769–75.

[18] Kehlet H, Jensen TS, Woolf CJ. Persistent postsurgical pain: risk factors and prevention. Lancet 2006;367(9522):1618–25.

[19] Guignard B, Bossard AE, Coste C, et al. Acute opioid tolerance: intraoperative remifentanil increases postoperative pain and morphine requirement. Anesthesiology 2000;93(2):409–17.

[20] Chia YY, Liu K, Wang JJ, et al. Intraoperative high dose fentanyl induces postoperative fentanyl tolerance. Can J Anaesth 1999;46(9):872–7.

[21] Kehlet H, Dahl JB. The value of "multimodal" or "balanced analgesia" in postoperative pain treatment. Anesth Analg 1993;77(5):1048–56.

[22] Baum C, Kennedy DL, Forbes MB. Utilization of nonsteroidal antiinflammatory drugs. Arthritis Rheum 1985;28(6):686–92.

[23] Dahl JB, Kehlet H. Non-steroidal anti-inflammatory drugs: rationale for use in severe postoperative pain. Br J Anaesth 1991;66(6):703–12.

[24] Laine L. Approaches to nonsteroidal anti-inflammatory drug use in the high-risk patient. Gastroenterology 2001;120(3):594–606.

[25] Vane JR, Botting RM. Mechanism of action of nonsteroidal anti-inflammatory drugs. Am J Med 1998;104(3A):2S–8S [discussion: 21S–2S].

[26] McCormack K. The spinal actions of nonsteroidal anti-inflammatory drugs and the dissociation between their anti-inflammatory and analgesic effects. Drugs 1994;47(Suppl 5):28–45 [discussion: 46–7].

[27] Cashman JN. The mechanisms of action of NSAIDs in analgesia. Drugs 1996;52(Suppl 5):13–23.

[28] Lanza FL. A review of gastric ulcer and gastroduodenal injury in normal volunteers receiving aspirin and other non-steroidal anti-inflammatory drugs. Scand J Gastroenterol Suppl 1989;163:24–31.

[29] Elia N, Lysakowski C, Tramer MR. Does multimodal analgesia with acetaminophen, nonsteroidal antiinflammatory drugs, or selective cyclooxygenase-2 inhibitors and

patient-controlled analgesia morphine offer advantages over morphine alone? Meta-analyses of randomized trials. Anesthesiology 2005;103(6):1296–304.

[30] Ready LB, Brown CR, Stahlgren LH, et al. Evaluation of intravenous ketorolac administered by bolus or infusion for treatment of postoperative pain. A double-blind, placebo-controlled, multicenter study. Anesthesiology 1994;80(6):1277–86.

[31] Stephens J, Laskin B, Pashos C, et al. The burden of acute postoperative pain and the potential role of the COX-2-specific inhibitors. Rheumatology (Oxford) 2003;42(Suppl 3): iii40–52.

[32] Balestrieri P, Simmons G, Hill D, et al. The effect of intravenous ketorolac given intraoperatively versus postoperatively on outcome from gynecologic abdominal surgery. J Clin Anesth 1997;9(5):358–64.

[33] Bo J, Sudmann E, Marton PF. Effect of indomethacin on fracture healing in rats. Acta Orthop Scand 1976;47(6):588–99.

[34] Kehlet H, Dahl JB. Are perioperative nonsteroidal anti-inflammatory drugs ulcerogenic in the short term? Drugs 1992;44(Suppl 5):38–41.

[35] Glassman SD, Rose SM, Dimar JR, et al. The effect of postoperative nonsteroidal anti-inflammatory drug administration on spinal fusion. Spine 1998;23(7):834–8.

[36] Munir MA, Enany N, Zhang JM. Nonopioid analgesics. Med Clin North Am 2007;91(1): 97–111.

[37] Vane JR, Botting RM. The mechanism of action of aspirin. Thromb Res 2003;110(5–6): 255–8.

[38] Edwards JE, Oldman AD, Smith LA, et al. Oral aspirin in postoperative pain: a quantitative systematic review. Pain 1999;81(3):289–97.

[39] Rees JOA, Smith LA, Collins S, et al. Single dose oral aspirin for acute pain. Cochrane Database Syst Rev 1999;(2):CD002067.

[40] Laska EM, Sunshine A, Wanderling JA, et al. Quantitative differences in aspirin analgesia in three models of clinical pain. J Clin Pharmacol 1982;22(11–12):531–42.

[41] Barden J, Edwards JE, McQuay HJ, et al. Pain and analgesic response after third molar extraction and other postsurgical pain. Pain 2004;107(1–2):86–90.

[42] Cooper S. Single dose analgesic studies: the upside and downside sensitivity. In: Max MPR, editor. Advances in pain research and therapy. New York: Raven Press; 1991. p. 117–24.

[43] Olson NZ, Sunshine A, Zighelboim I, et al. Onset and duration of analgesia of diclofenac potassium in the treatment of postepisiotomy pain. Am J Ther 1997;4(7–8):239–46.

[44] Available at: http://www.medicine.ox.ac.uk/bandolier/booth/painpag. Accessed February 27, 2009.

[45] Dahl V, Hagen IE, Sveen AM, et al. High-dose diclofenac for postoperative analgesia after elective caesarean section in regional anaesthesia. Int J Obstet Anesth 2002;11(2):91–4.

[46] Hynes D, McCarroll M, Hiesse-Provost O. Analgesic efficacy of parenteral paracetamol (propacetamol) and diclofenac in post-operative orthopaedic pain. Acta Anaesthesiol Scand 2006;50(3):374–81.

[47] Barden J, Edwards J, Moore RA, et al. Single dose oral diclofenac for postoperative pain. Cochrane Database Syst Rev 2004;(2):CD004768.

[48] Burke Anne SE, FitzGerald Garret A. Analgesic-antipyretic and antiinflammatory agents; pharmacotherapy of gout. 11th edition. New York: The McGraw-Hill Companies, Inc; 2006.

[49] Gillis JC, Brogden RN. Ketorolac. A reappraisal of its pharmacodynamic and pharmacokinetic properties and therapeutic use in pain management. Drugs 1997;53(1):139–88.

[50] Buckley MM, Brogden RN. Ketorolac. A review of its pharmacodynamic and pharmacokinetic properties, and therapeutic potential. Drugs 1990;39(1):86–109.

[51] Morley-Forster P, Newton PT, Cook MJ. Ketorolac and indomethacin are equally efficacious for the relief of minor postoperative pain. Can J Anaesth 1993;40(12):1126–30.

[52] Zhou TJ, Tang J, White PF. Propacetamol versus ketorolac for treatment of acute postoperative pain after total hip or knee replacement. Anesth Analg 2001;92(6):1569–75.

[53] McQuay HJ, Poppleton P, Carroll D, et al. Ketorolac and acetaminophen for orthopedic postoperative pain. Clin Pharmacol Ther 1986;39(1):89–93.

[54] Smith LA, Carroll D, Edwards JE, et al. Single-dose ketorolac and pethidine in acute postoperative pain: systematic review with meta-analysis. Br J Anaesth 2000;84(1):48–58.

[55] Cepeda MS, Carr DB, Miranda N, et al. Comparison of morphine, ketorolac, and their combination for postoperative pain: results from a large, randomized, double-blind trial. Anesthesiology 2005;103(6):1225–32.

[56] Picard P, Bazin JE, Conio N, et al. Ketorolac potentiates morphine in postoperative patient-controlled analgesia. Pain 1997;73(3):401–6.

[57] Macario A, Lipman AG. Ketorolac in the era of cyclo-oxygenase-2 selective nonsteroidal antiinflammatory drugs: a systematic review of efficacy, side effects, and regulatory issues. Pain Med 2001;2(4):336–51.

[58] Graham GG, Scott KF. Mechanism of action of paracetamol. Am J Ther 2005;12(1): 46–55.

[59] Munsterhjelm E, Munsterhjelm NM, Niemi TT, et al. Dose-dependent inhibition of platelet function by acetaminophen in healthy volunteers. Anesthesiology 2005;103(4):712–7.

[60] Strassels SA, McNicol E, Suleman R. Postoperative pain management: a practical review, part 1. Am J Health Syst Pharm 2005;62(18):1904–16.

[61] White PF. The changing role of non-opioid analgesic techniques in the management of postoperative pain. Anesth Analg 2005;101(5 suppl):S5–22.

[62] Flouvat B, Leneveu A, Fitoussi S, et al. Bioequivalence study comparing a new paracetamol solution for injection and propacetamol after single intravenous infusion in healthy subjects. Int J Clin Pharmacol Ther 2004;42(1):50–7.

[63] Schug SA, Sidebotham DA, McGuinnety M, et al. Acetaminophen as an adjunct to morphine by patient-controlled analgesia in the management of acute postoperative pain. Anesth Analg 1998;87(2):368–72.

[64] Hyllested M, Jones S, Pedersen JL, et al. Comparative effect of paracetamol, NSAIDs or their combination in postoperative pain management: a qualitative review. Br J Anaesth 2002;88(2):199–214.

[65] Delbos A, Boccard E. The morphine-sparing effect of propacetamol in orthopedic postoperative pain. J Pain Symptom Manage 1995;10(4):279–86.

[66] Remy C, Marret E, Bonnet F. Effects of acetaminophen on morphine side-effects and consumption after major surgery: meta-analysis of randomized controlled trials. Br J Anaesth 2005;94(4):505–13.

[67] Oscier CD, Milner QJ. Peri-operative use of paracetamol. Anaesthesia 2009;64(1): 65–72.

[68] Kehlet H, Wilkinson RC, Fischer HB, et al. PROSPECT: evidence-based, procedure-specific postoperative pain management. Best Pract Res Clin Anaesthesiol 2007;21(1):149–59.

[69] Oxford League table of analgesics in acute pain. Available at: http://www. medicine.ox.ac.uk/bandolier/booth/painpag/Acutrev/Analgesics/Leagtab.html. Accessed February 25, 2009.

[70] FitzGerald GA, Patrono C. The coxibs, selective inhibitors of cyclooxygenase-2. N Engl J Med 2001;345(6):433–42.

[71] Clemett D, Goa KL. Celecoxib: a review of its use in osteoarthritis, rheumatoid arthritis and acute pain. Drugs 2000;59(4):957–80.

[72] Gajraj NM, Joshi GP. Role of cyclooxygenase-2 inhibitors in postoperative pain management. Anesthesiol Clin North America 2005;23(1):49–72.

[73] Buvanendran A, Kroin JS, Tuman KJ, et al. Cerebrospinal fluid and plasma pharmacokinetics of the cyclooxygenase 2 inhibitor rofecoxib in humans: single and multiple oral drug administration. Anesth Analg 2005;100(5):1320–4, table of contents.

[74] Huang YM, Wang CM, Wang CT, et al. Perioperative celecoxib administration for pain management after total knee arthroplasty—a randomized, controlled study. BMC Musculoskelet Disord 2008;9:77.

[75] Derry S, Barden J, McQuay HJ, et al. Single dose oral celecoxib for acute postoperative pain in adults. Cochrane Database Syst Rev 2008;(4):CD004233.

[76] Collins SL, Moore RA, McQuay HJ, et al. Single dose oral ibuprofen and diclofenac for postoperative pain. Cochrane Database Syst Rev 2000;(2):CD001548.

[77] Chou R, Helfand M, Peterson K, et al. Comparative effectiveness and safety of analgesics for osteoarthritis. Comparative effectiveness review no. 4. Portland (OR): Agency for Healthcare Research and Quality; 2006.

[78] Vonkeman HE, van de Laar MA. Nonsteroidal anti-inflammatory drugs: adverse effects and their prevention. Semin Arthritis Rheum 2008; epub ahead of print.

[79] Eisenach JC. Data fabrication and article retraction: how not to get lost in the woods. Anesthesiology 2009;110(5):955–6.

[80] Shafer SL. Notice of retraction. Anesth Analg 2009;108(4):1350.

[81] Shafer SL. Notice of retraction. Anesth Analg 2009;108(6):1953.

[82] Shafer SL. Tattered threads. Anesth Analg 2009;108(5):1361–3.

[83] White PF, Kehlet H, Liu S. Perioperative analgesia: what do we still know? Anesth Analg 2009;108(5):1364–7.

[84] Nicoll R. Introduction to the pharmacology of CNS drugs. In: Katzung B, editor. Basic & clinical pharmacology. 10th edition. New York: The McGraw-Hill Companies, Inc; 2007.

[85] Petrenko AB, Yamakura T, Baba H, et al. The role of N-methyl-D-aspartate (NMDA) receptors in pain: a review. Anesth Analg 2003;97(4):1108–16.

[86] Weinbroum AA, Gorodezky A, Niv D, et al. Dextromethorphan attenuation of postoperative pain and primary and secondary thermal hyperalgesia. Can J Anaesth 2001;48(2):167–74.

[87] Woolf CJ, Thompson SW. The induction and maintenance of central sensitization is dependent on N-methyl-D-aspartic acid receptor activation; implications for the treatment of post-injury pain hypersensitivity states. Pain 1991;44(3):293–9.

[88] Kiefer RT, Rohr P, Ploppa A, et al. Efficacy of ketamine in anesthetic dosage for the treatment of refractory complex regional pain syndrome: an open-label phase II study. Pain Med 2008;9(8):1173–201.

[89] Himmelseher S, Durieux ME. Ketamine for perioperative pain management. Anesthesiology 2005;102(1):211–20.

[90] Urban MK, Ya Deau JT, Wukovits B, et al. Ketamine as an adjunct to postoperative pain management in opioid tolerant patients after spinal fusions: a prospective randomized trial. HSS J 2008;4(1):62–5.

[91] Weinbroum AA, Gorodetzky A, Nirkin A, et al. Dextromethorphan for the reduction of immediate and late postoperative pain and morphine consumption in orthopedic oncology patients: a randomized, placebo-controlled, double-blind study. Cancer 2002;95(5):1164–70.

[92] Kohrs R, Durieux ME. Ketamine: teaching an old drug new tricks. Anesth Analg 1998;87(5):1186–93.

[93] Cohen SP, Verdolin MH, Chang AS, et al. The intravenous ketamine test predicts subsequent response to an oral dextromethorphan treatment regimen in fibromyalgia patients. J Pain 2006;7(6):391–8.

[94] Himmelseher S, Pfenninger E, Georgieff M. The effects of ketamine-isomers on neuronal injury and regeneration in rat hippocampal neurons. Anesth Analg 1996;83(3):505–12.

[95] Zakine J, Samarcq D, Lorne E, et al. Postoperative ketamine administration decreases morphine consumption in major abdominal surgery: a prospective, randomized, double-blind, controlled study. Anesth Analg 2008;106(6):1856–61.

[96] Kollender Y, Bickels J, Stocki D, et al. Subanaesthetic ketamine spares postoperative morphine and controls pain better than standard morphine does alone in orthopaedic-oncological patients. Eur J Cancer 2008;44(7):954–62.

[97] Guillou N, Tanguy M, Seguin P, et al. The effects of small-dose ketamine on morphine consumption in surgical intensive care unit patients after major abdominal surgery. Anesth Analg 2003;97(3):843–7.

[98] Suzuki M, Tsueda K, Lansing PS, et al. Small-dose ketamine enhances morphine-induced analgesia after outpatient surgery. Anesth Analg 1999;89(1):98–103.

[99] Fu ES, Miguel R, Scharf JE. Preemptive ketamine decreases postoperative narcotic requirements in patients undergoing abdominal surgery. Anesth Analg 1997;84(5):1086–90.

[100] Bell RF, Dahl JB, Moore RA, et al. Perioperative ketamine for acute postoperative pain. Cochrane Database Syst Rev 2006;(1):CD004603.

[101] Carpenter CL, Marks SS, Watson DL, et al. Dextromethorphan and dextrorphan as calcium channel antagonists. Brain Res 1988;439(1–2):372–5.

[102] Sang CN, Booher S, Gilron I, et al. Dextromethorphan and memantine in painful diabetic neuropathy and postherpetic neuralgia: efficacy and dose-response trials. Anesthesiology 2002;96(5):1053–61.

[103] Carlsson KC, Hoem NO, Moberg ER, et al. Analgesic effect of dextromethorphan in neuropathic pain. Acta Anaesthesiol Scand 2004;48(3):328–36.

[104] Raffa RB. A novel approach to the pharmacology of analgesics. Am J Med 1996;101(1A): 40S–6S.

[105] Helmy SA, Bali A. The effect of the preemptive use of the NMDA receptor antagonist dextromethorphan on postoperative analgesic requirements. Anesth Analg 2001;92(3): 739–44.

[106] McCartney CJ, Sinha A, Katz J. A qualitative systematic review of the role of N-methyl-D-aspartate receptor antagonists in preventive analgesia. Anesth Analg 2004;98(5): 1385–400, table of contents.

[107] Wadhwa A, Clarke D, Goodchild CS, et al. Large-dose oral dextromethorphan as an adjunct to patient-controlled analgesia with morphine after knee surgery. Anesth Analg 2001;92(2):448–54.

[108] Duedahl TH, Romsing J, Moiniche S, et al. A qualitative systematic review of peri-operative dextromethorphan in post-operative pain. Acta Anaesthesiol Scand 2006;50(1):1–13.

[109] Buvanendran A, McCarthy RJ, Kroin JS, et al. Intrathecal magnesium prolongs fentanyl analgesia: a prospective, randomized, controlled trial. Anesth Analg 2002;95(3): 661–6, table of contents.

[110] Koinig H, Wallner T, Marhofer P, et al. Magnesium sulfate reduces intra- and postoperative analgesic requirements. Anesth Analg 1998;87(1):206–10.

[111] Tramer MR, Schneider J, Marti RA, et al. Role of magnesium sulfate in postoperative analgesia. Anesthesiology 1996;84(2):340–7.

[112] Seyhan TO, Tugrul M, Sungur MO, et al. Effects of three different dose regimens of magnesium on propofol requirements, haemodynamic variables and postoperative pain relief in gynaecological surgery. Br J Anaesth 2006;96(2):247–52.

[113] Rosenstock J, Tuchman M, LaMoreaux L, et al. Pregabalin for the treatment of painful diabetic peripheral neuropathy: a double-blind, placebo-controlled trial. Pain 2004;110(3):628–38.

[114] Freynhagen R, Strojek K, Griesing T, et al. Efficacy of pregabalin in neuropathic pain evaluated in a 12-week, randomised, double-blind, multicentre, placebo-controlled trial of flexible- and fixed-dose regimens. Pain 2005;115(3):254–63.

[115] Backonja M, Beydoun A, Edwards KR, et al. Gabapentin for the symptomatic treatment of painful neuropathy in patients with diabetes mellitus: a randomized controlled trial. JAMA 1998;280(21):1831–6.

[116] Keskinbora K, Pekel AF, Aydinli I. Gabapentin and an opioid combination versus opioid alone for the management of neuropathic cancer pain: a randomized open trial. J Pain Symptom Manage 2007;34(2):183–9.

[117] Rowbotham M, Harden N, Stacey B, et al. Gabapentin for the treatment of postherpetic neuralgia: a randomized controlled trial. JAMA 1998;280(21):1837–42.

[118] Serpell MG. Gabapentin in neuropathic pain syndromes: a randomised, double-blind, placebo-controlled trial. Pain 2002;99(3):557–66.

[119] Werner MU, Perkins FM, Holte K, et al. Effects of gabapentin in acute inflammatory pain in humans. Reg Anesth Pain Med 2001;26(4):322–8.

[120] Gee NS, Brown JP, Dissanayake VU, et al. The novel anticonvulsant drug, gabapentin (Neurontin), binds to the alpha2delta subunit of a calcium channel. J Biol Chem 1996;271(10):5768–76.

[121] Tiippana EM, Hamunen K, Kontinen VK, et al. Do surgical patients benefit from perioperative gabapentin/pregabalin? A systematic review of efficacy and safety. Anesth Analg 2007;104(6):1545–56, table of contents.

[122] Luo ZD, Chaplan SR, Higuera ES, et al. Upregulation of dorsal root ganglion (alpha)2(delta) calcium channel subunit and its correlation with allodynia in spinal nerve-injured rats. J Neurosci 2001;21(6):1868–75.

[123] Zahn PK, Brennan TJ. Primary and secondary hyperalgesia in a rat model for human postoperative pain. Anesthesiology 1999;90(3):863–72.

[124] Dirks J, Fredensborg BB, Christensen D, et al. A randomized study of the effects of single-dose gabapentin versus placebo on postoperative pain and morphine consumption after mastectomy. Anesthesiology 2002;97(3):560–4.

[125] Dierking G, Duedahl TH, Rasmussen ML, et al. Effects of gabapentin on postoperative morphine consumption and pain after abdominal hysterectomy: a randomized, double-blind trial. Acta Anaesthesiol Scand 2004;48(3):322–7.

[126] Turan A, Karamanlioglu B, Memis D, et al. Analgesic effects of gabapentin after spinal surgery. Anesthesiology 2004;100(4):935–8.

[127] Pandey CK, Priye S, Singh S, et al. Preemptive use of gabapentin significantly decreases postoperative pain and rescue analgesic requirements in laparoscopic cholecystectomy. Can J Anaesth 2004;51(4):358–63.

[128] Pandey CK, Sahay S, Gupta D, et al. Preemptive gabapentin decreases postoperative pain after lumbar discoidectomy. Can J Anaesth 2004;51(10):986–9.

[129] Seib RK, Paul JE. Preoperative gabapentin for postoperative analgesia: a meta-analysis. Can J Anaesth 2006;53(5):461–9.

[130] Ho KY, Gan TJ, Habib AS. Gabapentin and postoperative pain—a systematic review of randomized controlled trials. Pain 2006;126(1–3):91–101.

[131] Fink K, Dooley DJ, Meder WP, et al. Inhibition of neuronal Ca(2+) influx by gabapentin and pregabalin in the human neocortex. Neuropharmacology 2002;42(2):229–36.

[132] Shneker BF, McAuley JW. Pregabalin: a new neuromodulator with broad therapeutic indications. Ann Pharmacother 2005;39(12):2029–37.

[133] Field MJ, Holloman EF, McCleary S, et al. Evaluation of gabapentin and S-(+)-3-isobutyl-gaba in a rat model of postoperative pain. J Pharmacol Exp Ther 1997;282(3):1242–6.

[134] Paech MJ, Goy R, Chua S, et al. A randomized, placebo-controlled trial of preoperative oral pregabalin for postoperative pain relief after minor gynecological surgery. Anesth Analg 2007;105(5):1449–53, table of contents.

[135] Jokela R, Ahonen J, Tallgren M, et al. A randomized controlled trial of perioperative administration of pregabalin for pain after laparoscopic hysterectomy. Pain 2008;134(1-2):106–12.

[136] Agarwal A, Gautam S, Gupta D, et al. Evaluation of a single preoperative dose of pregabalin for attenuation of postoperative pain after laparoscopic cholecystectomy. Br J Anaesth 2008;101(5):700–4.

[137] Hill CM, Balkenohl M, Thomas DW, et al. Pregabalin in patients with postoperative dental pain. Eur J Pain 2001;5(2):119–24.

[138] Mathiesen O, Jacobsen LS, Holm HE, et al. Pregabalin and dexamethasone for postoperative pain control: a randomized controlled study in hip arthroplasty. Br J Anaesth 2008;101(4):535–41.

[139] Mathiesen O, Rasmussen ML, Dierking G, et al. Pregabalin and dexamethasone in combination with paracetamol for postoperative pain control after abdominal hysterectomy. A randomized clinical trial. Acta Anaesthesiol Scand 2009;53(2):227–35.

[140] De Kock M, Crochet B, Morimont C, et al. Intravenous or epidural clonidine for intra- and postoperative analgesia. Anesthesiology 1993;79(3):525–31.

[141] Guo TZ, Jiang JY, Buttermann AE, et al. Dexmedetomidine injection into the locus ceruleus produces antinociception. Anesthesiology 1996;84(4):873–81.

[142] Gurbet A, Basagan-Mogol E, Turker G, et al. Intraoperative infusion of dexmedetomidine reduces perioperative analgesic requirements. Can J Anaesth 2006;53(7):646–52.

[143] Buvanendran A, Kroin JS. Useful adjuvants for postoperative pain management. Best Pract Res Clin Anaesthesiol 2007;21(1):31–49.

[144] Unnerstall JR, Kopajtic TA, Kuhar MJ. Distribution of alpha 2 agonist binding sites in the rat and human central nervous system: analysis of some functional, anatomic correlates of the pharmacologic effects of clonidine and related adrenergic agents. Brain Res 1984;319(1):69–101.

[145] Buerkle H, Yaksh TL. Pharmacological evidence for different alpha 2-adrenergic receptor sites mediating analgesia and sedation in the rat. Br J Anaesth 1998;81(2):208–15.

[146] Habib AS, Gan TJ. Role of analgesic adjuncts in postoperative pain management. Anesthesiol Clin North America 2005;23(1):85–107.

[147] Maze M, Tranquilli W. Alpha-2 adrenoceptor agonists: defining the role in clinical anesthesia. Anesthesiology 1991;74(3):581–605.

[148] Davies DS, Wing AM, Reid JL, et al. Pharmacokinetics and concentration-effect relationships of intervenous and oral clonidine. Clin Pharmacol Ther 1977;21(5):593–601.

[149] Park J, Forrest J, Kolesar R, et al. Oral clonidine reduces postoperative PCA morphine requirements. Can J Anaesth 1996;43(9):900–6.

[150] Dyck JB, Maze M, Haack C, et al. The pharmacokinetics and hemodynamic effects of intravenous and intramuscular dexmedetomidine hydrochloride in adult human volunteers. Anesthesiology 1993;78(5):813–20.

[151] Bhana N, Goa KL, McClellan KJ. Dexmedetomidine. Drugs 2000;59(2):263–8 [discussion: 269–70].

[152] Jeffs SA, Hall JE, Morris S. Comparison of morphine alone with morphine plus clonidine for postoperative patient-controlled analgesia. Br J Anaesth 2002;89(3):424–7.

[153] Bernard JM, Kick O, Bonnet F. [Which way for the administration of alpha 2-adrenergic agents to obtain the best analgesia?]. Cah Anesthesiol 1994;42(2):223–8.

[154] Bernard JM, Kick O, Bonnet F. Comparison of intravenous and epidural clonidine for postoperative patient-controlled analgesia. Anesth Analg 1995;81(4):706–12.

[155] Lin TF, Yeh YC, Lin FS, et al. Effect of combining dexmedetomidine and morphine for intravenous patient-controlled analgesia. Br J Anaesth 2009;102(1):117–22.

[156] Dholakia C, Beverstein G, Garren M, et al. The impact of perioperative dexmedetomidine infusion on postoperative narcotic use and duration of stay after laparoscopic bariatric surgery. J Gastrointest Surg 2007;11(11):1556–9.

[157] Unlugenc H, Gunduz M, Guler T, et al. The effect of pre-anaesthetic administration of intravenous dexmedetomidine on postoperative pain in patients receiving patient-controlled morphine. Eur J Anaesthesiol 2005;22(5):386–91.

[158] Gomez-Vazquez ME, Hernandez-Salazar E, Hernandez-Jimenez A, et al. Clinical analgesic efficacy and side effects of dexmedetomidine in the early postoperative period after arthroscopic knee surgery. J Clin Anesth 2007;19(8):576–82.

[159] Rhen T, Cidlowski JA. Antiinflammatory action of glucocorticoids—new mechanisms for old drugs. N Engl J Med 2005;353(16):1711–23.

[160] Brodner G, Pogatzki E, Van Aken H, et al. A multimodal approach to control postoperative pathophysiology and rehabilitation in patients undergoing abdominothoracic esophagectomy. Anesth Analg 1998;86(2):228–34.

[161] Pedersen JL, Crawford ME, Dahl JB, et al. Effect of preemptive nerve block on inflammation and hyperalgesia after human thermal injury. Anesthesiology 1996;84(5):1020–6.

[162] Wang JJ, Ho ST, Tzeng JI, et al. The effect of timing of dexamethasone administration on its efficacy as a prophylactic antiemetic for postoperative nausea and vomiting. Anesth Analg 2000;91(1):136–9.

[163] Holte K, Kehlet H. Perioperative single-dose glucocorticoid administration: pathophysiologic effects and clinical implications. J Am Coll Surg 2002;195(5):694–712.

[164] Masferrer JL, Zweifel BS, Manning PT, et al. Selective inhibition of inducible cyclooxygenase 2 in vivo is antiinflammatory and nonulcerogenic. Proc Natl Acad Sci U S A 1994;91(8):3228–32.

[165] Romundstad L, Breivik H, Niemi G, et al. Methylprednisolone intravenously 1 day after surgery has sustained analgesic and opioid-sparing effects. Acta Anaesthesiol Scand 2004;48(10):1223–31.

[166] Feo CV, Sortini D, Ragazzi R, et al. Randomized clinical trial of the effect of preoperative dexamethasone on nausea and vomiting after laparoscopic cholecystectomy. Br J Surg 2006;93(3):295–9.

[167] Kardash KJ, Sarrazin F, Tessler MJ, et al. Single-dose dexamethasone reduces dynamic hip pain after total hip arthroplasty. Anesth Analg 2008;106(4):1253–7.

Advances in Anesthesia 27 (2009) 143–165

ADVANCES IN ANESTHESIA

Evidence-Based Update and Controversies in the Treatment and Prevention of Postoperative Nausea and Vomiting

Ashraf S. Habib, MBBCh, MSc, FRCA[a],*,
Tong J. Gan, MB, FRCA, FFARSC(I)[a]

[a]Department of Anesthesiology, Duke University Medical Center, Durham, Box 3094, NC 27710, USA

P ostoperative nausea and vomiting (PONV) are frequent and unpleasant side effects of surgery. The overall incidence of PONV has decreased from 60% when ether and cyclopropane were used, to approximately 30% nowadays, [1,2] although in certain high-risk patients the incidence is still as high as 70% [3,4]. PONV can increase medical costs from delayed recovery room discharge or unplanned admissions after outpatient surgery [5]. One study estimated that the cost of PONV to a busy ambulatory surgical unit ranged from $0.25 million to $1.5 million in lost surgical revenue [6].

For patients, nausea and vomiting are among the most unpleasant experiences associated with surgery and one of the most common reasons for poor patient satisfaction rating in the postoperative period [7]. Philip reported that patients ranked the absence of PONV as more important than earlier discharge from an ambulatory surgical unit [8]. Macario and colleagues [9] quantified patients' preferences for postoperative outcomes. PONV were among the 10 most undesirable outcomes following surgery, with vomiting being the most undesirable outcome. Patients allocated the highest amount (about $30) to avoid PONV out of a total of $100 they were allowed to spend to avoid all complications. Gan and colleagues [10] also reported that surgical patients were willing to pay up to $100, at their own expense, to avoid PONV.

PONV may be associated with serious complications such as wound dehiscence, pulmonary aspiration of gastric contents, hematoma formation beneath skin flaps, dehydration, electrolyte disturbances, Mallory-Weiss tear, and esophageal rupture [11–13]. Intraocular hemorrhage resulting in loss of vision, [14] and subcutaneous emphysema causing airway compromise as a result of prolonged postoperative vomiting (POV) have also been reported [15,16].

This article discusses identification of patients at risk for PONV, highlights current options for the prophylaxis and treatment of PONV (with emphasis

*Corresponding author. E-mail address: habib001@mc.duke.edu (A.S. Habib).

0737-6146/09/$ – see front matter
doi:10.1016/j.aan.2009.07.002

on new and recent advances in this field), and presents management recommendations.

RISK FACTORS FOR POSTOPERATIVE NAUSEA AND VOMITING

Because only 30% of patients will experience PONV, and because of the costs and side effects associated with antiemetics, it is recommended that prophylaxis is targeted to those patients who are at risk for developing PONV [17,18]. Understanding of the risk factors for PONV is incomplete partly because of its multifactorial etiology. Numerous patient-, anesthesia-, and surgery-related risk factors have been identified: well-established patient-related risk factors include female gender, nonsmoking status, and history of PONV or motion sickness [4,19–21]; increasing duration of surgery [19,21], use of volatile agents [22], nitrous oxide [23–25], and opioids [4,26] are well-established surgery- and anesthesia-related risk factors. The incidence of PONV increases after the age of 3 years, with a peak incidence of about 40% in the 11- to 14-year age group [19,27,28]. Gender differences for POV before puberty have not been identified [18].

There is a debate about other risk factors. For instance, although type of surgery has been identified as an independent risk factor in several studies, the type of surgery associated with increased risk varied among the studies. Types of surgery that might be associated with increased risk include abdominal, laparoscopic, major gynecologic, orthopedic, ear, nose, and throat, breast, plastic surgery, neurosurgery, and, in children, hernia repair, adenotonsillectomy, strabismus repair, penile surgery, and orchiopexy [2,19–23,27,29–32]. However, only 3 of 8 published PONV risk scoring systems included type of surgery as a risk factor [19,29,32]. It has been suggested that scores incorporating type of surgery do not perform better than operation-independent models [33]. One study suggested that risk factors for postoperative nausea might be different from those for vomiting. The authors reported that female gender, nonsmoking status, and general anesthesia increase PONV, whereas a history of migraine and type of surgery tend to influence only nausea [20]. Other possible risk factors include preoperative anxiety [29], and large doses of neostigmine for reversal of neuromuscular blockade [34]. The degree of expression and activity of the cytochrome P450 (CYP450) enzyme has also been suggested to affect the individual's risk for PONV [35,36]. CYP450 enzyme synthesis might be affected by smoking, alcohol consumption, medications such as cimetidine and erythromycin, vegetables such as cabbage and cauliflower, gender, and ethnicity [35,37,38].

Several previously suggested risk factors have also been disproved, including early stage of menstrual cycle [39], obesity [40], and high inspired oxygen concentration [41]. One small study suggested that the use of remifentanil rather than fentanyl for intraoperative analgesia might be associated with a reduced incidence of PONV [42], but this has not been confirmed in subsequent studies [23,43].

Several PONV scoring systems have been developed, most of which include mainly patient-related factors. However, given the gaps in knowledge of PONV risk factors, those scoring systems have shown only poor to moderate accuracy with areas under the receiver operating characteristic curve ranging from 0.56 to 0.785 [2,4,19,21,29,32,44]. This means that those scoring systems achieve only a 12% to 57% relative improvement compared with pure guessing. However, using those scoring systems to identify patients at risk for PONV and tailor antiemetic prophylaxis accordingly has been shown to significantly reduce the overall incidence of PONV, particularly in high-risk patients [45–47]. Studies have shown that the more user-friendly simplified scoring systems that omit constants and coefficients derived from logistic regression modeling do not seem to diminish the accuracy of the prediction [4,21,32]. Therefore, despite their moderate predictive accuracy, the simplified scores developed by Apfel and Eberhart are the current preferred choices for use in inpatient adults and children, respectively. The Apfel score consists of four predictors: female gender, history of motion sickness or PONV, nonsmoking status, and the use of opioids for postoperative analgesia. If none, one, two, three, or four of these risk factors were present, the incidences of PONV were 10, 21, 39, 61, and 79% respectively [4]. Similarly, the Eberhart score, which was developed for children, includes four risk factors: duration of surgery 30 minutes or longer, age 3 years or older, strabismus surgery, and history of POV in the child or POV/PONV in a parent or sibling. If 0, 1, 2, 3, or 4 of these risk factors were present, the incidences of PONV were 9%, 10%, 30%, 55%, and 70%, respectively [32].

CURRENTLY AVAILABLE ANTIEMETICS

Several receptor systems are involved in the pathogenesis of PONV. These include the dopaminergic D_2 receptors, the cholinergic muscarinic receptors, the histaminergic H_1 receptors, the serotonergic 5-hydroxytryptamine$_3$ (5-HT$_3$) receptors, and the neurokinin 1 (NK$_1$) receptors. Traditionally, antagonists on the first 4 receptor subtypes were the mainstay of PONV management. Several antiemetics have been investigated in systematic reviews. Table 1 shows the number needed to treat (NNT) of commonly used doses of antiemetics that were included in meta-analyses. Table 2 summarizes the advantages and side effects of different classes of antiemetics.

Dopamine receptor antagonists

Metoclopramide and droperidol are the most commonly studied dopamine receptor antagonists. Although metoclopramide has prokinetic effects, its antiemetic effects in a dose of 10 mg are uncertain, with approximately 50% of studies reporting this dose to be no more effective than placebo [18,58]. One study, however, suggested that 20 mg might be an efficacious dose [59]. A more recent study also reported that metoclopramide in doses of 25 mg and 50 mg was effective for PONV prophylaxis and resulted in a relative risk reduction of 26% to 37% [60].

Table 1
Number needed to treat with 95% confidence intervals for antiemetics studied in systematic reviews

	Early nausea	Late nausea	Early vomiting	Late vomiting
Anticholinergics				
Scopolamine [48]		5 (3.2 to 11.1)		5.9 (4.2 to 11.1)
Antihistamines				
Dimenhydrinate [49]	8 (3 to 20)	6 (3 to 33)	7 (4 to 50)	5 (3 to 8)
Buterophenones				
Droperidol 0.5–0.75 mg [50]	4.8 (3.0 to 12)	11 (6.9 to 25)	10 (4.6 to 51)	3.4 (2.4 to 5.7)
Droperidol 1–1.25 mg [50]	6.1 (4.5 to 9.4)	6.8 (5.2 to 9.7)	7.6 (5.8 to 11)	8.2 (5.6 to 15)
Droperidol in PCA morphine [51]		5.1 (3.1 to 15)		3.1 (2.3 to 4.8)
5-HT₃ receptor antagonists				
Ondansetron				
Ondansetron 4 mg [52]	5.6 (4 to 9)	4.6 (4 to 5.5)	5.5 (4.4 to 7.5)	6.4 (5.3 to 7.9)
Ondansetron 8 mg [52]	11 (4.2 to ∞)	6.4 (4.6 to 10)	6.4 (4.7 to 10)	5.0 (4.0 to 6.7)
Ondansetron in PCA morphine [51]		−67 (−5.8 to ∞)		5.1 (2.8 to 23)
Trapisetron				
Trapisetron 2–5 mg [53]		6.7 (4.8 to 11.1)		5 (3.6 to 8.3)
Benzamides				
Metoclopramide 10 mg [54]	16 (7.5 to −210)	12 (6 to −1587)	9.1 (5.5 to 27)	10 (6 to 41)
Propofol				
Propofol induction [55]	9.3 (6.1 to 19.4)	50.1 (7.6 to ∞)	13.7 (8.1 to 45.4)	14.9 (6 to ∞)
Propofol maintenance [55]	8 (6.4 to 10.8)	5.8 (4.2 to 9.4)	9.2 (7.6 to 11.7)	10.1 (6.2 to 28.8)
Steroids				
Dexamethasone 8 mg [56]	5 (2.2 to −21)	4.3 (2.3 to 26)	3.6 (2.3 to 8)	4.3 (2.6 to 12)
Other interventions				
Omitting nitrous oxide [25]	30 (13.5 to ∞) −636	36.9 (11.8 to ∞) 14	11.8 (8.5 to 19.4) 417	13.8 (8.8 to 31.6) 23
Omitting reversal of neuromuscular blockade [34]				
Nonpharmacologic techniques (0–48 h) [57]	4 (3 to 6)		5 (4 to 8)	14 (6 to ∞)

Table 2
Advantages and side effects of different classes of antiemetics

Class of antiemetics	Advantages	Side effects
Dopamine receptor antagonists:		
Phenothiazines (eg, promethazine, prochlorperazine)	Long duration of action	Sedation, extrapyramidal side effects, hypotension, restlessness, anticholinergic syndrome
Buterophenones (eg, droperidol, haloperidol)	Improved prophylaxis against nausea	Sedation with high doses, hypotension, extrapyramidal side effects, neuroleptic malignant syndrome, droperidol has an FDA black box warning regarding prolongation of QTc, although the risk is considered minimal with antiemetic doses
Benzamides (eg, metoclopramide)	Have prokinetic effects	Sedation, restlessness, extrapyramidal side effects
Anticholinergics (eg, scopolamine)	Effective against motion sickness Transdermal preparation with a long duration of action available	Sedation, blurred vision, dry mouth, restlessness, central cholinergic syndrome
Antihistamines (eg, dimenhydrinate, cyclizine)	Effective against motion sickness Effective for PONV after middle ear surgery	Sedation, dry mouth, restlessness
5-HT$_3$ receptor antagonists (eg, ondansetron, dolasetron, granisetron)	Specific for PONV Do not have sedative side effects Long duration of action	Headache, constipation, elevated liver enzymes
NK$_1$ receptor antagonists (eg, aprepitant)	Improved efficacy against vomiting Do not have sedative side effects	Headache, constipation
Corticosteroids (eg, dexamethasone)	Do not have sedative side effects Long duration of action	No data available regarding side effects following single dose for PONV prophylaxis, hyperglycemia especially in diabetic and obese patients

Droperidol in a dose of 0.625 mg to 1.25 mg has been demonstrated to be highly effective for the prophylaxis of PONV [50]. It has a long duration of action (as long as 24 hours following administration) probably because of its strong binding affinity to the emetic receptors, although its half-life is relatively short (3 hours) [61]. In a large multicenter study, the 1.25-mg dose was superior to ondansetron 4 mg for the prevention of nausea, and was not associated with increased sedation [62]. Cost-effectiveness studies recommended that droperidol should be used as first line agent for PONV prophylaxis [63,64]. However, in December 2001 the US Food and Drug Administration (FDA) issued a black box warning on droperidol because of concerns about QT interval prolongation following its administration. The FDA noted that it has been associated with corrected QT (QTc) interval prolongation or torsades de pointes, and in some cases resulted in fatal cardiac arrhythmias. The warning was based on 273 cases reported in a 4-year period, of which 127 resulted in serious adverse outcomes. A cardiac event occurred in 74 of those cases. A total of 89 deaths were reported, but the dose of droperidol was 2.5 mg or less in only 2 deaths. The majority of deaths involved droperidol doses that ranged from 25 to 250 mg. A total of 5 patients receiving droperidol 2.5 mg or less experienced ventricular tachycardia or torsades [65]. Analysis of the 10 cases in which the dose of droperidol used was 0.625 to 1.25 mg showed that there were several confounding factors that made it impossible to determine the precise cause of the adverse cardiac events.[66] Although the decision by the FDA was criticized by many experts in the field because droperidol is well studied and has a long record of safety when antiemetic doses are used [67–70]. there was a significant decline in the use of this agent, [66] despite 92% of respondents in one survey believing the black box warning was not justified [71]. Although the cost advantage of droperidol compared with ondansetron is now no longer applicable since ondansetron became generic, the superior antinausea efficacy of droperidol has caused continued interest in this agent [50].

There is no doubt that QT prolongation occurs with higher doses of droperidol [72,73]. but it was not clear whether the low doses used in the management of PONV are associated with a similar risk. Therefore several recent studies have investigated this issue. White and colleagues [74] reported that the maximum prolongation of the QT interval occurred 3 to 6 min after the prophylactic administration of droperidol 0.625 mg and 1.25 mg during desflurane- remifentanil-based anesthesia. The average prolongation was not different compared with patients who received placebo and returned to baseline by 2 hours after arrival at the postanesthesia care unit (PACU). In another study, Charbit and colleagues [75] reported that QTc was significantly prolonged after administration of droperidol 0.75 mg or ondansetron 4 mg for the treatment of established PONV with no significant differences between the groups. The QTc was significantly prolonged compared with baseline until 5 minutes after administration, and was lower compared with predrug administration by 90 minutes. Similar results were reported by Chan and colleagues, [76] who measured the QTc at 5 minutes and 2 to 3 hours after the administration of droperidol 1.25 mg, ondansetron 4 mg, and the combination of both drugs. The combination did not result in any greater QTc prolongation compared with each drug alone. In a more recent small study involving 16 volunteers, Charbit and colleagues [77] reported significant prolongation of QTc following droperidol 1 mg, ondansetron 4 mg, and the combination of both agents when compared with placebo. The mean maximal prolongation with droperidol and of the combination was about 8 to 11 milliseconds longer than the prolongation with ondansetron alone. No arrhythmias were experienced by any subject in any of those studies.

Therefore it appears that QTc is prolonged in a dose-related manner after the administration of droperidol. When given at doses less than 2.5 mg, this prolongation is modest and transient, and unlikely to induce arrhythmias [77]. However, because droperidol is generic, the manufacturer did not respond to the FDA's request to submit data (either from the existing literature or from new studies) to support a labeling indicating droperidol for the management of PONV at doses less than 2.5 mg [78]. As a result of this black box warning and lack of clarification regarding the applicability of this warning to doses less than 2.5 mg (2.5 mg is the FDA-approved dose), the use of this effective antiemetic continues to decline.

Recently, it was suggested that haloperidol in a dose of 1 to 2 mg might be a suitable alternative to droperidol [79–84]. However, there is a lack of large well-conducted studies investigating the safety and efficacy of haloperidol in this setting. The only advantage of haloperidol compared with droperidol is the lack of the black box warning [85].

Anticholinergics

Scopolamine is an anticholinergic agent that was widely used with opioid premedication. Transdermal scopolamine (TDS) 1.5 mg was shown to be effective for PONV prophylaxis in several settings, including outpatient laparoscopy and after epidural morphine administration [65,86]. There has recently been renewed interest in studying this transdermal preparation, with a recent study reporting similar efficacy to ondansetron 4 mg and droperidol 1.25 mg [87]. In a quantitative systemic review, the number needed to harm for the most commonly reported side effects with scopolamine was 5.6 for dry mouth, 12.5 for visual disturbances, 50 for dizziness, and 100 for agitation [48]. In a more recent randomized double-blind clinical trial, controlled-released TDS in combination with ondansetron 4 mg demonstrated no difference in the frequency of anticholinergic-related side effects (7.1% vs 6.8%) compared with the ondansetron 4 mg only [88].

Antihistamines

The antihistamines include the ethanolamines (dimenhydrinate, diphenhydramine) and the piperazines (cyclizine, hydroxyzine, meclizine). Their major disadvantages are sedation, dry mouth, blurred vision, urinary retention, and delayed recovery room discharge [89]. Although these agents have not been well studied, a systematic review suggested that dimenhydrinate is effective for PONV prophylaxis with an overall NNT of 5 [49]. Promethazine is an effective antiemetic with a long duration of action. In a dose of 12.5 to 25 mg given toward the end of surgery, it has been shown to be effective for PONV management [90]. However, its use is limited by sedation and prolonged recovery from anesthesia [58]. There is also a black box warning about the risk of respiratory depression in children younger than 2 years [91]. However, one study did not show increased awakening time or duration of PACU stay when compared with ondansetron and placebo in patients undergoing middle ear surgery [90]. Recently, the use of low-dose promethazine (6.25 mg) was shown to be as effective as higher doses, with a possible association with less sedation [91–93]. Promethazine is buffered with acetic acid–sodium acetate and has a pH between 4.0 and 5.5. There are reports in the literature of necrosis and gangrene after inadvertent intra-arterial injection or extravasation of peripheral intravenous lines associated with the use of promethazine [94–96].

Serotonin receptor antagonists

The 5-HT$_3$ receptor antagonists are highly specific and selective for nausea and vomiting. Their antivomiting efficacy is better than their antinausea efficacy [52]. Antagonists in this group exert their effects by binding to the 5-HT$_3$ receptor in the chemoreceptor trigger zone and at vagal afferents in the gastrointestinal tract. Their favorable side-effect profile, and in particular the lack of sedation, make them popular and suitable for ambulatory surgery. First-generation 5-HT$_3$ receptor antagonists include ondansetron, granisetron, dolasetron, and tropisetron. There is no evidence that there is any difference in efficacy or side-effect profile between the various 5-HT$_3$ receptor antagonists, when appropriate doses are used for the management of PONV. Therefore, acquisition cost is the main factor that differentiates the 5-HT$_3$ compounds [97]. Ondansetron, the most commonly studied agent in this group, has recently become generic. The 5-HT$_3$ receptor antagonists are extensively metabolized by CYPP450. The highly genetically polymorphic 2D6 isoform of CYP (CYP2D6) is involved in the metabolism of ondansetron, tropisetron, and dolasetron. However, the metabolism of granisetron involves the 3A4 isoform of CYP [98]. CYP2D6 has many genetic polymorphisms that affect enzyme activity and result in patients being poor, intermediate, extensive, or ultrarapid metabolizers [99,100]. Ultrarapid metabolizers have an increased incidence of therapeutic failures after treatment with ondansetron, dolasetron, and tropisetron [101–103].

Other antiemetic interventions

Dexamethasone has also proved effective for the prophylaxis of PONV. In a dose of 4 mg, it has comparable efficacy to ondansetron 4 mg and droperidol 1.25 mg [23]. It is most effective when administered at induction of anesthesia [104]. Advantages of dexamethasone include lack of sedation, and prolonged duration of action.[56] Although there are no reports of significant adverse effects associated with a single intraoperative dose, hyperglycemia has been reported, especially in obese and diabetic patients [105,106].

Other effective antiemetic interventions include total intravenous anesthesia with propofol [55], and nonpharmacologic techniques such as stimulation of the P6 (Neiguan) acupoint [57]. The latter modality is particularly effective for prophylaxis against nausea [107–109]. The use of opioid antagonists such as low-dose naloxone (0.25 µg/kg/h) [110,111], nalmefene [112], and alvimopan [113] significantly reduced the incidence of opioid-related side effects associated with patient-controlled analgesia, including nausea, vomiting, and pruritus. Other therapies that might be of benefit include benzodiazepines [114,115], ephedrine [116,117], and aggressive intravenous hydration [118].

Newer generation antiemetics

Palonosetron

Palonosetron is a second-generation 5-HT$_3$ receptor antagonist that is approved by the FDA for the prevention of acute and delayed chemotherapy-induced nausea and vomiting (CINV) at a dose of 0.25 mg intravenously (IV) and for the prevention of PONV at a dose of 0.075 mg administered IV over 10 seconds immediately before the induction of anesthesia.

Palonosetron exhibits several different characteristics that distinguish it from other 5-HT$_3$ receptor antagonists. For instance, palonosetron has a significantly different chemical structure compared with other agents in this class. Although the other 5-HT$_3$ receptor antagonists are based on a 3-substituted indole structure that mimics the structure of serotonin [119], palonosetron has a 3-member ring moiety attached to a quinuclidine ring [120]. Palonosetron also has about 30-fold greater binding affinity for the receptor than other antagonists (pK$_i$ = 10.45) [121], and a substantially longer half-life exceeding 40 hours [122], compared with 5 to 12 hours with the other agents in this class. Palonosetron exhibits unique molecular interactions with the 5-HT$_3$ receptor [123]. For instance, ondansetron and granisetron produce competitive antagonism of the 5-HT$_3$ receptor by competing directly with serotonin for the same binding site on the receptor. In contrast, palonosetron produces allosteric inhibition of the receptor and binds to a site different from the binding site for serotonin and other 5-HT$_3$ receptor antagonists such as ondansetron and granisetron [123]. Binding of palonosetron to the 5-HT$_3$ receptor induces a conformational change such that the endogenous ligand cannot bind and the affinity of other bound 5-HT$_3$ receptor antagonists such as ondansetron and granisetron is reduced. Palonosetron also exhibits positive cooperativity, wherein the binding of the first molecule causes a conformational change to the structure of the receptor that increases the affinity between the receptor and other palonosetron molecules. In contrast, ondansetron and granisetron exhibit simple bimolecular interactions. Palonosetron also produces significant inhibition of serotonin-induced calcium influx, an effect that is absent with ondansetron and minimal with granisetron. Palonosetron binding at an allosteric site may also induce internalization of the 5-HT$_3$

receptor, thereby providing fewer available receptor sites and decreasing agonist responses to a greater extent than simple reversible antagonism [123]. The long plasma half-life of palonosetron combined with the unique receptor-binding characteristics may result in long-lasting inhibition of the serotonin receptor, and an extended duration of action.

Palonosetron has been shown to be superior to older-generation $5\text{-}HT_3$ receptor antagonists for the prophylaxis of acute and delayed CINV [124–127]. Compared with dolasetron 100 mg, the complete response rate (no emesis and no rescue) with palonosetron 0.25 mg was 63% (vs 52.9%) in the acute phase, and 54% (vs 38.7%) in the delayed phase [124]. In another study comparing palonosetron 0.25 mg with ondansetron 32 mg, the complete response rate during the acute phase and delayed periods was 81% versus 68.6% and 74.1% versus 55.1%, respectively [125]. Similarly, after dexamethasone pretreatment, reduction of emesis was significantly higher for 5 days post chemotherapy with palonosetron 0.25 mg (53.3%) compared with ondansetron 32 mg (33.3%) [126]. In a more recent study, the combination of palonosetron with dexamethasone achieved significantly higher complete response rate compared with a combination of granisetron and dexamethasone during delayed CINV (56.8% vs 44.5%) [127]. Furthermore, palonosetron was significantly more effective against nausea compared with other $5\text{-}HT_3$ receptor antagonists [125,128,129].

The efficacy of palonosetron for the prophylaxis of PONV was evaluated in 2 recent studies. Both studies were placebo controlled, included 3 doses of palonosetron administered before induction of anesthesia (0.025 mg, 0.050 mg, or 0.075 mg), and evaluated the antiemetic effect of palonosetron for 72 hours after surgery [130,131]. The highest dose studied (0.075 mg) was the only dose significantly more effective than placebo in both studies. Both studies showed improved efficacy with this dose compared with placebo up to 72 hours after surgery, but the results were statistically significant for the entire 72-hour duration in one study [131], which was seen as a trend in the second study but with statistical significance only for the first 24 hours [130]. The first study included women undergoing elective inpatient gynecologic or breast surgery [131]. The complete response rate (no emesis and no use of rescue medications) was significantly higher with palonosetron 0.075 mg compared with placebo (56% vs 36% at 0–24 hours, 70 % vs 52% for 24–72 hours, and 52% vs 36% for 0–72 hours postoperative interval). The incidence of nausea and vomiting at 0 to 24 hours was significantly reduced with palonosetron 0.075 mg compared with placebo (50% vs 71% and 40% vs 60%, respectively). Palonosetron also reduced the severity of nausea during the first 24 hours, and significantly prolonged time to emesis (> 72 hours vs 3.9 hours, $P = .002$). The second study included patients undergoing outpatient abdominal or gynecologic laparoscopic surgery [130]. In that study, the complete response rate with palonosetron was significantly higher than placebo for the 0- to 24-hour time period (43% vs 26%), but not for the 24 to 72-hour observation period (41% vs 49%). The incidence of vomiting was lower with palonosetron at 0 to 24 hours, but the difference was not statistically significant (33% vs 44%, $P = .075$). The incidence and severity of nausea were significantly lower with palonosetron in the first 24 hours, and the reduction in severity was also apparent for the entire 72-hour duration of the study. The authors also reported a significant reduction in the impact of PONV on patient function in the first 24 hours with palonosetron 0.075 mg. The most common side effects reported in both studies were headache and constipation; the incidence of both was low and not different from placebo. There were no prolongations of QTc interval compared with placebo.

Studies comparing palonosetron with other commonly used antiemetics and studies investigating the use of palonosetron in combination with other agents and as part of a multimodal approach are needed. The unique binding characteristics and long duration of action of palonosetron might confer advantages when used in the treatment of established PONV, and this needs to be investigated in future trials. It has also been suggested that 0.075 mg might not be the optimal dose for prophylaxis [132], and future studies will need to assess if higher doses would increase efficacy for PONV prevention.

Nk_1 receptor antagonists

Substance P belongs to a family of neuropeptides known as tachykinins. The most common mammalian tachykinins include substance P, neurokinin A, and neurokinin B. Their actions are mediated through specific cell surface receptors known as NK_1, NK_2, and NK_3, with substance P being the preferred agonist for NK_1 receptors. These receptors belong to the family of G-protein coupled receptors and are coupled to the inositol phosphate and signal transduction pathway [133].

Substance P is the most abundant and widely distributed tachykinin in the mammalian CNS [134]. Extensive substance P-like immunoreactivity has been demonstrated in key brain areas associated with emesis, such as the nucleus tractus solitarius (NTS) and area postrema [134]. Substance P is excitatory when applied to neurons in the area postrema of the dog [135], and is able to evoke emesis when injected directly into the brain stem in ferrets [136]. Autoradiographic mapping demonstrated a high concentration of NK_1 receptors in brain stem nuclei of the dorsal vagal complex, such as the NTS, which receives central emetic signals from the area postrema and peripheral vagal afferents [134]. Depletion of substance P in the NTS prevented the responses to peripheral and central emetogenic stimuli secondary to reduced activation of neurons [137]. Selective NK_1 receptor antagonists that cross the blood-brain barrier were therefore developed and investigated for their antiemetic effects. In slices of ferret brain stem, action potentials of single NTS neurons induced by substance P were inhibited by HSP-117, an NK_1 receptor antagonist with potent antiemetic activity [138]. Similarly, positron emission tomography studies in rhesus monkeys suggest that NK_1 receptor antagonists exert their main antiemetic effect centrally by depressing the neural activity of the NTS [139]. A peripheral mechanism of action on the NK_1 receptor located on vagal terminals in the gut was also suggested, because peripheral injection of a peptide-based NK_1 receptor antagonist in the ferret was effective against cisplatin-induced emesis [140].

Animal studies demonstrated broader spectrum antiemetic activity of NK_1 receptor antagonists compared with the $5-HT_3$ receptor antagonists [141]. In humans, NK_1 receptor antagonists were effective for the prophylaxis and treatment of PONV. In one study in females undergoing gynecologic surgery, the NK_1 receptor antagonist CP-122,721 provided better prophylaxis against vomiting compared with ondansetron. The combination of both agents also significantly prolonged the time to administration of rescue antiemetics compared with either drug alone, and was associated with a very low incidence of emesis (2%). However, the incidence of nausea was not different between the groups [142]. Another NK_1 receptor antagonist, GR20517, was also more effective than placebo for the treatment of established emesis [143]. Casopitant is another NK_1 receptor antagonist that was investigated in a dose of 50 mg orally and compared with placebo given 60 minutes before anesthesia together with ondansetron 4 mg IV given before induction of anesthesia. The complete response rate was higher with casopitant compared with placebo (57% vs 43%), but there was no difference in nausea between the groups [144]. In a more recent multicenter study in 805 patients receiving general anesthesia for open abdominal surgery, the NK_1 antagonist aprepitant was compared with intravenous ondansetron 4 mg for the prophylaxis of PONV. Aprepitant, which has a long half-life of 9 to 12 hours, was administered orally in a dose of 40 mg or 125 mg 1 to 3 hours before induction of anesthesia. The incidence of no vomiting (0–24 hours) was significantly higher with aprepitant 125 mg (95%) and aprepitant 40 mg (90%) versus ondansetron (74%). Both aprepitant doses also had higher incidences of no vomiting for 0 to 48 hours (93% and 85% versus 67% with ondansetron, $P < .001$). However, nausea incidence and severity, need for rescue antiemetics, and complete response were not different across the 3 groups [145]. In another study with a similar design, aprepitant was significantly more effective than ondansetron in preventing vomiting at 24 and 48 hours (percentage of patients with no vomiting at 0–24 hours/0–48 hours: 86/85%, 84/82%, and 71/66% with aprepitant 40 mg, aprepitant 125 mg, and ondansetron 4 mg, respectively). In this study the severity of nausea was lower in the aprepitant groups in the first 48 hours postoperatively [146]. The most commonly reported adverse events were fever, constipation, and headache with no differences between the groups. Pooled data from these two studies showed that aprepitant 40 mg was more effective than ondansetron in achieving no significant nausea (56.4% vs 48.1%), no nausea (39.6% vs 33.1%), no vomiting (86.7% vs 72.4%), and no rescue (37.9% vs 31.2%) [147]. The 40-mg dose of aprepitant was approved for the prophylaxis of PONV and is the only NK_1 receptor antagonist currently available for the management of PONV in the United States.

In summary, NK_1 receptor antagonists have a long duration of action, and a favorable side- effect profile. They seem to be particularly effective for prophylaxis against vomiting. Studies investigating the combination of those agents with other antiemetics, and studies examining the efficacy of those agents for the prophylaxis against postdischarge nausea and vomiting, and for the treatment of established PONV are warranted.

Combination therapy and the multimodal approach

Several randomized controlled trials have been published that compare combination versus single agents for PONV prophylaxis. Most of these studies demonstrate improved prophylaxis using a combination of two or more agents acting at different receptor sites [148]. This has been confirmed in systematic reviews [56,149]. Another meta-analysis reported that a combination of two antiemetics was more effective for the prophylaxis against postdischarge nausea and vomiting, compared with monotherapy. In that analysis, the NNT to prevent postdischarge nausea following ambulatory surgery was 12.9, 12.2, and 5.2 after the prophylactic administration of ondansetron, dexamethasone, and a combination of two antiemetics, respectively. For postdischarge vomiting, the NNT was 13.8 for ondansetron and 5 for combination treatment [150].

The most commonly studied combinations have included a 5-HT$_3$ receptor antagonist with droperidol or dexamethasone and the combination of droperidol with dexamethasone. These combination regimens appear to be equally efficacious [23,149,151]. The combination of scopolamine with ondansetron was also recently shown to be safe and effective for the prophylaxis of PONV [88].

In addition to using a combination of antiemetics acting at different receptor sites, the multifactorial etiology of PONV might be better addressed by the adoption of a multimodal approach. This is especially important in patients at high risk for PONV. This approach incorporates a combination of antiemetics and strategies for keeping the baseline risk of PONV low (Table 3). For instance, there is an 11-fold increased risk for PONV in patients receiving

---

Table 3
Strategies to keep the baseline risk of postoperative nausea and vomiting low

(A) Use of regional anesthesia [19]
(B) Avoid emetogenic stimuli:
- Nitrous oxide [4,25,152]
- Inhalational agents [153]
(C) Minimize the following:
- Intraoperative and postoperative opioids [4,30,153–155]
- The dose of neostigmine [34]
(D) Multimodal therapy:
- Total intravenous anesthesia with propofol [55]
- Adequate hydration [118], especially with
   colloids [156]
- Anxiolytics (eg, benzodiazepines) [114,115,157]
- Nonpharmacologic techniques (eg, acupuncture) [57]
- α_2-adrenergic agonists (eg, clonidine) [158,159]

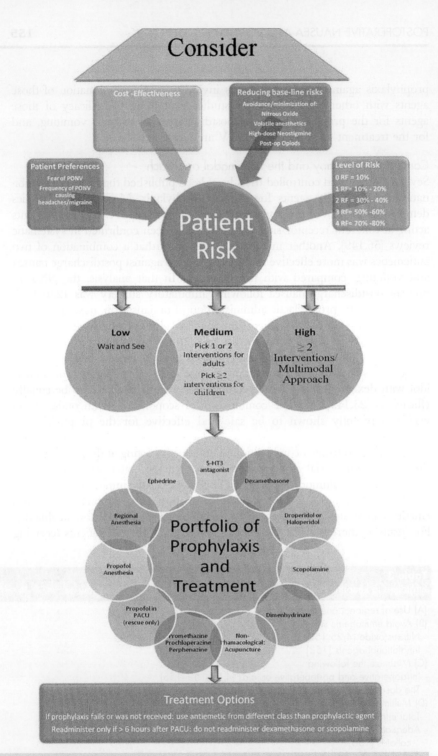

Fig. 1. Algorithm for the management of PONV. (*Modified from* Gan TJ, Meyer TA, Apfel CC, et al. Society for ambulatory anesthesia guidelines for the management of postoperative nausea and vomiting. Anesth Analg 2007;105:1615–28.)

general anesthesia compared with those receiving a regional anesthetic [19]. Total intravenous anesthesia with propofol has been shown to reduce the incidence of PONV, especially in the early postoperative period [55]. Avoidance of nitrous oxide (which increases POV) and volatile agents (which cause PONV for up to 2 hours postoperatively), and minimizing intraoperative and postoperative opiates, also reduce the incidence of PONV [4,22,25,30,153–155]. Large doses of neostigmine (>2.5 mg) increase the risk of PONV [34]. Other strategies that might reduce the incidence of PONV include adequate hydration especially using colloids [118,156] anxiolysis with benzodiazepines [160], and the use of α_2-agonists [158,159].

Scuderi and colleagues [161] tested a multimodal approach to the management of PONV in females undergoing outpatient laparoscopy. Their multimodal regimen consisted of total intravenous anesthesia with propofol and remifentanil, no nitrous oxide, no neuromuscular blockade, aggressive intravenous hydration (25 mL/kg), triple prophylactic antiemetics (ondansetron 1 mg, droperidol 0.625 mg, and dexamethasone 10 mg), and ketorolac 30 mg. Control groups included standard balanced outpatient anesthetic with or without 4 mg ondansetron prophylaxis. Multimodal management resulted in a 98% complete response rate (no PONV and no antiemetic rescue) in PACU. No patient in this group vomited before discharge, compared with 7% of patients in the ondansetron group ($P = .07$) and 22% of patients in the placebo group ($P = .0003$). Subsequently, more studies confirmed the efficacy of a multimodal approach, especially in high-risk patients [23,160–165].

RECOMMENDATIONS FOR THE PROPHYLAXIS AND TREATMENT OF POSTOPERATIVE NAUSEA AND VOMITING

A multidisciplinary panel of experts has issued guidelines for the management of PONV (Fig. 1) [18]. The panel recommended that a risk-adapted strategy for the prophylaxis for PONV should be adopted, using one or two interventions in adults at moderate risk for PONV, and more than two interventions or a multimodal approach for patients deemed at high risk for PONV. Furthermore, the panel recommended strategies for the reduction of baseline risk for PONV. For the treatment of established PONV, an agent from a pharmacologic class different from the agent used for prophylaxis should be used. For instance, low-dose promethazine (6.25 mg) has been shown to be more effective for the treatment of PONV after ondansetron failure compared with a repeat dose of ondansetron [93,165]. If no prophylaxis was given, treatment with a low-dose 5-HT_3 receptor antagonist is recommended. The doses of 5-HT_3 receptor antagonists needed for treatment are smaller than those used for prophylaxis [166].

SUMMARY

PONV is a significant problem after anesthesia and surgery. Better understanding of risk factors for PONV might help target aggressive prophylaxis to high-risk patients. Communication with patients is essential to establish the level of PONV risk and patient preference regarding PONV management. More studies are needed to investigate whether the use of novel antiemetics with a long duration of action and unique characteristics in combination with other antiemetic interventions can further improve our management of PONV.

References

[1] Bonica J, Crepps W, Monk B, et al. Post-anesthetic nausea, retching and vomiting. Anesthesiology 1958;19:532–40.

[2] Cohen MM, Duncan PG, DeBoer DP, et al. The postoperative interview: assessing risk factors for nausea and vomiting. Anesth Analg 1994;78:7–16.

[3] Gan TJ, Ginsberg B, Grant AP, et al. Double-blind, randomized comparison of ondansetron and intraoperative propofol to prevent postoperative nausea and vomiting. Anesthesiology 1996;85:1036–42.

[4] Apfel CC, Laara E, Koivuranta M, et al. A simplified risk score for predicting postoperative nausea and vomiting: conclusions from cross-validations between two centers. Anesthesiology 1999;91:693–700.

[5] Gold BS, Kitz DS, Lecky JH, et al. Unanticipated admission to the hospital following ambulatory surgery. JAMA 1989;262:3008–10.

[6] Hirsch J. Impact of postoperative nausea and vomiting in the surgical setting. Anaesthesia 1994;49:30–3.

[7] Myles PS, Williams DL, Hendrata M, et al. Patient satisfaction after anaesthesia and surgery: results of a prospective survey of 10,811 patients. Br J Anaesth 2000;84:6–10.

[8] Philip BK. Patients' assessment of ambulatory anesthesia and surgery. J Clin Anesth 1992;4:355–8.

[9] Macario A, Weinger M, Carney S, et al. Which clinical anesthesia outcomes are important to avoid? The perspective of patients. Anesth Analg 1999;89:652–8.

[10] Gan T, Sloan F, Dear Gde L, et al. How much are patients willing to pay to avoid postoperative nausea and vomiting? Anesth Analg 2001;92:393–400.

[11] Watcha MF, White PF. Postoperative nausea and vomiting. Its etiology, treatment, and prevention. Anesthesiology 1992;77:162–84.

[12] Wilder-Smith OH, Martin NC, Morabia A. Postoperative nausea and vomiting: a comparative survey of the attitudes, perceptions, and practice of Swiss anesthesiologists and surgeons. Anesth Analg 1997;84:826–31.

[13] Kapur PA. The big "Little problem". Anesth Analg 1991;73:243–5.

[14] Zhang GS, Mathura JR Jr. Images in clinical medicine. Painless loss of vision after vomiting. N Engl J Med 2005;352:e16.

[15] Schumann R, Polaner DM. Massive subcutaneous emphysema and sudden airway compromise after postoperative vomiting. Anesth Analg 1999;89:796–7.

[16] Toprak V, Keles GT, Kaygisiz Z, et al. Subcutaneous emphysema following severe vomiting after emerging from general anesthesia. Acta Anaesthesiol Scand 2004;48:917–8.

[17] Habib AS, Gan TJ. Evidence-based management of postoperative nausea and vomiting: a review. Can J Anaesth 2004;51:326–41.

[18] Gan TJ, Meyer TA, Apfel CC, et al. Society for ambulatory anesthesia guidelines for the management of postoperative nausea and vomiting. Anesth Analg 2007;105:1615–28.

[19] Sinclair DR, Chung F, Mezei G. Can postoperative nausea and vomiting be predicted? Anesthesiology 1999;91:109–18.

[20] Stadler M, Bardiau F, Seidel L, et al. Difference in risk factors for postoperative nausea and vomiting. Anesthesiology 2003;98:46–52.

[21] Koivuranta M, Laara E, Snare L, et al. A survey of postoperative nausea and vomiting. Anaesthesia 1997;52:443–9.

[22] Apfel CC, Kranke P, Katz MH, et al. Volatile anaesthetics may be the main cause for early but not delayed postoperative vomiting: a randomized controlled trial of factorial design. Br J Anaesth 2002;88:659–68.

[23] Apfel CC, Korttila K, Abdalla M, et al. A factorial trial of six interventions for the prevention of postoperative nausea and vomiting. N Engl J Med 2004;350:2441–51.

[24] Myles PS, Leslie K, Chan MT, et al. Avoidance of nitrous oxide for patients undergoing major surgery: a randomized controlled trial. Anesthesiology 2007;107:221–31.

[25] Tramer M, Moore A, McQuay H. Omitting nitrous oxide in general anaesthesia: meta-analysis of intraoperative awareness and postoperative emesis in randomized controlled trials. Br J Anaesth 1996;76:186–93.

[26] Roberts GW, Bekker TB, Carlsen HH, et al. Postoperative nausea and vomiting are strongly influenced by postoperative opioid use in a dose-related manner. Anesth Analg 2005;101:1343–8.

[27] Lerman J. Surgical and patient factors involved in postoperative nausea and vomiting. Br J Anaesth 1992;69:24S–32S.

[28] Rowley MP, Brown TC. Postoperative vomiting in children. Anaesth Intensive Care 1982;10:309–13.

[29] Van den Bosch JE, Moons KG, Bonsel GJ, et al. Does measurement of preoperative anxiety have added value for predicting postoperative nausea and vomiting? Anesth Analg 2005;100:1525–32, table of contents.

[30] Apfel CC, Kranke P, Eberhart LHJ, et al. Comparison of predictive models for postoperative nausea and vomiting. Br J Anaesth 2002;88:234–40.

[31] Rose JB, Watcha MF. Postoperative nausea and vomiting in paediatric patients. Br J Anaesth 1999;83:104–17.

[32] Eberhart LH, Geldner G, Kranke P, et al. The development and validation of a risk score to predict the probability of postoperative vomiting in pediatric patients. Anesth Analg 2004;99:1630–7.

[33] Apfel CC, Greim CA, Haubitz I, et al. The discriminating power of a risk score for postoperative vomiting in adults undergoing various types of surgery. Acta Anaesthesiol Scand 1998;42:502–9.

[34] Tramer MR, Fuchs-Buder T. Omitting antagonism of neuromuscular block: effect on postoperative nausea and vomiting and risk of residual paralysis. A systematic review. Br J Anaesth 1999;82:379–86.

[35] Sweeney BP. Why does smoking protect against PONV? Br J Anaesth 2002;89:810–3.

[36] Gan TJ. Risk factors for postoperative nausea and vomiting. Anesth Analg 2006;102:1884–98.

[37] Brockmoller J, Kirchheiner J, Meisel C, et al. Pharmacogenetic diagnostics of cytochrome p450 polymorphisms in clinical drug development and in drug treatment. Pharmacogenomics 2000;1:125–51.

[38] Stern RM. The psychophysiology of nausea. Acta Biol Hung 2002;53:589–99.

[39] Eberhart LH, Morin AM, Georgieff M. The menstruation cycle in the postoperative phase. Its effect of the incidence of nausea and vomiting. Anaesthesist 2000;49:532–5 [in German].

[40] Kranke P, Apfel CC, Papenfuss T, et al. An increased body mass index is no risk factor for postoperative nausea and vomiting. A systematic review and results of original data. Acta Anaesthesiol Scand 2001;45:160–6.

[41] Orhan-Sungur M, Kranke P, Sessler D, et al. Does supplemental oxygen reduce postoperative nausea and vomiting? A meta-analysis of randomized controlled trials. Anesth Analg 2008;106:1733–8.

[42] Rama-Maceiras P, Ferreira TA, Molins N, et al. Less postoperative nausea and vomiting after propofol + remifentanil versus propofol + fentanyl anaesthesia during plastic surgery. Acta Anaesthesiol Scand 2005;49:305–11.

[43] Habib AS, Muir HA, Schultz JR, et al. Postoperative nausea and vomiting following the use of fentanyl or remifentanil in ambulatory gynecologic laparoscopic surgery: a prospective randomized trial. Ambul Surg 2007;13:69–84.

[44] Palazzo M, Evans R. Logistic regression analysis of fixed patient factors for postoperative sickness: a model for risk assessment. Br J Anaesth 1993;70:135–40.

[45] Rusch D, Eberhart L, Biedler A, et al. Prospective application of a simplified risk score to prevent postoperative nausea and vomiting. Can J Anaesth 2005;52:478–84.

[46] Biedler A, Wermelt J, Kunitz O, et al. A risk adapted approach reduces the overall institutional incidence of postoperative nausea and vomiting. Can J Anaesth 2004;51:13–9.

[47] Pierre S, Corno G, Benais H, et al. A risk score-dependent antiemetic approach effectively reduces postoperative nausea and vomiting – a continuous quality improvement initiative. Can J Anaesth 2004;51:320–5.

[48] Kranke P, Morin AM, Roewer N, et al. The efficacy and safety of transdermal scopolamine for the prevention of postoperative nausea and vomiting: a quantitative systematic review. Anesth Analg 2002;95:133–43.

[49] Kranke P, Morin AM, Roewer N, et al. Dimenhydrinate for prophylaxis of postoperative nausea and vomiting: a meta-analysis of randomized controlled trials. Acta Anaesthesiol Scand 2002;46:238–44.

[50] Henzi I, Sonderegger J, Tramer MR. Efficacy, dose-response, and adverse effects of droperidol for prevention of postoperative nausea and vomiting. Can J Anaesth 2000;47:537–51.

[51] Tramer MR, Walder B. Efficacy and adverse effects of prophylactic antiemetics during patient-controlled analgesia therapy: a quantitative systematic review. Anesth Analg 1999;88:1354–61.

[52] Tramer MR, Reynolds DJ, Moore RA, et al. Efficacy, dose-response, and safety of ondansetron in prevention of postoperative nausea and vomiting: a quantitative systematic review of randomized placebo-controlled trials. Anesthesiology 1997;87:1277–89.

[53] Kranke P, Eberhart LH, Apfel CC, et al. Tropisetron for prevention of postoperative nausea and vomiting: a quantitative systematic review. Anaesthesist 2002;51:805–14 [in German].

[54] Henzi I, Walder B, Tramer MR. Metoclopramide in the prevention of postoperative nausea and vomiting: a quantitative systematic review of randomized, placebo-controlled studies. Br J Anaesth 1999;83:761–71.

[55] Tramer M, Moore A, McQuay H. Propofol anaesthesia and postoperative nausea and vomiting: quantitative systematic review of randomized controlled studies. Br J Anaesth 1997;78:247–55.

[56] Henzi I, Walder B, Tramer MR. Dexamethasone for the prevention of postoperative nausea and vomiting: a quantitative systematic review. Anesth Analg 2000;90:186–94.

[57] Lee A, Done ML. The use of nonpharmacologic techniques to prevent postoperative nausea and vomiting: a meta-analysis. Anesth Analg 1999;88:1362–9.

[58] Rowbotham DJ. Current management of postoperative nausea and vomiting. Br J Anaesth 1992;69:46S–59S.

[59] Quaynor H, Raeder JC. Incidence and severity of postoperative nausea and vomiting are similar after metoclopramide 20 mg and ondansetron 8 mg given by the end of laparoscopic cholecystectomies. Acta Anaesthesiol Scand 2002;46:109–13.

[60] Wallenborn J, Gelbrich G, Bulst D, et al. Prevention of postoperative nausea and vomiting by metoclopramide combined with dexamethasone: Randomised double blind multicentre trial. Br Med J 2006;333:324.

[61] Fischler M, Bonnet F, Trang H, et al. The pharmacokinetics of droperidol in anesthetized patients. Anesthesiology 1986;64:486–9.

[62] Fortney JT, Gan TJ, Graczyk S, et al. A comparison of the efficacy, safety, and patient satisfaction of ondansetron versus droperidol as antiemetics for elective outpatient surgical procedures. S3a-409 and s3a-410 study groups. Anesth Analg 1998;86:731–8.

[63] Hill RP, Lubarsky DA, Phillips-Bute B, et al. Cost-effectiveness of prophylactic antiemetic therapy with ondansetron, droperidol, or placebo. Anesthesiology 2000;92:958–67.

[64] Tang J, Watcha MF, White PF. A comparison of costs and efficacy of ondansetron and droperidol as prophylactic antiemetic therapy for elective outpatient gynecologic procedures. Anesth Analg 1996;83:304–13.

[65] Bailey PL, Streisand JB, Pace NL, et al. Transdermal scopolamine reduces nausea and vomiting after outpatient laparoscopy. Anesthesiology 1990;72:977–80.

[66] Habib AS, Gan TJ. Food and Drug Administration black box warning on the perioperative use of droperidol: a review of the cases. Anesth Analg 2003;96:1377–9.

[67] Gan TJ, White PF, Scuderi PE, et al. FDA "black box" warning regarding use of droperidol for postoperative nausea and vomiting: Is it justified? Anesthesiology 2002;97:287.

[68] White PF. Droperidol: a cost-effective antiemetic for over thirty years. Anesth Analg 2002;95:789–90.

[69] Habib AS, Gan TJ. Pro: the food and drug administration black box warning on droperidol is not justified. Anesth Analg 2008;106:1414–7.

[70] Bailey P, Norton R, Karan S. The FDA droperidol warning: Is it justified? Anesthesiology 2002;97:288–9.

[71] Habib AS, Gan TJ. The use of droperidol before and after the food and drug administration black box warning: a survey of the members of the society of ambulatory anesthesia. J Clin Anesth 2008;20:35–9.

[72] Lischke V, Behne M, Doelken P, et al. Droperidol causes a dose-dependent prolongation of the qt interval. Anesth Analg 1994;79:983–6.

[73] Guy JM, Andre-Fouet X, Porte J, et al. Torsades de pointes and prolongation of the duration of QT interval after injection of droperidol. Ann Cardiol Angeiol (Paris) 1991;40:541–5 [in French].

[74] White PF, Song D, Abrao J, et al. Effect of low-dose droperidol on the QT interval during and after general anesthesia: A placebo-controlled study. Anesthesiology 2005;102:1101–5.

[75] Charbit B, Albaladejo P, Funck-Brentano C, et al. Prolongation of QTc interval after postoperative nausea and vomiting treatment by droperidol or ondansetron. Anesthesiology 2005;102:1094–100.

[76] Chan MT, Choi KC, Gin T, et al. The additive interactions between ondansetron and droperidol for preventing postoperative nausea and vomiting. Anesth Analg 2006;103:1155–62.

[77] Charbit B, Alvarez JC, Dasque E, et al. Droperidol and ondansetron-induced QT interval prolongation: a clinical drug interaction study. Anesthesiology 2008;109:206–12.

[78] Ludwin DB, Shafer SL. Con. the black box warning on droperidol should not be removed (but should be clarified!). Anesth Analg 2008;106:1418–20.

[79] Buttner M, Walder B, von Elm E, et al. Is low-dose haloperidol a useful antiemetic?: a meta-analysis of published and unpublished randomized trials. Anesthesiology 2004;101:1454–63.

[80] Wang TF, Liu YH, Chu CC, et al. Low dose haloperidol prevents postoperative nausea and vomiting after ambulatory laparoscopic surgery. Acta Anaesthesiol Scand 2008;52:280–4.

[81] Parlow JL, Costache I, Avery N, et al. Single-dose haloperidol for the prophylaxis of postoperative nausea and vomiting after intrathecal morphine. Anesth Analg 2004;98:1072–6.

[82] Lee Y, Wang PK, Lai HY, et al. Haloperidol is as effective as ondansetron for preventing postoperative nausea and vomiting. Can J Anaesth 2007;54:349–54.

[83] Rosow CE, Haspel KL, Smith SE, et al. Haloperidol versus ondansetron for prophylaxis of postoperative nausea and vomiting. Anesth Analg 2008;106:1407–9.

[84] Grecu L, Bittner EA, Kher J, et al. Haloperidol plus ondansetron versus ondansetron alone for prophylaxis of postoperative nausea and vomiting. Anesth Analg 2008;106:1410–3.

[85] Habib AS, Gan TJ. Haloperidol for postoperative nausea and vomiting: are we reinventing the wheel? Anesth Analg 2008;106:1343–5.

[86] Loper KA, Ready LB, Dorman BH. Prophylactic transdermal scopolamine patches reduce nausea in postoperative patients receiving epidural morphine. Anesth Analg 1989;68:144–6.

[87] White PF, Tang J, Song D, et al. Transdermal scopolamine: an alternative to ondansetron and droperidol for the prevention of postoperative and postdischarge emetic symptoms. Anesth Analg 2007;104:92–6.

[88] Gan TJ, Sinha AC, Kovac AL, et al. A randomized, double-blind, multicenter trial comparing transdermal scopolamine plus ondansetron to ondansetron alone for the prevention of postoperative nausea and vomiting in the outpatient setting. Anesth Analg 2009;108:1498–504.

[89] Dundee JW, Loan WB, Morrison JD. A comparison of the efficacy of cyclizine and perhenazine in reducing the emetic effects of morphine and pethidine. Br J Clin Pharmacol 1975;2:81–5.

[90] Khalil S, Philbrook L, Rabb M, et al. Ondansetron/promethazine combination or promethazine alone reduces nausea and vomiting after middle ear surgery. J Clin Anesth 1999;11:596–600.

[91] Habib AS, Breen TW, Gan TJ. Comment: promethazine adverse events after implementation of a medication shortage interchange. Ann Pharmacother 2005;39:1370 [author reply: 1370–71].

[92] Chia YY, Lo Y, Liu K, et al. The effect of promethazine on postoperative pain: a comparison of preoperative, postoperative, and placebo administration in patients following total abdominal hysterectomy. Acta Anaesthesiol Scand 2004;48:625–30.

[93] Habib AS, Reuveni J, Taguchi A, et al. A comparison of ondansetron with promethazine for treating postoperative nausea and vomiting in patients who received prophylaxis with ondansetron: a retrospective database analysis. Anesth Analg 2007;104:548–51.

[94] Foret AL, Bozeman AP, Floyd WE 3rd. Necrosis caused by intra-arterial injection of promethazine: case report. J Hand Surg Am 2009;34:919–23.

[95] Keene JR, Buckley KM, Small S, et al. Accidental intra-arterial injection: a case report, new treatment modalities, and a review of the literature. J Oral Maxillofac Surg 2006;64:965–8.

[96] Paparella S. The dangers of intravenous promethazine administration. J Emerg Nurs 2007;33:53–6, quiz 92.

[97] Gan TJ, Meyer T, Apfel CC, et al. Consensus guidelines for managing postoperative nausea and vomiting. Anesth Analg 2003;97:62–71.

[98] Gan TJ. Selective serotonin 5-HT3 receptor antagonists for postoperative nausea and vomiting: are they all the same? CNS Drugs 2005;19:225–38.

[99] Kim MK, Cho JY, Lim HS, et al. Effect of the CYP2D6 genotype on the pharmacokinetics of tropisetron in healthy Korean subjects. Eur J Clin Pharmacol 2003;59:111–6.

[100] Blower PR. 5-HT3-receptor antagonists and the cytochrome P450 system: clinical implications. Cancer J 2002;8:405–14.

[101] Candiotti KA, Birnbach DJ, Lubarsky DA, et al. The impact of pharmacogenomics on postoperative nausea and vomiting: do CYP2D6 allele copy number and polymorphisms affect the success or failure of ondansetron prophylaxis? Anesthesiology 2005;102:543–9.

[102] Janicki PK, Schuler HG, Jarzembowski TM, et al. Prevention of postoperative nausea and vomiting with granisetron and dolasetron in relation to CYP2D6 genotype. Anesth Analg 2006;102:1127–33.

[103] Kaiser R, Sezer O, Papies A, et al. Patient-tailored antiemetic treatment with 5-hydroxytryptamine type 3 receptor antagonists according to cytochrome P-450 2D6 genotypes. J Clin Oncol 2002;20:2805–11.

[104] Wang JJ, Ho ST, Tzeng JI, et al. The effect of timing of dexamethasone administration on its efficacy as a prophylactic antiemetic for postoperative nausea and vomiting. Anesth Analg 2000;91:136–9.

[105] Hans P, Vanthuyne A, Dewandre PY, et al. Blood glucose concentration profile after 10 mg dexamethasone in non-diabetic and type 2 diabetic patients undergoing abdominal surgery. Br J Anaesth 2006;97:164–70.

[106] Nazar CE, Lacassie HJ, Lopez RA, et al. Dexamethasone for postoperative nausea and vomiting prophylaxis: effect on glycaemia in obese patients with impaired glucose tolerance. Eur J Anaesthesiol 2009;26:318–21.

[107] White PF, Issioui T, Hu J, et al. Comparative efficacy of acustimulation (ReliefBand) versus ondansetron (Zofran) in combination with droperidol for preventing nausea and vomiting. Anesthesiology 2002;97:1075–81.

[108] Zarate E, Mingus M, White PF, et al. The use of transcutaneous acupoint electrical stimulation for preventing nausea and vomiting after laparoscopic surgery. Anesth Analg 2001;92:629–35.

[109] Gan TJ, Jiao KR, Zenn M, et al. A randomized controlled comparison of electro-acupoint stimulation or ondansetron versus placebo for the prevention of postoperative nausea and vomiting. Anesth Analg 2004;99:1070–5.

[110] Gan TJ, Ginsberg B, Glass PS, et al. Opioid-sparing effects of a low-dose infusion of naloxone in patient-administered morphine sulfate. Anesthesiology 1997;87: 1075–81.

[111] Maxwell LG, Kaufmann SC, Bitzer S, et al. The effects of a small-dose naloxone infusion on opioid-induced side effects and analgesia in children and adolescents treated with intravenous patient-controlled analgesia: a double-blind, prospective, randomized, controlled study. Anesth Analg 2005;100:953–8.

[112] Joshi GP, Duffy L, Chehade J, et al. Effects of prophylactic nalmefene on the incidence of morphine-related side effects in patients receiving intravenous patient-controlled analgesia. Anesthesiology 1999;90:1007–11.

[113] Taguchi A, Sharma N, Saleem RM, et al. Selective postoperative inhibition of gastrointestinal opioid receptors. N Engl J Med 2001;345:935–40.

[114] Splinter WM, MacNeill HB, Menard EA, et al. Midazolam reduces vomiting after tonsillectomy in children. Can J Anaesth 1995;42:201–3.

[115] Khalil SN, Berry JM, Howard G, et al. The antiemetic effect of lorazepam after outpatient strabismus surgery in children. Anesthesiology 1992;77:915–9.

[116] Rothenberg DM, Parnass SM, Litwack K, et al. Efficacy of ephedrine in the prevention of postoperative nausea and vomiting. Anesth Analg 1991;72:58–61.

[117] Naguib K, Osman HA, Al-Khayat HC, et al. Prevention of post-operative nausea and vomiting following laparoscopic surgery – ephedrine vs propofol. Middle East J Anesthesiol 1998;14:219–30.

[118] Yogendran S, Asokumar B, Cheng DC, et al. A prospective randomized double-blinded study of the effect of intravenous fluid therapy on adverse outcomes on outpatient surgery. Anesth Analg 1995;80:682–6.

[119] Gaster LM, King FD. Serotonin 5-HT3 and 5-HT4 receptor antagonists. Med Res Rev 1997;17:163–214.

[120] Wong EH, Clark R, Leung E, et al. The interaction of rs 25259-197, a potent and selective antagonist, with 5-HT3 receptors, in vitro. Br J Pharmacol 1995;114:851–9.

[121] Aapro MS. Palonosetron as an anti-emetic and anti-nausea agent in oncology. Ther Clin Risk Manag 2007;3:1009–20.

[122] Stoltz R, Cyong JC, Shah A, et al. Pharmacokinetic and safety evaluation of palonosetron, a 5-hydroxytryptamine-3 receptor antagonist, in U.S. and Japanese healthy subjects. J Clin Pharmacol 2004;44:520–31.

[123] Rojas C, Stathis M, Thomas AG, et al. Palonosetron exhibits unique molecular interactions with the 5-HT3 receptor. Anesth Analg 2008;107:469–78.

[124] Eisenberg P, Figueroa-Vadillo J, Zamora R, et al. Improved prevention of moderately emetogenic chemotherapy-induced nausea and vomiting with palonosetron, a pharmacologically novel 5-HT3 receptor antagonist: results of a phase III, single-dose trial versus dolasetron. Cancer 2003;98:2473–82.

[125] Gralla R, Lichinitser M, Van Der Vegt S, et al. Palonosetron improves prevention of chemotherapy-induced nausea and vomiting following moderately emetogenic chemotherapy: results of a double-blind randomized phase III trial comparing single doses of palonosetron with ondansetron. Ann Oncol 2003;14:1570–7.

[126] Aapro MS, Grunberg SM, Manikhas GM, et al. A phase III, double-blind, randomized trial of palonosetron compared with ondansetron in preventing chemotherapy-induced nausea and vomiting following highly emetogenic chemotherapy. Ann Oncol 2006;17:1441–9.

[127] Saito M, Aogi K, Sekine I, et al. Palonosetron plus dexamethasone versus granisetron plus dexamethasone for prevention of nausea and vomiting during chemotherapy: a double-blind, double-dummy, randomised, comparative phase III trial. Lancet Oncol 2009;10: 115–24.

[128] Decker GM, DeMeyer ES, Kisko DL. Measuring the maintenance of daily life activities using the functional living index-emesis (FLIE) in patients receiving moderately emetogenic chemotherapy. J Support Oncol 2006;4:35–41, 52.

[129] Grunberg SM, Deuson RR, Mavros P, et al. Incidence of chemotherapy-induced nausea and emesis after modern antiemetics. Cancer 2004;100:2261–8.

[130] Candiotti KA, Kovac AL, Melson TI, et al. A randomized, double-blind study to evaluate the efficacy and safety of three different doses of palonosetron versus placebo for preventing postoperative nausea and vomiting. Anesth Analg 2008;107:445–51.

[131] Kovac AL, Eberhart L, Kotarski J, et al. A randomized, double-blind study to evaluate the efficacy and safety of three different doses of palonosetron versus placebo in preventing postoperative nausea and vomiting over a 72-hour period. Anesth Analg 2008;107:439–44.

[132] Lichtor JL, Glass PS. We're tired of waiting. Anesth Analg 2008;107:353–5.

[133] Otsuka M, Yoshioka K. Neurotransmitter functions of mammalian tachykinins. Physiol Rev 1993;73:229–308.

[134] Leslie RA. Neuroactive substances in the dorsal vagal complex of the medulla oblongata: nucleus of the tractus solitarius, area postrema, and dorsal motor nucleus of the vagus. Neurochem Int 1985;7:191–211.

[135] Carpenter DO, Briggs DB, Strominger N. Responses of neurons of canine area postrema to neurotransmitters and peptides. Cell Mol Neurobiol 1983;3:113–26.

[136] Gardner CJ, Twissell DJ, Dale TJ, et al. The broad-spectrum anti-emetic activity of the novel non-peptide tachykinin NK1 receptor antagonist GR203040. Br J Pharmacol 1995;116: 3158–63.

[137] Andrews PL, Bhandari P. Resinferatoxin, an ultrapotent capsaicin analogue, has anti-emetic properties in the ferret. Neuropharmacology 1993;32:799–806.

[138] Saito R, Suehiro Y, Ariumi H, et al. Anti-emetic effects of a novel NK-1 receptor antagonist HSP-117 in ferrets. Neurosci Lett 1998;254:169–72.

[139] Bergstrom M, Fasth KJ, Kilpatrick G, et al. Brain uptake and receptor binding of two [11C]labelled selective high affinity NK1-antagonists, GR203040 and GR205171–pet studies in rhesus monkey. Neuropharmacology 2000;39:664–70.

[140] Minami M, Endo T, Kikuchi K, et al. Antiemetic effects of sendide, a peptide tachykinin NK1 receptor antagonist, in the ferret. Eur J Pharmacol 1998;363:49–55.

[141] Gardner CJ, Armour DR, Beattie DT, et al. GR205171: A novel antagonist with high affinity for the tachykinin NK1 receptor, and potent broad-spectrum anti-emetic activity. Regul Pept 1996;65:45–53.

[142] Gesztesi Z, Scuderi PE, White PF, et al. Substance P (neurokinin-1) antagonist prevents postoperative vomiting after abdominal hysterectomy procedures. Anesthesiology 2000;93:931–7.

[143] Diemunsch P, Schoeffler P, Bryssine B, et al. Antiemetic activity of the NK1 receptor antagonist GR205171 in the treatment of established postoperative nausea and vomiting after major gynaecological surgery. Br J Anaesth 1999;82:274–6.

[144] Chung F, Singla N, Singla S, et al. Casopitant for preventing postoperative vomiting in patients receiving opioids: pooled data analysis [abstract]. Anesthesiology 2006;105:206.

[145] Gan TJ, Apfel CC, Kovac A, et al. A randomized, double-blind comparison of the NK1 antagonist, aprepitant, versus ondansetron for the prevention of postoperative nausea and vomiting. Anesth Analg 2007;104:1082–9, tables of contents.

[146] Diemunsch P, Gan TJ, Philip BK, et al. Single-dose aprepitant vs ondansetron for the prevention of postoperative nausea and vomiting: a randomized, double-blind phase III trial in patients undergoing open abdominal surgery. Br J Anaesth 2007;99:202–11.

[147] Diemunsch P, Apfel C, Gan TJ, et al. Preventing postoperative nausea and vomiting: post hoc analysis of pooled data from two randomized active-controlled trials of aprepitant. Curr Med Res Opin 2007;23:2559–65.

[148] Habib AS, Gan TJ. Combination therapy for postoperative nausea and vomi[tin]g – a more effective prophylaxis? Ambul Surg 2001;9:59–71.

[149] Habib AS, El-Moalem HE, Gan TJ. The efficacy of the 5-HT(3) receptor antagonists combined with droperidol for PONV prophylaxis is similar to their combination with dexamethasone. A meta-analysis of randomized controlled trials. Can J Anaesth 2004;51:311–9.

[150] Gupta AM, Wu CL, Elkassabany N, et al. Does the routine prophylactic use of antiemetics affect the incidence of postdischarge nausea and vomiting following ambulatory surgery? A systematic review of randomized controlled trials. Anesthesiology 2003;99:488–95.

[151] Sanchez-Ledesma MJ, Lopez-Olaondo L, Pueyo FJ, et al. A comparison of three antiemetic combinations for the prevention of postoperative nausea and vomiting. Anesth Analg 2002;95:1590–5.

[152] Tramer M, Moore A, McQuay H. Meta-analytic comparison of prophylactic antiemetic efficacy for postoperative nausea and vomiting: Propofol anaesthesia vs omitting nitrous oxide vs total I.V. Anaesthesia with propofol. Br J Anaesth 1997;78:256–9.

[153] Sukhani R, Vazquez J, Pappas AL, et al. Recovery after propofol with and without intraoperative fentanyl in patients undergoing ambulatory gynecologic laparoscopy. Anesth Analg 1996;83:975–81.

[154] Moiniche S, Romsing J, Dahl JB, et al. Nonsteroidal antiinflammatory drugs and the risk of operative site bleeding after tonsillectomy: a quantitative systematic review. Anesth Analg 2003;96:68–77.

[155] Polati E, Verlato G, Finco G, et al. Ondansetron versus metoclopramide in the treatment of postoperative nausea and vomiting. Anesth Analg 1997;85:395–9.

[156] Moretti EW, Robertson KM, El-Moalem H, et al. Intraoperative colloid administration reduces postoperative nausea and vomiting and improves postoperative outcomes compared with crystalloid administration. Anesth Analg 2003;96:611–7.

[157] Splinter W, Noel LP, Roberts D, et al. Antiemetic prophylaxis for strabismus surgery. Can J Ophthalmol 1994;29:224–6.

[158] Mikawa K, Nishina K, Maekawa N, et al. Oral clonidine premedication reduces vomiting in children after strabismus surgery. Can J Anaesth 1995;42:977–81.

[159] Oddby-Muhrbeck E, Eksborg S, Bergendahl HT, et al. Effects of clonidine on postoperative nausea and vomiting in breast cancer surgery. Anesthesiology 2002;96:1109–14.

[160] Habib AS. Midazolam—an anti-emetic? [letter]. Anaesthesia 2002;57:725.

[161] Scuderi PE, James RL, Harris L, et al. Multimodal antiemetic management prevents early postoperative vomiting after outpatient laparoscopy. Anesth Analg 2000;91:1408–14.

[162] Hammas B, Thorn SE, Wattwil M. Superior prolonged antiemetic prophylaxis with a four-drug multimodal regimen - comparison with propofol or placebo. Acta Anaesthesiol Scand 2002;46:232–7.

[163] Eberhart LH, Mauch M, Morin AM, et al. Impact of a multimodal anti-emetic prophylaxis on patient satisfaction in high-risk patients for postoperative nausea and vomiting. Anaesthesia 2002;57:1022–7.

[164] Habib AS, White WD, Eubanks S, et al. A randomized comparison of a multimodal management strategy versus combination antiemetics for the prevention of postoperative nausea and vomiting. Anesth Analg 2004;99:77–81.

[165] Habib AS, Gan TJ. The effectiveness of rescue antiemetics after failure of prophylaxis with ondansetron or droperidol: a preliminary report. J Clin Anesth 2005;17:62–5.

[166] Kazemi-Kjellberg F, Henzi I, Tramer MR. Treatment of established postoperative nausea and vomiting: a quantitative systematic review. BMC Anaesthesiol 2001;1:2.

Advances in Anesthesia 27 (2009) 167–189

ADVANCES IN ANESTHESIA

ELSEVIER
MOSBY

Impact of Central Neuraxial Analgesia on the Progress of Labor

Christopher R. Cambic, MD[a], Cynthia A. Wong, MD[a,b,*]

[a]Department of Anesthesiology, Northwestern University Feinberg School of Medicine, 251 East Huron Street, F5-704, Chicago, IL 60611, USA
[b]Section of Obstetrical Anesthesiology, Northwestern University Feinberg School of Medicine, 251 East Huron Street F5-704, Chicago, IL 60611, USA

E pidural and spinal anesthesia have become the de facto gold standard for pain relief during labor and delivery. Multiple randomized controlled trials comparing epidural analgesia with systemic opioid analgesia or nitrous oxide have demonstrated lower pain scores and higher patient satisfaction with neuraxial analgesia [1–4]. Furthermore, neuraxial analgesia has been shown to impart significant safety and physiologic benefits to mother and fetus [5–8]. As such, the use of neuraxial techniques for labor analgesia has progressively increased over the past 3 decades. In the United States, the percentage of women receiving neuraxial analgesia for labor had risen to 77% in 2001 from 21% in 1981; in the United Kingdom, approximately 36% of parturients chose epidural analgesia for labor in 2007/2008 [9,10]. Despite the increased use and proposed benefits of neuraxial labor analgesia, there has been significant controversy regarding the impact of neuraxial analgesia on the progress of labor and mode of delivery. Although it seems at first glance that parturients who have neuraxial analgesia for labor have higher cesarean delivery rates, higher rates of instrumental vaginal delivery, and longer duration of labor, the cause-effect relationship of these associations remains controversial and unclear. The purpose of this article is to summarize the literature exploring this topic to arrive at a clearer understanding of how, and to what extent, neuraxial analgesia impacts labor and delivery.

DIFFICULTIES WITH DESIGNING AND CONDUCTING CLINICAL TRIALS

There are several inherent limitations in designing and conducting clinical trials investigating the effect of neuraxial analgesia on labor outcomes. In an ideal randomized clinical trial investigating this topic, the control group participants would receive no, or placebo, analgesia. However, this study design is not

*Corresponding author. E-mail address: c-wong2@northwestern.edu (C.A. Wong).

0737-6146/09/$ – see front matter
doi:10.1016/j.aan.2009.07.001

ethical, and even if it were to be performed, the crossover rate of the control group would likely be so high that it would render the data uninterpretable. Therefore, trials must compare neuraxial analgesia to another form of pain relief, for example, systemic opioids. However, this design, too, is prone to a high crossover rate due to the superior analgesia provided by neuraxial analgesia [4]. Moreover, the marked difference in analgesia between neuraxial and systemic techniques would nullify any attempts at maintaining blinding of group allocation, thereby potentially resulting in bias from the study participants, nurses, and obstetric and anesthetic providers. Finally, and perhaps most ironically, the effect of systemic opioids on the progress and outcome of labor has not been well investigated; there is even evidence for differences among the opioids [11,12].

The inherent difficulty in designing trials to investigate this topic is further compounded by the presence of multiple factors that can affect labor progress and outcome: obstetric provider and patient preferences, parity, rupture of membranes, use of oxytocin, and payer status. Nowhere was this difficulty better demonstrated than in a study by Nobel and colleagues [13], assessing obstetric outcomes in parturients randomized to receive epidural analgesia versus "conventional" analgesia. In this study, 43 of the 245 enrolled participants ultimately dropped out of the trial. Most of the patients who dropped out from the conventional analgesia group were nulliparous women who were in severe pain and whose fetuses presented in the occiput-posterior position. In contrast, most of the patients who dropped out from the epidural group were multiparous women whose labors progressed so rapidly that there was inadequate time to initiate epidural analgesia. Patients at low risk for operative delivery were therefore excluded from the epidural group, and patients at high risk for vaginal delivery were excluded from the systemic analgesia group, thereby making the results difficult to interpret. Moreover, this study illustrates the difficulty in controlling for factors that allow for adequate comparisons, especially among women with an increased risk of abnormal labor and operative delivery.

Ideally, all factors affecting labor progress and outcome should be controlled for in well-designed clinical studies. One such factor, which is especially difficult to control, is the obstetric provider. A retrospective study by Neuhoff and colleagues [14] found an overall lower incidence of cesarean delivery (5% vs 17%, $P<.001$) and a lower incidence of cesarean delivery for dystocia (0.5% vs 13.7%, $P<.001$) in patients whose care was primarily provided by residents, versus patients whose care was provided by a private obstetrician. Another study by Guillemette and Fraser [15] demonstrated significant variation in cesarean delivery rates among obstetric providers, despite similarities in the use of oxytocin and epidural analgesia. Furthermore, there is evidence that temporal variation in cesarean delivery incidence exists, possibly linked to obstetric provider convenience, and that fear of potential litigation or adverse outcomes may also play a role in obstetric provider management [16,17].

Ironically, the presence of labor pain itself may lead to selection bias and difficulty in interpreting the results. Women at increased risk for prolonged labor and operative delivery are more likely to experience severe labor pain, and therefore receive neuraxial labor analgesia, compared with women with rapid, uncomplicated labors [18]. Wuitchik and colleagues [18] observed that women experiencing higher levels of pain during the latent phase of labor not only underwent longer latent and active phases but also were twice as likely to require instrumental delivery. Similarly, Alexander and colleagues [19] found a significantly higher rate of cesarean delivery in women who self-administered 50 mg/h or more of patient-controlled intravenous meperidine analgesia than women who self-administered less than 50 mg/h (14% vs 1.4%). Hess and colleagues [20] found that women experiencing more breakthrough pain during low-dose bupivacaine/fentanyl epidural analgesia were more than twice as likely to undergo cesarean delivery than those with less breakthrough pain (odds ratio [OR], 2.62; 95% confidence interval [CI], 2.01–3.43) (Fig. 1). Finally, in a recent retrospective study of more than 2000 patients by Toledo and colleagues [21], women who experienced breakthrough pain during the first stage of labor were more likely to undergo instrumental vaginal delivery. These studies suggest that the early onset of severe pain and higher labor analgesia requirements predict an increased risk of dysfunctional labor and

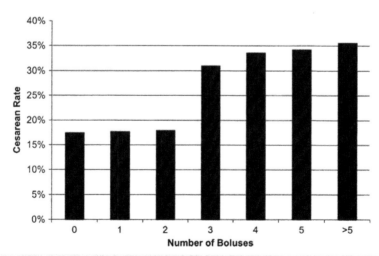

Fig. 1. The rate of cesarean delivery as a function of the incidence of breakthrough pain during epidural analgesia maintained with a continuous infusion of low-dose bupivacaine or bupivacaine-fentanyl. The need for supplemental bolus analgesia was considered a marker for breakthrough pain. The rate of cesarean delivery was more than twice as high in women who required 3 or more supplemental bolus doses than in women who required 2 or fewer bolus doses (OR, 2.62; 95% CI, 2.01–3.43). (*From* Hess PE, Pratt SD, Soni AK, et al. Association between severe labor pain and cesarean delivery. Anesth Analg 2000;90:883; with permission.)

operative delivery, thereby possibly explaining the observed association between neuraxial analgesia and operative delivery.

THE EFFECT OF NEURAXIAL ANALGESIA ON CESAREAN DELIVERY RATES

Randomized controlled trials

Multiple randomized controlled trials have investigated the effect of neuraxial analgesia on cesarean delivery rates compared with systemic analgesia [4,22–37]. A 2005 meta-analysis by Halpern and Leighton [38] included a total of 17 studies involving 6701 women. The OR for cesarean delivery was 1.03 (95% CI, 0.86–1.22) for systemic opioid compared with neuraxial analgesia. Although differing in many variables (eg, parity, type of neuraxial analgesia, crossover rate, labor management), all of the studies analyzed in this systematic review, except one, found no difference in cesarean delivery rates between women who received neuraxial versus systemic analgesia.

The single dissenting study was by Thorp and colleagues [37], in which 93 nulliparous women were randomized to receive either epidural analgesia or systemic meperidine analgesia. Twelve (25%) of the women in the epidural group underwent cesarean delivery, compared with 1 (2%) patient in the meperidine group. Several factors, however, in the study design and results are of concern. First, there was an anomalous outcome in the cesarean delivery rate for both groups: the cesarean delivery rate in the epidural group was significantly higher, and that in the meperidine group significantly lower, than the historical norm (15%) for the study institution. Second, the investigators were ultimately responsible for deciding the method of delivery, which has obvious bias implications. Third, there was no standardization between groups of other factors known to influence labor outcomes, specifically timing and dose of oxytocin, and timing of rupture of membranes.

Investigators from the Parkland Hospital of the University of Texas Southwestern in Dallas performed 4 randomized trials investigating this topic [4,24,35,36]. This institution is unique in that the patient population is composed primarily of indigent, Hispanic parturients, whose labor is managed by the same group of resident physicians and midwives, supervised by the same core group of attending obstetricians, who all work in shifts. As such, this distinctive organizational structure minimizes the impact of several factors that are known to confound results of similar studies (ie, patient and obstetric provider variability, and style of labor management).

Their first study investigated 1330 women of mixed parity who were randomized to receive either epidural bupivacaine-fentanyl or intravenous meperidine for labor analgesia. The investigators reported a cesarean delivery rate of 9.0% in the epidural group versus 3.9% in the meperidine groups [4]. However, a major flaw of this study was a lack of an intent-to-treat analysis of the data and a high crossover rate: approximately one-third of the women in each group did not receive the treatment to which they were randomized. Therefore, at a later date, the investigators performed a secondary analysis of their data with an intent-to-treat analysis, which revealed a cesarean delivery rate of 6% in both groups [39]. The investigators, in hopes of decreasing the crossover rate of the meperidine group, designed a second study in which meperidine was administered by patient-controlled intravenous analgesia (PCIA) [35]. Although, because of rapid labor, a significant number of women did not receive the treatment to which they were randomized, only 5 of 357 patients in the PCIA group crossed over to the epidural group. Again, after using an intent-to-treat analysis, the investigators found a cesarean delivery rate of 4% in the epidural group versus 5% in the PCIA group.

In a third randomized trial, the Parkland investigators compared cesarean delivery rates in women of mixed parity who were randomized to receive combined spinal-epidural (CSE) analgesia (intrathecal sufentanil 10 µg, followed by epidural bupivacaine with fentanyl at the second request for analgesia) or intravenous meperidine (50 mg every hour on request) [24]. Although only 60% of the patients received the treatment to which they were allocated, an intent-to-treat analysis of the data revealed a cesarean delivery rate of 6% in the CSE group versus 5.5% in the meperidine group. Finally, an individual patient meta-analysis of the Parkland Hospital studies (n = 4465) produced an OR for cesarean delivery of 1.04 (95% CI, 0.81–1.34) for epidural compared with systemic meperidine analgesia (Fig. 2) [40]. The results of these studies suggest that the administration of neuraxial analgesia, by itself, does not increase the risk of cesarean delivery.

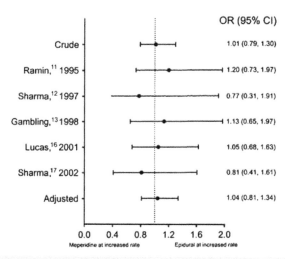

Fig. 2. Meta-analysis of studies from Parkland Hospital investigating cesarean delivery rates in women randomly assigned to neuraxial or systemic meperidine analgesia. The ORs with 95% CIs for each randomized study, and the overall crude and adjusted ORs with 95% CIs are shown. An OR less than 1 favored epidural more than meperidine analgesia. (*From* Sharma SK, McIntire DD, Wiley J, et al. Labor analgesia and cesarean delivery: an individual patient meta-analysis of nulliparous women. Anesthesiology 2004;100:146; with permission.)

Dose-response studies have been performed to determine whether the concentration of local anesthetic would have any impact on cesarean delivery rates. One such study, the COMET study, randomized 1054 women to 1 of 3 labor analgesia regimens: (1) high-dose epidural (intermittent boluses of bupivacaine 0.25%); (2) low-dose epidural (intermittent boluses of bupivacaine 0.1% and fentanyl 2 μg/mL); or (3) low-dose CSE analgesia (intrathecal bupivacaine 2.5 mg/fentanyl 25 μg, followed by intermittent boluses of bupivacaine 0.1% and fentanyl 2 μg/mL) [41]. The investigators found no difference in the cesarean delivery rate among the 3 groups. Three other randomized controlled trials comparing different concentrations of local anesthetic also found no difference between groups in terms of cesarean delivery rates [42–44]. These results suggest that that there is no dose-response effect of local anesthetic concentrations on cesarean delivery rates. Furthermore, these results suggest that the mode of neuraxial analgesia imparts no effect on cesarean delivery rates because several of these studies also compared the effect of CSE analgesia versus epidural analgesia.

Impact studies

Impact studies are a second type of study design used to investigate the effect of a specific treatment modality on patient outcomes. Also known as before-after studies, these studies are designed to assess the incidence of a patient outcome before and after the implementation of a specific treatment. A benefit of this type of study design is that it eliminates the crossover rate between treatment groups, because the control group is the time period before the treatment implementation. Furthermore, the results of these studies may have more external validity, as patients have not chosen to participate in a study, and therefore may present a more realistic representation of the general population. However, in interpreting the results from these types of studies, one must assume that there were no other changes in the medical or obstetric management of patients between the "before" and "after" time periods.

The largest impact study investigating the impact of neuraxial labor analgesia on cesarean delivery rates was a 1999 study by Yancey and colleagues [45], in which cesarean delivery rates at the Tripler Army Hospital in Hawaii were compared before and after 1993. Before 1993, the rate of epidural analgesia at this hospital was less than 1%. However, in 1993, a policy change within the United States Department of Defense mandated the on-demand availability of neuraxial analgesia for labor in military hospitals. This change resulted in an increase in the rate of epidural labor analgesia to 80% over a 1-year period. Yet, during this same period, the cesarean delivery rate in nulliparous patients in spontaneous labor remained unchanged (19.0% versus 19.4%). Several other impact studies have also shown no association with cesarean delivery rates and rates of epidural administration [46–51]. These findings were further confirmed in a meta-analysis which included 9 impact studies of more than 37,000 patients. Again, there was no increase in the rate of cesarean delivery in a period of increased rate of use of epidural analgesia compared with a historical control period (Fig. 3) [52]. These results further support the results of randomized controlled trials in refuting the hypothesis that neuraxial labor analgesia increases the risk of cesarean delivery.

Timing of initiation of neuraxial analgesia

For several years, the American College of Obstetricians and Gynecologists (ACOG) recommended that women delay requesting epidural analgesia, "when feasible, until the cervix is dilated to 4 to 5 cm" [53]. This recommendation was primarily based on data from observational studies, suggesting an association between cesarean delivery and the initiation of neuraxial analgesia during early labor (defined as cervical dilation less than 4–5 cm) [54,55]. However, similar to the cause-and-effect question raised earlier regarding neuraxial analgesia and cesarean delivery, a similar question is whether early initiation of neuraxial labor analgesia causes an increase in the rate of cesarean delivery or is merely associated with an increased risk of cesarean delivery.

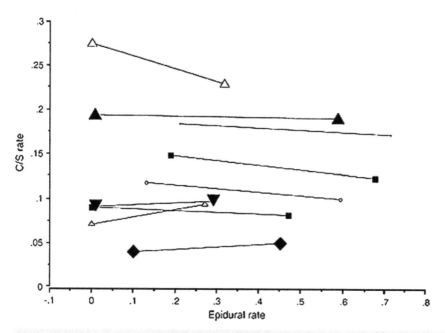

Fig. 3. Rates of cesarean delivery during periods of higher and lower availability of epidural analgesia in 9 studies (n = 37,753) subjected to meta-analysis. Each pair of symbols shows data from 1 investigation (the left symbol is the epidural analgesia rate and cesarean rate during the period of low epidural availability and the right symbol is the epidural analgesia rate and cesarean delivery rate during the period of high epidural availability). The size of the plot symbol is proportional to the number of patients included in the analysis. (*From* Segal S, Su M, Gilbert P. The effect of a rapid change in availability of epidural analgesia on the cesarean delivery rate: A meta-analysis. Am J Obstet Gynecol 2000;183:976; with permission.)

Several randomized controlled trials have addressed this issue by comparing early-labor neuraxial analgesia to systemic opioid analgesia followed by neuraxial analgesia at cervical dilation of 4 to 5 cm [56–60]. Two studies by Chestnut and colleagues [56,57] randomized nulliparous women in spontaneous labor or those receiving oxytocin to 1 of 2 groups: early epidural analgesia or early intravenous nalbuphine analgesia followed by epidural analgesia when cervical dilation reached 5 cm. The investigators found no difference between groups in the cesarean delivery rate, but the median cervical dilation at the time of initiation of analgesia was 3.5 to 4.0 cm. However, many women, especially those undergoing induction of labor, request analgesia at a smaller cervical dilation. Wong and colleagues and Ohel and colleagues [59,60] reported randomized trials of early-labor neuraxial analgesia compared with systemic opioid analgesia in which the median cervical dilation at initiation of analgesia was 2 cm. Similar to the results of the previous studies, there was no difference in the rate of cesarean delivery in the 2 groups, nor was there a difference in the rate of instrumental vaginal delivery. The results of these studies prompted the ACOG, in 2006, to publish an updated committee opinion entitled *Analgesia and Cesarean Delivery Rates*, recommending that:

> In the absence of a medical contraindication, maternal request is a sufficient medical indication for pain relief during labor. The fear of unnecessary cesarean delivery should not influence the method of pain relief that women can choose during labor [61].

Finally, a 2007 meta-analysis of 8 randomized controlled trials and cohort studies of early labor versus late labor initiation of neuraxial analgesia (n = 3320) confirmed this recommendation by demonstrating that early initiation of neuraxial analgesia does not cause an increase in the rate of cesarean delivery (Fig. 4)[62].

THE EFFECT OF NEURAXIAL ANESTHESIA ON THE INSTRUMENTAL VAGINAL DELIVERY RATE

There are observational data linking neuraxial labor analgesia and an increased rate of instrumental vaginal delivery (ie, forceps delivery or vacuum extraction). Although assessed as a secondary outcome in numerous trials, no randomized clinical trial has assessed the effect of neuraxial analgesia on mode of vaginal delivery as its primary outcome. However, similar to the data of the studies investigating the effect of neuraxial analgesia on cesarean delivery rates, interpretation of these data is difficult because of the presence of multiple confounding factors: station and position of the fetal vertex, maternal pain and the urge to bear down, and neuraxial analgesia-induced motor blockade. The contribution of these factors to the mode of vaginal delivery, and their interactions, are not well understood, and have not been well controlled in many studies.

Nevertheless, most systematic reviews have concluded that epidural analgesia is associated with an increased risk of instrumental vaginal delivery

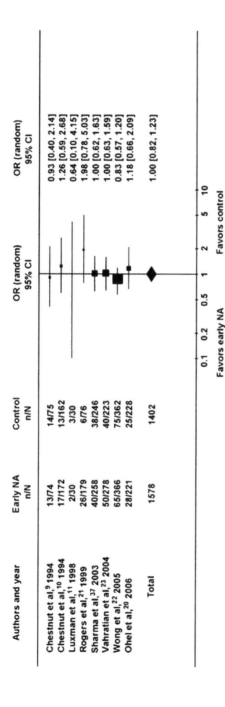

Authors and year	Early NA n/N	Control n/N	OR (random) 95% CI	OR (random) 95% CI
Chestnut et al,[9] 1994	13/74	14/75		0.93 [0.40, 2.14]
Chestnut et al,[10] 1994	17/172	13/162		1.26 [0.59, 2.68]
Luxman et al,[11] 1998	2/30	3/30		0.64 [0.10, 4.15]
Rogers et al,[21] 1999	26/179	6/76		1.98 [0.78, 5.03]
Sharma et al,[37] 2003	40/258	38/246		1.00 [0.62, 1.63]
Vahratian et al,[23] 2004	50/278	40/223		1.00 [0.63, 1.59]
Wong et al,[22] 2005	65/366	75/362		0.83 [0.57, 1.20]
Ohel et al,[20] 2006	28/221	25/228		1.18 [0.66, 2.09]
Total	1578	1402		1.00 [0.82, 1.23]

0.1 0.2 0.5 1 2 5 10

Favors early NA   Favors control

Fig. 4. Meta-analysis of rates of cesarean delivery for individual studies comparing early-labor initiation of neuraxial analgesia with control (initiation of neuraxial analgesia at cervical dilation of 4–5 cm). The size of the box at the point estimate for each study is proportional to the number of patients in the study. The diamond represents the point estimate of the pooled OR and the length of the diamond is proportional to the CI. n, number of events (cesarean delivery) in the treatment or control group; N, total number of patients in the treatment or control group; NA, neuraxial analgesia. (From Marucci M, Cinnella G, Perchiazzi G, et al. Patient-requested neuraxial analgesia for labor: impact on rates of cesarean and instrumental vaginal delivery. Anesthesiology 2007;106:1041; with permission.)

compared with systemic analgesia [38,40]. For example, in the most recent meta-analysis of 17 studies by Halpern and Leighton [38], the OR for instrumental vaginal delivery in women randomized to receive epidural, compared with systemic, opioid analgesia was 1.92 (95% CI, 1.52–2.42). Similarly, in the individual patient meta-analysis reported by Sharma and colleagues [40], and a 2004 meta-analysis by Liu and colleagues [63], the adjusted ORs were 1.86 (95% CI, 1.43–2.40) and 1.63 (95% CI, 1.12–2.37), respectively.

In contrast to the results of these studies, many impact studies have observed no difference in the instrumental vaginal delivery rate before and after the availability of neuraxial analgesia [45,48,50,64]. For example, the rate of instrumental vaginal delivery did not change at Tripler Army Hospital (11.1% vs 11.9%), despite the large increase in epidural analgesia rate [45]. These results were further confirmed in a systematic review of 7 impact studies involving more than 28,000 patients, which also showed no difference in instrumental vaginal delivery rates (mean change, 0.76%; 95% CI, –1.2% to 2.8%) [52].

These conflicting results underscore the potential impact of multiple confounding factors on data interpretation for this topic. The density of neuraxial analgesia during the second stage of labor has been implicated as one confounding factor. Theoretically, there are several reasons why this makes sense. First, high concentrations of epidural local anesthetic may result in maternal motor blockade, resulting in relaxation of pelvic and pelvic floor musculature, which, in turn, may interfere with fetal rotation during descent. Second, abdominal wall muscle relaxation secondary to local anesthetic-induced motor blockade may decrease the effectiveness of maternal expulsive efforts. Third, dense sensory blockade of the uterus may decrease maternal ability to coordinate expulsive efforts with uterine contractions. Finally, obstetricians may be more likely to perform elective instrumental vaginal deliveries in patients with effective second-stage analgesia than in patients without analgesia.

Adding even more confusion to this topic is the fact that the density of neuraxial analgesia is, in turn, influenced by several other factors, including specific analgesic technique, local anesthetic concentration, total dose of local anesthetic, and degree of motor blockade, all of which overlap and are difficult to study. Several randomized studies have investigated the effect of bupivacaine concentrations on the rate of instrumental vaginal delivery, with conflicting outcomes [41,43,44,65]. For example, in a large study (n = 1000) by Olofsson and colleagues [44], women randomized to low-dose bupivacaine 0.125% with sufentanil had a lower instrumental vaginal delivery rate than those who received high-dose bupivacaine 0.25% with epinephrine. In contrast, Collis and colleagues [42] found no difference in the instrumental vaginal delivery rate between parturients randomized to receive low-dose CSE (intrathecal bupivacaine/fentanyl followed by intermittent boluses of epidural bupivacaine 0.1%/fentanyl 2 µg/mL) versus traditional high-dose epidural (0.25% bupivacaine).

Even more puzzling were the results from the COMET study, in which a lower rate of instrumental vaginal delivery was noted in the groups randomized to receive either the low-dose epidural or CSE technique, compared with the group who received 0.25% bupivacaine [41]. However, the total bupivacaine dose in the high-dose epidural group did not differ from the low-dose epidural group because the former was given by intermittent injection and the latter by continuous infusion. On the other hand, the total bupivacaine dose in the CSE group was significantly lower.

To add further uncertainty to the picture, the method of maintenance of epidural analgesia (ie, continuous infusion versus intermittent boluses) affects the density of the neuraxial blockade. In general, continuous infusion techniques result in higher total doses of bupivacaine (and, thus, a greater degree of motor blockade) compared with intermittent bolus techniques. However, the relationship between motor blockade and instrumental vaginal delivery is inconsistent. A randomized trial of 57 parturients by Smedstad and Morison [66] demonstrated a higher incidence of instrumental vaginal delivery when bupivacaine 0.25% was administered as a continuous epidural infusion compared with intermittent bolus injections. However, 2 later studies (a 2006 study by Wong and colleagues [67] and the COMET study) noted no difference in the instrumental vaginal delivery rate between groups who received low-dose bupivacaine/fentanyl either by intermittent bolus or continuous infusion [41]. Furthermore, a meta-analysis comparing patient-controlled epidural analgesia (PCEA, without background infusions) with continuous epidural infusions found lower doses of bupivacaine and less-dense motor blockade in the PCEA group, but no difference in the rate of instrumental vaginal delivery [68]. The inconsistency in the results among studies may be explained by the actual absolute difference in bupivacaine doses/concentrations (0.25% and 0.125% vs 0.125% and 0.0625%) and motor blockade.

A recent study by Cappiello and colleagues [69] demonstrated, as a secondary outcome, a higher incidence of instrumental vaginal delivery in patients who received a dura-arachnoid puncture with a 25-gauge spinal needle without intrathecal medication before epidural drug administration compared with patients who received epidural analgesia without a dura-arachnoid puncture. Although the total dose of bupivacaine between the 2 groups was not different, the potentially higher intrathecal exposure of local anesthetics may have contributed to this result. However, a recent prospective randomized trial by Kamiya and colleagues [70] demonstrated that lidocaine concentrations in cerebrospinal fluid were similar with or without a prior dura-arachnoid puncture, when the cerebrospinal fluid collection site was only 1 interspace from the epidural lidocaine administration site. The results of this study suggest that, although a small amount of local anesthetic does cross through a dural hole during epidural administration, the amount is trivial compared with the amount crossing through the intact dura-arachnoid. Moreover, the results of the COMET study demonstrate no difference in instrumental delivery rates between the low-dose epidural infusion group and CSE group, also suggesting that the presence of a dura-arachnoid puncture does not play a major role [41].

Further studies are needed to determine whether the presence of a dural puncture influences the rate of instrumental vaginal delivery.

If effective neuraxial analgesia prolongs the second stage of labor and increases the risk of instrumental vaginal delivery, one could speculate that discontinuation of neuraxial analgesia during the second stage of labor would result in less time in second stage and a lower instrumental vaginal delivery rate. Several studies have specifically assessed the effect of maintenance of neuraxial analgesia until delivery with regard to the duration and outcome of the second stage of labor, with conflicting results [71–76]. Nevertheless, discontinuation of second-stage neuraxial analgesia may theoretically pose more of a risk than a benefit to the mother and fetus. First, ineffective sacral analgesia may result in decreased maternal expulsive efforts secondary to severe pain. Second, discontinuing the maintenance of neuraxial analgesia may result in difficulty in reestablishing analgesia or anesthesia for operative delivery (especially in emergent situations) or for postpartum perineal repairs. Third, decreases in maintenance analgesia rates have been shown to be associated with higher rates of instrumental vaginal delivery. A recent study by Abenhaim and Fraser [77] found that suboptimal epidural analgesia during the second stage of labor was associated with an increased risk of adverse obstetric outcomes, including cesarean delivery, midpelvic procedures, low pelvic rotations, and third- or fourth-degree perineal tears. As such, the benefits of discontinuing or decreasing the rate of maintenance neuraxial analgesia during the second stage of labor must be weighed against the potential risks on a case-by-case basis.

As stated earlier, the available evidence suggests that effective second-stage neuraxial labor analgesia results in an increased risk of instrumental vaginal delivery. Increased rates of instrumental vaginal delivery are important to mothers and obstetric anesthesia providers because they may be associated with an increase in risk for short-term and long-term neonatal and maternal morbidity. Minimizing the risk of instrumental vaginal delivery while maximizing patient comfort is an art and a science, requiring the attention of the anesthesia provider to the individual needs of each patient. As such, a single analgesic technique or single dose/concentration of drug(s) will not work for everyone. However, based on the available evidence, the best technique to achieve these goals involves the use of PCEA using a dilute solution of local anesthetic with an opioid.

THE EFFECT OF NEURAXIAL ANALGESIA ON THE DURATION OF LABOR
First stage of labor
Similar to studies addressing the impact of neuraxial labor analgesia on instrumental delivery rates, no randomized controlled trials to date have investigated the effect of neuraxial analgesia on the duration of the first stage of labor as a primary outcome. However, studies that have treated this parameter as a secondary outcome have conflicting results, primarily due to variations in study design and the impact of confounding factors influencing uterine activity.

Determining the duration of labor requires documentation of a start and end time. Although the end time to the first stage of labor is clearly defined as a cervical dilation of 10 cm, the definition of the start time varies among studies (but is usually consistent between groups within a study). Yet even the determination of complete cervical dilation is influenced by variations in study protocols regarding frequency of cervical examinations. Most studies do not require regular cervical examinations, or, if they do, the intervals are usually far apart. As such, full cervical dilation is often diagnosed with a cervical examination only when the patient complains of rectal or vaginal pressure, which is likely to occur at a later time in women with effective neuraxial analgesia than in women with systemic opioid analgesia. Therefore, the duration of the first stage of labor may be artificially prolonged simply because of the presence of effective labor analgesia.

Changes in uterine activity are known to significantly impact the duration of the first stage of labor. Studies have observed increases and decreases in uterine activity with neuraxial labor analgesia [78–83]. However, there are several confounding factors which can increase or decrease uterine activity. Cheek and colleagues [84] and Zamoroa and colleagues [85] demonstrated decreased uterine activity after the intravenous administration of 1 L of crystalloid solution, but not after infusion of 0.5 L. One hypothesis to explain this observation is that a fluid bolus may inhibit the release of antidiuretic hormone from the posterior pituitary gland, which in turn may also transiently result in decreased production of oxytocin, which is also released by this organ. Because fluid boluses are routinely administered during neuraxial analgesia placement, this may partially explain the decrease in uterine activity with neuraxial analgesia.

Furthermore, epidural analgesia has itself been suggested to result in decreased levels of hormones known to increase uterine activity. In a prospective, nonrandomized study by Rahm and colleagues [82], epidural analgesia (bupivacaine with sufentanil) was associated with a decline in plasma oxytocin levels 60 minutes after initiation of analgesia, compared with patients who did not receive epidural analgesia. Furthermore, Behrens and colleagues [78] observed decreased plasma levels of prostaglandin $F_{2\alpha}$ in patients who received epidural analgesia during the first stage of labor. Therefore, these results suggest that epidural analgesia may play a role in decreasing uterine activity during the first stage of labor.

However, increased uterine activity after neuraxial analgesia has also been reported [79] Initiation of neuraxial analgesia is associated with an acute decrease in maternal plasma concentrations of epinephrine due to sympathectomy and acute pain relief [8]. Epinephrine is a tocolytic agent due to its effects on β-adrenergic receptors. An acute decrease in maternal epinephrine concentrations may result in increased uterine activity. In a 2009 randomized, double-blind, controlled trial by Abráo and colleagues [86], parturients who received CSE analgesia for labor had a higher incidence of uterine tachysystole (hypertonus) compared with women receiving a traditional epidural analgesia. Although maternal plasma epinephrine concentrations were not obtained in this study, the hypothesis proposed by the investigators to explain these findings was that the quicker onset of pain relief and sympathectomy in the CSE group caused a more precipitous decrease in maternal epinephrine concentrations, resulting in uterine tachysystole. However, the duration of the first stage of labor was not assessed as an outcome in this study, and other randomized controlled trials of CSE versus epidural technique have not found a difference in the duration of the first stage of labor [41,43,87]. Moreover, other studies have suggested that the addition of epinephrine 1.25 to 5 μg/mL (1:800,000 to 1:200,000) to epidural anesthetic solutions does not affect the progress of labor, despite systemic absorption of the medication [88–93].

Even more confusingly, randomized controlled trials specifically investigating first stage of labor duration as a secondary outcome have also reported conflicting results. In their trials examining the impact of early neuraxial analgesia administration during labor, Wong and colleagues [60] and Ohel and colleagues [59] found that the duration of the first stage of labor was significantly reduced in women randomized to receive early-labor neuraxial analgesia compared with systemic opioid analgesia. In contrast, a meta-analysis of 9 studies by Halpern and Leighton [38] found no difference between parturients randomized to receive epidural or systemic opioid labor analgesia. A 2005 Cochrane review of 9 studies (n = 2328) reported no difference in the duration of the first stage of labor among women receiving epidural labor analgesia and those receiving systemic opioid analgesia or no analgesia [1]. Yet meta-analysis of the Parkland Hospital data demonstrated prolongation of the first stage of labor by approximately 30 minutes in nulliparous women receiving neuraxial compared with systemic opioid analgesia [40].

The data suggest that neuraxial labor analgesia has a variable effect on the duration of the first stage of labor: it may prolong it in some patients, but shorten it in others. However, in those studies that have shown an association with prolongation of the first stage of labor and neuraxial analgesia, there has been no increase in adverse maternal or neonatal outcomes due to increased labor time.

Second stage of labor
The consensus among obstetric and anesthesia providers is that effective neuraxial analgesia prolongs the second stage of labor. Multiple meta-analyses of randomized controlled trials of neuraxial versus systemic opioid analgesia in which duration of the second stage of labor was assessed as a secondary outcome variable support this consensus opinion, demonstrating a mean second-stage duration approximately 15 minutes longer in women receiving neuraxial analgesia [38,40]. As such, the ACOG has incorporated the presence or absence of neuraxial analgesia into their definition of second-stage dystocia [94]. However, the ACOG also states that the need for intervention (instrumental or surgical) should not be mandated solely on second-stage duration, especially if progress is being made. Paterson and colleagues [95] evaluated the second stage of labor in 25,069 women who delivered an infant of at least

37 weeks' gestation, with a vertex presentation, after the spontaneous onset of labor. The investigators concluded that, for parous women not using epidural analgesia, the likelihood of spontaneous vaginal delivery after 1 hour in the second stage was low, but in parous women using epidural analgesia, and in all nulliparae, there was no clear cut-off point for expectation of spontaneous delivery. Moreover, several studies suggest that a prolonged second stage of labor does not result in adverse maternal or fetal outcomes, provided that fetal status is reassuring, the mother is well hydrated and has adequate analgesia, and there is progress in fetal head descent [96–98].

One potential factor influencing the length and outcome of the second stage of labor is the decision as to whether patients should begin pushing as soon as full cervical dilation is diagnosed or delay until the fetus reaches a lower station. Although several studies have investigated the impact of immediate and delayed pushing on second-stage labor duration and outcomes in women with neuraxial analgesia, the data are conflicting. The Pushing Early or Pushing Late with Epidural (PEOPLE) study, published in 2000, was a large (n = 1862), randomized, multicenter, controlled trial that demonstrated increased rate of spontaneous vaginal delivery, shorter duration of pushing, and lower incidence of midrotational forceps delivery in women randomized to delayed pushing, compared with women in the immediate pushing group [99]. However, the duration of second-stage labor was longer in the delayed pushing group. These results are in contrast to a 2004 meta-analysis of 9 studies (n = 3000), which concluded that delayed pushing did not decrease the rate of instrumental vaginal delivery or cesarean delivery, but did decrease the rate of midpelvic rotational forceps deliveries (Fig. 5) [100]. Therefore, delayed pushing does not seem to impart any major maternal or neonatal benefits, although it is not unreasonable to delay pushing until the fetus has descended from a high fetal station.

Third stage of labor
Only 1 study reviewed the impact of neuraxial analgesia on the duration of the third stage of labor. In a 3-year retrospective study (n = 7468) by Rosaeg and colleagues [101], epidural analgesia was not associated with a prolonged third stage of labor in parturients with spontaneous or expressed placental delivery. However, the duration of the third stage of labor was shorter in women who received epidural analgesia and underwent manual removal of the placenta. The investigators concluded that epidural analgesia facilitated earlier manual removal secondary to improved pain control.

OXYTOCIN ADMINISTRATION AND AMBULATION
Oxytocin
The use of high-dose oxytocin to treat ineffective uterine contractions has become a key component in the active management of labor. Several randomized controlled trials comparing neuraxial analgesia with systemic opioid have noted a higher rate of oxytocin augmentation [4,40,102]. However, the

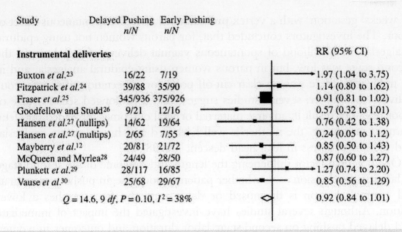

Fig. 5. Meta-analysis of the effect of delayed versus early pushing on the rate of instrumental vaginal delivery among women with neuraxial analgesia. The size of the box at the point estimate for each study is proportional to the number of patients in the study. The diamond represents the point estimate of the pooled relative risk (RR) and the length of the diamond is proportional to the CI. n, number of events (instrumental vaginal delivery) in the treatment or control group; N, total number of patients in the treatment or control group; RR, relative risk; CI, confidence interval. (*From* Roberts CL, Torvaldsen S, Cameron CA, et al. Delayed versus early pushing in women with epidural analgesia: a systemic review and meta-analysis. BJOG 2004;111:1335; with permission.)

relationship between neuraxial labor analgesia, oxytocin administration, and labor outcomes remains unclear, primarily because of a lack of control of oxytocin management in study designs.

Kotaska and colleagues [103] hypothesized that the negative results of studies comparing labor outcome in women randomized to neuraxial versus systemic opioid analgesia depend on the manner in which oxytocin is used. In a review of the literature, they identified 18 randomized controlled trials comparing epidural analgesia with systemic opioid. In 8 of these studies the labor outcomes and management protocols were well-described [103]. The investigators found that 7 out of the 8 trials used active management of labor protocols with high-dose oxytocin, with each trial demonstrating no difference in cesarean delivery rates. The eighth trial used a low-dose oxytocin regimen and found a higher rate of cesarean delivery in the neuraxial analgesia group [37]. Based on this analysis, the investigators concluded that epidural analgesia in the setting of low-dose oxytocin administration likely increases the rate of cesarean delivery. However, this conclusion is suspect, as it is based on the results of a single study, a study which other systemic reviews have identified as the only randomized controlled trial with a higher cesarean delivery rate in the epidural group than in the systemic opioid group. Furthermore, the remaining 11 studies not included in the analysis because of a lack of description of the labor management protocol, most likely used low-dose oxytocin protocols, which Kotaska and colleagues [103] found to be the most common method of oxytocin administration in North America. As such, these excluded studies most likely demonstrated no difference in cesarean delivery rates between neuraxial and systemic labor analgesia (the studies were not cited by the authors), despite the use of low-dose oxytocin.

Further evidence supporting a negligible effect of oxytocin administration in labor outcomes in patients receiving neuraxial labor analgesia can be found in studies evaluating the impact of early versus late neuraxial analgesia. Two parallel studies by Chestnut and colleagues [56,57] (one evaluating the incidence of cesarean delivery in women without prior or planned oxytocin administration, and the other evaluating the incidence of operative delivery in women receiving oxytocin induction or augmentation), yielded similar results in terms of operative delivery rates, despite differences in oxytocin usage. In a 2005 study by Wong and colleagues [60] early and late neuraxial groups had high oxytocin use rates (93%). However, the early systemic opioid group had a higher mean maximum oxytocin infusion rate than the neuraxial analgesia group, despite having a median duration of labor that was 90 minutes longer. Similarly, in a 2006 study by Ohel and colleagues [59] the duration of labor was shorter in the early neuraxial analgesia group, even though there was a low rate of oxytocin use in both groups (29% in the early group vs 27% in the late group).

As such, it seems that oxytocin does not play a major role in studies investigating the impact of neuraxial analgesia on labor outcomes, despite a lack of control for this factor in many study designs. In fact, the ACOG supports the use of oxytocin for management of first- or second-stage labor dystocia, regardless of whether the patient is receiving neuraxial analgesia [94].

Ambulation
Several randomized controlled trials investigating the impact of ambulation versus bed rest during the first stage of labor in women receiving neuraxial labor analgesia do not demonstrate any benefit with ambulation [43,104–107]. These results are further supported by a meta-analysis of 5 randomized controlled trials (n = 1161) which found no difference in the duration of labor between women randomized to ambulate or not [108].

SUMMARY
Neuraxial labor analgesia has some effects on the course, duration, and outcome of labor. The data clearly show that neuraxial labor analgesia does not increase the risk of cesarean delivery compared with systemic analgesia. In addition, initiation of neuraxial analgesia early in labor (ie, cervical dilation less than 4 cm) does not increase the rate of cesarean delivery or prolong the duration of labor. However, effective neuraxial analgesia prolongs the second stage of labor and, more than likely, increases the risk of instrumental vaginal delivery.

Ideally, a labor analgesia technique would provide continuous, reliable analgesia, with no or minimal risk to mother and fetus, and have no detrimental effects on the progress of labor. Unfortunately, no single, universal method of managing labor pain exists that also meets these requirements. Multiple obstetric and anesthetic factors exist that require tailoring of management of labor analgesia to individual patient needs. Ultimately, it is each anesthetic provider's responsibility to take these factors into account to provide safe and effective neuraxial analgesia for each laboring parturient, while minimizing the risk of operative delivery.

References

[1] Anim-Somuah M, Smyth RMD, Howell CJ. Epidural versus non-epidural or no analgesia in labour. Cochrane Database of Systematic Reviews 2005;(4):CD000331.

[2] Howell CJ, Chalmers I. A review of prospectively controlled comparisons of epidural with non-epidural forms of pain relief during labour. Int J Obstet Anesth 1992;1:93–110.

[3] Paech MJ. The King Edward Memorial Hospital 1,000 mother survey of methods of pain relief in labour. Anaesth Intensive Care 1991;19:393–9.

[4] Ramin SM, Gambling DR, Lucas MJ, et al. Randomized trial of epidural versus intravenous analgesia during labor. Obstet Gynecol 1995;86:783–9.

[5] Jouppila R, Hollmen A. The effect of segmental epidural analgesia on maternal and foetal acid-base balance, lactate, serum potassium and creatine phosphokinase during labour. Acta Anaesthesiol Scand 1976;20:259–68.

[6] Lederman RP, Lederman E, Work B, et al. Anxiety and epinephrine in multiparous labor: relationship to duration of labor and fetal heart rate pattern. Am J Obstet Gynecol 1985;153:870–7.

[7] Levinson G, Shnider SM, deLorimier AA, et al. Effects of maternal hyperventilation on uterine blood flow and fetal oxygenation and acid-base status. Anesthesiology 1974;40:340–7.

[8] Shnider SM, Abboud T, Artal R, et al. Maternal catecholamines decrease during labor after lumbar epidural analgesia. Am J Obstet Gynecol 1983;147:13–5.

[9] National Health Service Maternity Statistics 2007–08. Available at: http://www.ic.nhs.uk/statistics-and-data-collections/hospital-care/maternity/nhs-maternity-statistics-england:-2007-08. Accessed June 01, 2009.

[10] Bucklin BA, Hawkins JL, Anderson JR, et al. Obstetric anesthesia workforce survey: twenty-year update. Anesthesiology 2005;103:645–53.

[11] Sivalingam T, Pleuvry BJ. Actions of morphine, pethidine and pentazocine on the oestrus and pregnant rat uterus in vitro. Br J Anaesth 1985;57:430–3.

[12] Yoo KY, Lee J, Kim HS, et al. The effects of opioids on isolated human pregnant uterine muscles. Anesth Analg 2001;92:1006–9.

[13] Noble AD, Craft IL, Bootes JA, et al. Continuous lumbar epidural analgesia using bupivacaine: a study of the fetus and newborn child. J Obstet Gynaecol Br Commonw 1971;78:559–63.

[14] Neuhoff D, Burke MS, Porreco RP. Cesarean birth for failed progress in labor. Obstet Gynecol 1989;73:915–20.

[15] Guillemette J, Fraser WD. Differences between obstetricians in caesarean section rates and the management of labour. BJOG 1992;99:105–8.

[16] de Regt RH, Minkoff HL, Feldman J, et al. Relation of private or clinic care to the cesarean birth rate. N Engl J Med 1986;315:619–24.

[17] Fraser W, Usher RH, McLean FH, et al. Temporal variation in rates of cesarean section for dystocia: does "convenience" play a role? Am J Obstet Gynecol 1987;156:300–4.

[18] Wuitchik M, Bakal D, Lipshitz J. The clinical significance of pain and cognitive activity in latent labor. Obstet Gynecol 1989;73:35–42.

[19] Alexander JM, Sharma SK, McIntire DD, et al. Intensity of labor pain and cesarean delivery. Anesth Analg 2001;92:1524–8.

[20] Hess PE, Pratt SD, Soni AK, et al. An association between severe labor pain and cesarean delivery. Anesth Analg 2000;90:881–6.

[21] Toledo P, McCarthy RJ, Ebarvia MJ, et al. A retrospective case-controlled study of the association between request to discontinue second stage labor epidural analgesia and risk of instrumental vaginal delivery. Int J Obstet Anesth 2008;17: 304–8.

[22] Bofill JA, Vincent RD, Ross EL, et al. Nulliparous active labor, epidural analgesia, and cesarean delivery for dystocia. Am J Obstet Gynecol 1997;177:1465–70.

[23] Clark A, Carr D, Loyd G, et al. The influence of epidural analgesia on cesarean delivery rates: a randomized, prospective clinical trial. Am J Obstet Gynecol 1998;179:1527–33.

[24] Gambling DR, Sharma SK, Ramin SM, et al. A randomized study of combined spinal-epidural analgesia versus intravenous meperidine during labor: impact on cesarean delivery rate. Anesthesiology 1998;89:1336–44.

[25] Halpern SH, Breen TW, Campbell DC, et al. A multicenter, randomized, controlled trial comparing bupivacaine with ropivacaine for labor analgesia. Anesthesiology 2003;98:1431–5.

[26] Head BB, Owen J, Vincent RD Jr, et al. A randomized trial of intrapartum analgesia in women with severe preeclampsia. Obstet Gynecol 2002;99:452–7.

[27] Howell CJ, Kidd C, Roberts W, et al. A randomised controlled trial of epidural compared with non-epidural analgesia in labour. BJOG 2001;108:27–33.

[28] Jain S, Arya VK, Gopalan S, et al. Analgesic efficacy of intramuscular opioids versus epidural analgesia in labor. Int J Gynaecol Obstet 2003;83:19–27.

[29] Loughnan BA, Carli F, Romney M, et al. Randomized controlled comparison of epidural bupivacaine versus pethidine for analgesia in labour. Br J Anaesth 2000;84:715–9.

[30] Lucas MJ, Sharma SK, McIntire DD, et al. A randomized trial of labor analgesia in women with pregnancy-induced hypertension. Am J Obstet Gynecol 2001;185:970–5.

[31] Nikkola EM, Ekblad UU, Kerno PO, et al. Intravenous fentanyl PCA during labour. Can J Anaesth 1997;44:1248–55.

[32] Philipsen T, Jensen N H. Epidural block or parenteral pethidine as analgesic in labour: a randomized study concerning progress in labour and instrumental deliveries. Eur J Obstet Gynecol Reprod Biol 1989;30:27–33.

[33] Philipsen T, Jensen NH. Maternal opinion about analgesia in labour and delivery. A comparison of epidural blockade and intramuscular pethidine. Eur J Obstet Gynecol Reprod Biol 1990;34:205–10.

[34] Robinson JO, Rosen M, Evans JM, et al. Maternal opinion about analgesia for labour. A controlled trial between epidural block and intramuscular pethidine combined with inhalation. Anaesthesia 1980;35:1173–81.

[35] Sharma SK, Alexander JM, Messick G, et al. Cesarean delivery: a randomized trial of epidural analgesia versus intravenous meperidine analgesia during labor in nulliparous women. Anesthesiology 2002;96:546–51.

[36] Sharma SK, Sidawi JE, Ramin SM, et al. Cesarean delivery: a randomized trial of epidural versus patient-controlled meperidine analgesia during labor. Anesthesiology 1997;87: 487–94.

[37] Thorp JA, Hu DH, Albin RM, et al. The effect of intrapartum epidural analgesia on nulliparous labor: a randomized, controlled, prospective trial. Am J Obstet Gynecol 1993;169: 851–8.

[38] Halpern SH, Leighton BL. Epidural analgesia and the progress of labor. In: Halpern SH, Douglas MJ, editors. Evidence-based obstetric anesthesia. Oxford: Blackwell; 2005. p. 10–22.

[39] Sharma SK, Leveno KJ. Update: epidural analgesia does not increase cesarean births. Curr Anesthesiol Rep 2000;2:18–24.

[40] Sharma SK, McIntire DD, Wiley J, et al. Labor analgesia and cesarean delivery: an individual patient meta-analysis of nulliparous women. Anesthesiology 2004;100:142–8.

[41] Comparative Obstetric Mobile Epidural Trial Study Group UK. Effect of low-dose mobile versus traditional epidural techniques on mode of delivery: a randomised controlled trial. Lancet 2001;358:19–23.

[42] Collis RE, Davies DW, Aveling W. Randomised comparison of combined spinal-epidural and standard epidural analgesia in labour. Lancet 1995;345:1413–6.

[43] Nageotte MP, Larson D, Rumney PJ, et al. Epidural analgesia compared with combined spinal-epidural analgesia during labor in nulliparous women. N Engl J Med 1997;337: 1715–9.

[44] Olofsson C, Ekblom A, Ekman-Ordeberg G, et al. Obstetric outcome following epidural analgesia with bupivacaine-adrenaline 0.25% or bupivacaine 0.125% with sufentanil– a prospective randomized controlled study in 1000 parturients. Acta Anaesthesiol Scand 1998;42:284–92.

[45] Yancey MK, Pierce B, Schweitzer D, et al. Observations on labor epidural analgesia and operative delivery rates. Am J Obstet Gynecol 1999;180:353–9.

[46] Fogel ST, Shyken JM, Leighton BL, et al. Epidural labor analgesia and the incidence of Cesarean delivery for dystocia. Anesth Analg 1998;87:119–23.

[47] Gribble RK, Meier PR. Effect of epidural analgesia on the primary cesarean rate. Obstet Gynecol 1991;78:231–4.

[48] Impey L, MacQuillan K, Robson M. Epidural analgesia need not increase operative delivery rates. Am J Obstet Gynecol 2000;182:358–63.

[49] Johnson S, Rosenfield JA. The effect of epidural anesthesia on the length of labor. J Fam Pract 1995;40:244–7.

[50] Lyon DS, Knuckles G, Whitaker E, et al. The effect of instituting an elective labor epidural program on the operative delivery rate. Obstet Gynecol 1997;90:135–41.

[51] Socol ML, Garcia PM, Peaceman AM, et al. Reducing cesarean births at a primarily private university hospital. Am J Obstet Gynecol 1993;168:1748–58.

[52] Segal S, Su M, Gilbert P. The effect of a rapid change in availability of epidural analgesia on the cesarean delivery rate: a meta-analysis. Am J Obstet Gynecol 2000;183:974–8.

[53] American College of Obstetricians and Gynecology. ACOG practice bulletin obstetric analgesia and anesthesia no. 36 July 2002 American College of Obstetricians and Gynecology. Int J Gynaecol Obstet; 2002 100:177–191.

[54] Lieberman E, Lang JM, Cohen A, et al. Association of epidural analgesia with cesarean delivery in nulliparas. Obstet Gynecol 1996;88:993–1000.

[55] Thorp JA, Eckert LO, Ang MS, et al. Epidural analgesia and cesarean section for dystocia: risk factors in nulliparas. Am J Perinatol 1991;8:402–10.

[56] Chestnut DH, McGrath JM, Vincent RD, et al. Does early administration of epidural analgesia affect obstetric outcome in nulliparous women who are in spontaneous labor? Anesthesiology 1994;80:1201–8.

[57] Chestnut DH, Vincent RD, McGrath JM, et al. Does early administration of epidural analgesia affect obstetric outcome in nulliparous women who are receiving intravenous oxytocin? Anesthesiology 1994;90:1193–200.

[58] Luxman D, Wolman I, Groutz A, et al. The effect of early epidural block administration on the progression and outcome of labor. Int J Obstet Anesth 1998;7:161–4.

[59] Ohel G, Gonen R, Vaida S, et al. Early versus late initiation of epidural analgesia in labor: does it increase the risk of cesarean section? A randomized trial. Am J Obstet Gynecol 2006;194:600–5.

[60] Wong CA, Scavone BM, Peaceman AM, et al. The risk of cesarean delivery with neuraxial analgesia given early versus late in labor. N Engl J Med 2005;352: 655–65.

[61] American College of Obstetricians and Gynecologists Committee on Obstetric Practice. ACOG Committee Opinion No. 339 analgesia and cesarean delivery rates. Obstet Gynecol 2006;107:1487–8.

[62] Marucci M, Cinnella G, Perchiazzi G, et al. Patient-requested neuraxial analgesia for labor: impact on rates of cesarean and instrumental vaginal delivery. Anesthesiology 2007;106:1035–45.

[63] Liu EH, Sia AT, Liu EHC, et al. Rates of caesarean section and instrumental vaginal delivery in nulliparous women after low concentration epidural infusions or opioid analgesia: systematic review. BMJ 2004;328:1410–5.

[64] Zhang J, Yancey MK, Klebanoff MA, et al. Does epidural analgesia prolong labor and increase risk of cesarean delivery? A natural experiment. Am J Obstet Gynecol 2001;185:128–34.

[65] James KS, McGrady E, Quasim I, et al. Comparison of epidural bolus administration of 0.25% bupivacaine and 0.1% bupivacaine with 0.0002% fentanyl for analgesia during labour. Br J Anaesth 1998;81:501–10.

[66] Smedstad KG, Morison DH. A comparative study of continuous and intermittent epidural analgesia for labour and delivery. Can J Anaesth 1988;35:234–41.

[67] Wong CA, Ratliff JT, Sullivan JT, et al. A randomized comparison of programmed intermittent epidural bolus with continuous epidural infusion for labor analgesia. Anesth Analg 2006;102:904–9.

[68] van der Vyver M, Halpern S, Joseph G. Patient-controlled epidural analgesia versus continuous infusion for labour analgesia: a meta-analysis. Br J Anaesth 2002;89:459–65.

[69] Cappiello E, O'Rourke N, Segal S, et al. A randomized trial of dural puncture epidural technique compared with the standard epidural technique for labor analgesia. Anesth Analg 2008;107:1646–51.

[70] Kamiya Y, Kikuchi T, Inagawa G, et al. Lidocaine concentration in cerebrospinal fluid after epidural administration: a comparison between epidural and combined spinal-epidural anesthesia. Anesthesiology 2009;110:1127–32.

[71] Chestnut DH, Bates JN, Choi WW. Continuous infusion epidural analgesia with lidocaine: efficacy and influence during the second stage of labor. Obstet Gynecol 1987;69:323–7.

[72] Chestnut DH, Laszewski LJ, Pollack KL, et al. Continuous epidural infusion of 0.0625% bupivacaine-0.0002% fentanyl during the second stage of labor. Anesthesiology 1990;72:613–8.

[73] Chestnut DH, Vandewalker GE, Owen CL, et al. The influence of continuous epidural bupivacaine analgesia on the second stage of labor and method of delivery in nulliparous women. Anesthesiology 1987;66:774–80.

[74] Johnsrud ML, Dale PO, Lovland B. Benefits of continuous infusion epidural analgesia throughout vaginal delivery. Acta Obstet Gynecol Scand 1988;67:355–8.

[75] Luxman D, Wolman I, Niv D, et al. Effect of second-stage 0.25% epidural bupivacaine on the outcome of labor. Gynecol Obstet Invest 1996;42:167–70.

[76] Phillips KC, Thomas TA. Second stage of labour with or without extradural analgesia. Anaesthesia 1983;38:972–6.

[77] Abenhaim HA, Fraser WD. Impact of pain level on second-stage delivery outcomes among women with epidural analgesia: results from the PEOPLE study. Am J Obstet Gynecol 2008;199(49):500. e1–6.

[78] Behrens O, Goeschen K, Luck HJ, et al. Effects of lumbar epidural analgesia on prostaglandin F2 alpha release and oxytocin secretion during labor. Prostaglandins 1993;45:285–96.

[79] Clarke VT, Smiley RM, Finster M. Uterine hyperactivity after intrathecal injection of fentanyl for analgesia during labor: a cause of fetal bradycardia? Anesthesiology 1994;81:1083.

[80] Miller BM. Epidural analgesia during labour. Br J Anaesth 1999;82:304.

[81] Nielsen PE, Abouleish E, Meyer BA, et al. Effect of epidural analgesia on fundal dominance during spontaneous active-phase nulliparous labor. Anesthesiology 1996;84:540–4.

[82] Rahm VA, Hallgren A, Hogberg H, et al. Plasma oxytocin levels in women during labor with or without epidural analgesia: a prospective study. Acta Obstet Gynecol Scand 2002;81:1033–9.

[83] Schellenberg JC. Uterine activity during lumbar epidural analgesia with bupivacaine. Am J Obstet Gynecol 1977;127:26–31.

[84] Cheek TG, Samuels P, Miller F, et al. Normal saline i.v. fluid load decreases uterine activity in active labour. Br J Anaesth 1996;77:632–5.

[85] Zamora JE, Rosaeg OP, Lindsay MP, et al. Haemodynamic consequences and uterine contractions following 0.5 or 1.0 litre crystalloid infusion before obstetric epidural analgesia. Can J Anaesth 1996;43:347–52.

[86] Abrao KC, Francisco RP, Miyadahira S, et al. Elevation of uterine basal tone and fetal heart rate abnormalities after labor analgesia: a randomized controlled trial. Obstet Gynecol 2009;113:41–7.

[87] Norris MC, Fogel ST, Conway-Long C. Combined spinal-epidural versus epidural labor analgesia. Anesthesiology 2001;95:913–20.

[88] Abboud TK, David S, Nagappala S, et al. Maternal, fetal, and neonatal effects of lidocaine with and without epinephrine for epidural anesthesia in obstetrics. Anesth Analg 1984;63: 973–9.

[89] Abboud TK, Sheik-ol-Eslam A, Yanagi T, et al. Safety of efficacy of epinephrine added to bupivacaine for lumbar epidural analgesia in obstetrics. Anesth Analg 1985;64:585–91.

[90] Craft JB Jr, Epstein BS, Coakley CS. Effect of lidocaine with epinephrine versus lidocaine (plain) on induced labor. Anesth Analg 1972;51:243–6.

[91] Eisenach JC, Grice SC, Dewan DM. Epinephrine enhances analgesia produced by epidural bupivacaine during labor. Anesth Analg 1987;66:447–51.

[92] Grice SC, Eisenach JC, Dewan DM. Labor analgesia with epidural bupivacaine plus fentanyl: enhancement with epinephrine and inhibition with 2-chloroprocaine. Anesthesiology 1990;72:623–8.

[93] Yau G, Gregory MA, Gin T, et al. Obstetric epidural analgesia with mixtures of bupivacaine, adrenaline and fentanyl. Anaesthesia 1990;45:1020–3.

[94] American College of Obstetricians and Gynecologists. ACOG Practice Bulletin No. 49, December 2003: Dystocia and augmentation of labor. Obstet Gynecol 2003;102: 1445–54.

[95] Paterson CM, Saunders NS, Wadsworth J. The characteristics of the second stage of labour in 25,069 singleton deliveries in the North West Thames Health Region, 1988. BJOG 1992;99:377–80.

[96] Derham RJ, Crowhurst J, Crowther C. The second stage of labour: durational dilemmas. Aust N Z J Obstet Gynaecol 1991;31:31–6.

[97] Menticoglou SM, Manning F, Harman C, et al. Perinatal outcome in relation to second-stage duration. Am J Obstet Gynecol 1995;173:906–12.

[98] Saunders NS, Paterson CM, Wadsworth J. Neonatal and maternal morbidity in relation to the length of the second stage of labour. BJOG 1992;99:381–5.

[99] Fraser WD, Marcoux S, Krauss I, et al. Multicenter, randomized, controlled trial of delayed pushing for nulliparous women in the second stage of labor with continuous epidural analgesia. The PEOPLE (Pushing Early or Pushing Late with Epidural) Study Group. Am J Obstet Gynecol 2000;182:1165–72.

[100] Roberts CL, Torvaldsen S, Cameron CA, et al. Delayed versus early pushing in women with epidural analgesia: a systematic review and meta-analysis. BJOG 2004;111:1333–40.

[101] Rosaeg OP, Campbell N, Crossan ML. Epidural analgesia does not prolong the third stage of labour. Can J Anaesth 2002;49:490–2.

[102] Leighton BL, Halpern SH. The effects of epidural analgesia on labor, maternal, and neonatal outcomes: a systematic review. Am J Obstet Gynecol 2002;186:S69–77.

[103] Kotaska AJ, Klein MC, Liston RM. Epidural analgesia associated with low-dose oxytocin augmentation increases cesarean births: a critical look at the external validity of randomized trials. Am J Obstet Gynecol 2006;194:809–14.

[104] Collis RE, Harding SA, Morgan BM. Effect of maternal ambulation on labour with low-dose combined spinal-epidural analgesia. Anaesthesia 1999;54:535–9.

[105] Frenea S, Chirossel C, Rodriguez R, et al. The effects of prolonged ambulation on labor with epidural analgesia. Anesth Analg 2004;98:224–9.

[106] Karraz MA. Ambulatory epidural anesthesia and the duration of labor. Int J Gynaecol Obstet 2003;80:117–22.

[107] Vallejo MC, Firestone LL, Mandell GL, et al. Effect of epidural analgesia with ambulation on labor duration. Anesthesiology 2001;95:857–61.

[108] Roberts CL, Algert CS, Olive E. Impact of first-stage ambulation on mode of delivery among women with epidural analgesia. Aust N Z J Obstet Gynaecol 2004;44:489–94.

Advances in Anesthesia 27 (2009) 191–222

ADVANCES IN ANESTHESIA

ELSEVIER
MOSBY

Regional Anesthesia in Trauma

Laura Clark, MD*, Marina Varbanova, MD

Department of Anesthesiology and Perioperative Medicine, University of Louisville Hospital, 530 South Jackson Street, Louisville, KY 40202, USA

Trauma is a major cause of morbidity and mortality worldwide. Each year more than 100,000 deaths in the United States and about 8% of all deaths worldwide are caused by traumatic injury [1]. It is the leading cause of death in persons younger than 30 years. Anesthesia for trauma patients is one of the greatest challenges in anesthesia. Critically ill patients must be treated whose history, status, and injuries are not well known. The pain management of a trauma patient, with their specific physical and emotional experience, imposes additional demands to anesthesiologists and critical care specialists. Many factors in the management of the trauma victim (hemodynamic fluctuations, respiratory depression, and level of consciousness) contribute to the difficulties faced in the pain control of these patients. In addition, the consequences of inadequate pain management after an injury are more than just psychologic. Acute pain is known to potentiate the physiologic stress response to trauma. The tissue damage and the dynamic of the central nervous system can engage mechanisms and create chronic pain problems that outlast the period of healing. Study results indicate that adequate analgesia is associated with improved results, whereas inadequate analgesia is associated with adverse outcomes [2–6]. Inadequate treatment of pain is reported to result in chronic pain syndromes in 69% of patients [7]. Unfortunately, trauma and orthopedic surgeons often underestimate the potential benefits of regional anesthesia and analgesia.

Multimodal therapy is increasingly recognized as the best pain management approach in the trauma patient [8]. It includes a wide range of measures, such as regional anesthesia procedures, opioids, nonsteroidal anti-inflammatory drugs, α_2 agonists, N-methyl-D-aspartate receptor blockers, anticonvulsants, and antidepressants to treat and modulate pain at its various sites of action. For these reasons, regional anesthesia can play an important role in the treatment of pain and promote favorable recovery from trauma.

*Corresponding author. E-mail address: mickai@aol.com (L. Clark).

0737-6146/09/$ – see front matter
doi:10.1016/j.aan.2009.08.001

This article reviews the importance of regional anesthesia with emphasis on its indications, benefits, and limitations when applied to the trauma patient. Some of the potential benefits of regional anesthesia include the following:

- Avoidance of a difficult airway
- Patient is awake and protective airway reflexes are intact
- Reduction of general anesthesia requirement, when given in combination with general anesthesia
- Reduction in postoperative pain scores
- Reduction in postoperative opioid consumption and opioid-related side effects, such as respiratory depression and postoperative nausea and vomiting
- Reduction in time in the postanesthesia care unit
- Decreased hospital length of stay
- Reduction in postoperative bleeding
- Decreased incidence of deep vein thrombosis
- Increased range of motion
- Decreased rehabilitation time
- Increased patient satisfaction

THE CONSEQUENCES OF TRAUMA AND THE ROLE OF THE ANESTHESIOLOGIST

Trauma is one of the five leading causes of death and disability worldwide, after cancer, ischemic heart disease, stroke, and diseases of the respiratory system. In the United States, injury fatalities are reported at almost 150,000 patients per year. According to the Centers for Disease Control and Prevention, an estimated 5.3 million people in the United States have long-term disabilities resulting from traumatic brain injury and another 200,000 from spinal cord injuries. The importance of trauma-related morbidity is a public health problem that is expected to grow. Researchers at the University of Washington in Seattle, who noted that postinjury pain could lead to disability, depression, and posttraumatic stress disorder, analyzed data from 3047 patients (ages 18–84) who were hospitalized for treatment of acute trauma and survived at least 1 year. At 12 months after injury, 62.7% of patients reported injury-related pain. Most patients had pain in more than one body region, and the mean (average) severity of pain in the previous month was 5.5 on a 10-point scale. The most common painful areas were joints and extremities (44.3%); back (26.2%); head (11.5%); neck (6.9%); abdomen (4.4%); chest (3.8%); and face (2.8%) [9].

The prevalence of pain reported in this study was similar to that found in previous studies of trauma patients. Castillo and colleagues [10] showed that among patients with serious lower extremity injuries, 73% of patients reported pain 7 years after injury, and Urquhart and colleagues [11] reported 37.2% of patients had moderate to severe pain 6 months after orthopedic trauma. Conversely, patients with chronic pain often report trauma as an important factor in their medical history. Trauma was the reported cause of pain in 18.7% of patients seeking care in 10 pain clinics in North Britain [12]. The conclusion of Castillo and colleagues [10] is that most trauma patients have moderately severe pain from their injuries 1 year later and that earlier and more intensive interventions to treat pain in trauma patients may be needed.

Anesthesiologists have particular skills in the provision of pain relief and this is of vital importance in the early and consequent management of the injured patient. Analgesia should be regarded as part of the resuscitation process because it not only brings pain relief, but also improves hemodynamic stability resulting in improved organ and tissue perfusion. Regional anesthesia and its techniques of pain control may have an important role in the regimen of pain relief and possibly, in this important subset of patients, in the prevention of chronic pain problems.

HISTORY OF PAIN RELIEF FOR THE TRAUMA PATIENT

Trauma has been a major cause of death and injury throughout human history. Early civilizations evidently tried to manage pain with opium or its derivatives. Opium poppy capsules dating from 4200 BC have been recovered, and ancient Sumer and other empires are known to have farmed opium. The use of opium-like preparations for anesthesia is recorded in the Ebers Papyrus of 1500 BC [13]. By 1100 BC poppies were scored for opium collection in Cyprus by methods similar to those used in the present day; a simple apparatus for smoking opium was found in a Minoan temple.

Opium was not introduced to India and China until 330 BC and between AD 600 and 1200, respectively, but these nations pioneered the use of cannabis for analgesia. In the second century, according to the Book of Later Han, the physician Hua Tuo performed abdominal surgery using an anesthetic substance called "mafeisan" (cannabis boil powder) dissolved in wine. Throughout Europe, Asia, and the Americas a variety of Solanum species containing potent alkaloids were used for the same purpose.

The first effective local anesthetic was cocaine, which was isolated in 1859. It was first used in 1884 as a topical solution for ophthalmic surgery by Karl Koller. Before that, a mixture of salt and ice was used for the numbing effects of cold. A spray of ether or ethyl chloride was also used to induce anesthesia. Another method tried was pressure on select nerves to numb an area. Around 2500 BC, the Egyptians were already compressing peripheral nerves to achieve localized anesthesia. By the eighteenth century, clamps had been developed that were screwed onto a limb to compress the main nerves. They were applied for at least half an hour before surgery and helped reduce the pain of amputation [14].

Throughout history attempts have been made to develop a method of injecting materials into the body for the relief of trauma pain. It did not become practical until Illinois physician Zophar Jayne invented the first true hypodermic syringe in 1841. Guido Fisher of Germany improved the syringe and introduced a model in 1906 that became the prototype for most modern syringes [15]. Infiltration anesthesia was introduced by Karl Schleich in 1892 when he described the use of a dilute solution of cocaine to block pain [16]. A number of cocaine derivatives and safer replacements were soon produced, including procaine (1905), eucaine, stovaine, and lidocaine (1943).

One of the most significant advances in regional anesthesia occurred when conduction anesthesia was discovered by William Halstead (1852–1922) [17]. The term "regional anesthesia" was first introduced by Harvey Cushing in 1901. Ansbro [18] performed the first continuous nerve block in 1946 with repeated supraclavicular injections of the brachial plexus to prolong the duration of anesthesia in patients undergoing upper extremity surgery. More than 30 years later Selander [19] published a study on 137 patients, in whom an axillary catheter was placed for hand surgery. Tuominen and colleagues [20] described the first reported use of continuous interscalene infusion for postoperative pain management in 1987 for shoulder surgery. The same group also evaluated the effects of a continuous interscalene block on the ventilatory function demonstrating paresis of the ipsilateral hemidiaphragm [21]. In 1997, Borgeat and colleagues [22] introduced patient controlled interscalene analgesia with 0.15% bupivacaine using a basal infusion rate of 5 mL·h^{-1} and bolus of 3 to 4 mL with a lock-out period of 20 minutes. This technique has proved to be safe and effective without symptoms of toxicity and provides superior pain management than does patient-controlled analgesia morphine.

The clinical history of neuraxial anesthesia dates back to August Bier and August Hildebrandt and their first attempt at spinal anesthesia on August 15, 1898. Epidural anesthesia by a caudal approach was known in the early twentieth century, but a well-defined technique using lumbar injection was not developed until the 1930s. In 1945 Tuohy introduced the needle, bearing his name, which is still the most commonly used needle for epidural anesthesia. Improvements in equipment, drugs, and technique have made epidural anesthesia a popular and versatile technique, with applications in surgery, obstetrics, and pain control [23], and the trauma patient.

Regional anesthesia in the battlefield

Treatment of traumatic pain relief in civilians has benefited tremendously from advances made in medicine on the battlefield. Although improvements in resuscitation methods have had the most impact on combat medicine, regional anesthesia methods are safe and effective in combat situations. A decrease in mortality from 46% to 12.5% was reported in World War II when spinal anesthesia replaced inhalational anesthesia for abdominal wound surgery [24]. Thompson and colleagues [25,26] were on the forefront of introducing the paresthesia technique for peripheral nerve blockade in the Vietnam War. Caudal anesthesia was used during the Falklands War [27], and one of the first articles on the safety and use of long-term continuous peripheral nerve catheters was published by Buckenmaier and coworkers [28] based on experience in Operation Iraqi Freedom. The military is currently making strides to establish regional anesthesia as a more available option in combat. Established in 2003, with the help of Congressman

John P. Murtha, the Army Regional Anesthesia and Pain Management Initiative seeks to improve the management of pain in military and civilian medicine and implement improvements in medical practice and technology that promote regional anesthesia and analgesia for the care of military beneficiaries [29].

NEUROCHEMISTRY OF NOCICEPTION IN TRAUMA

The sensation of pain involves a complex interaction of excitatory and inhibitory neurotransmitter mechanisms. Following trauma, injured tissues release local inflammatory mediators causing vasodilatation, erythema, and swelling in the involved area. Inflammatory mediators that are implicated in pain and hyperalgesia include bradykinins; potassium; cytokines (interleukin-1β, -8, and -6, and tumor necrosis factor-α); substance P; histamine; hydrogen ions; serotonin; leukotrienes; prostacyclin; and prostaglandins. Signals from noxious stimuli are transmitted along the axons of the primary afferent to their cell bodies in the dorsal root ganglia and then centrally by synapsing onto secondary neurons in the dorsal horns of the spinal cord. The nociceptive fibers (A-δ and C fibers) terminate in lamina I and II. Lamina II has the highest concentration of opioid receptors in the spinal cord. Laminas III and IV interneurons receive input from nociceptive and nonnociceptive fibers. The neurons in laminas I, V, VII, and VIII contain most of the cell bodies of spinothalamic tract neurons [30].

Changes in pain transmission can occur in the dorsal horns. Constant C-fiber nociceptive input to dorsal horn could result in more exaggerated response to subsequent C-fiber stimuli or peripheral tissue injury, a phenomenon known as "wind-up" or central hypersensitization. Some of the central changes associated with pain can possibly be pre-empted by blocking the afferents to the dorsal horn with local anesthetic technique [31]. Nociceptive information can be processed entirely in the spinal cord as in the case of spinal reflexes. Spinal reflexes can also be blocked at the level of the spinal cord (eg, with local anesthetics).

The somatosensory system is composed of two main signaling channels. The nociceptive information is transmitted from the spinal cord to the thalamus by the anterolateral system (spinothalamic tract) and the dorsal column–medial lemniscal system, a channel for innocuous stimuli. There are two sets of somatosensory input to the brain stem and diencephalon. First, many neurons from the ascending anterolateral spinal quadrant terminate in the nuclei of the brainstem and midbrain. The remainder of the anterolateral system fibers continues through the brainstem and the midbrain and terminates in the hypothalamus, and some of the lateral and medial thalamus regions. From the thalamus, nociceptive information can be transmitted to the cortex, resulting in subsequent response to the noxious stimulus [1]. The implications are that there are three sites (periphery, spinal cord, and brain) available for modulation by the different modalities of pain control.

Hormone release in the trauma patient

Traumatized tissue releases algesic agents that excite the primary afferent fibers and stimulate the hypothalamic-pituitary-adrenal axis. Hormones released as result of the stress response to trauma include corticotropin-releasing hormone, adrenocorticotropic hormone, β endorphins, epinephrine, norepinephrine, cortisol, antidiuretic hormone, vasopressin, aldosterone, glucagon, and growth hormone. As a result of the release of these hormones the patient can develop hypertension, tachycardia, increased oxygen consumption, increased catabolism, a hypercoagulable state, immune system suppression, decreased anabolism, and water and salt retention.

The "ebb phase" following acute trauma typically lasts 24 hours and is characterized by α receptor–mediated vasoconstriction, decreased urine flow and oxygen use, and elevated stress hormone levels. This phase is followed by the "flow phase," typically lasting 2 to 5 days and involving an increase of cardiac output, elevation of oxygen consumption, β adrenoreceptor–mediated increases in regional blood flow, and a hypermetabolic state. The hypermetabolic response to trauma involves increased lipolysis and ketogenesis, increased muscle proteolysis, increased gluconeogenesis and glycogenolysis, insulin resistance, and increased lactate production in skeletal muscle. The primary injury phase in the posttrauma response is followed by an inflammatory phase associated with the release of the traditional inflammatory mediators and cytokines, leukotrienes, neuropeptides, nitric oxide, and nerve growth factor. This "inflammatory soup" may cause sensitization of nociceptors and provide persistent input to the spinal cord that contributes to the pain pattern in the postinjury phase even after the stimulus has receded [32].

Benefits of regional anesthesia and analgesia on the stress response in the trauma patient

Uncontrolled pain may contribute to morbidity through activation of the sympathetic nervous system, the stress response, and the coagulation cascade. Increased sympathetic nervous system activity increases myocardial oxygen demand by increasing heart rate, contractility, and systemic vascular resistance. In addition, it can enhance hypercoagulability, which contributes to vasospasm and thrombosis and is especially not desirable in the trauma patient. Experimental data suggest that thoracic epidural anesthesia with local anesthetics can reduce sympathetic activation and provide a favorable balance of oxygen supply and demand to the myocardium [33]. The relief of pain with neuraxial or peripheral nerve block, when indicated, can be a key in the successful management of the trauma victim.

The beneficial effect of regional anesthesia in trauma is most likely the modulation of pain and the subsequent sympathetic response. In addition, a sympathetic blockade (specifically with neuraxial anesthesia and local anesthetics) allows parasympathetic (vagal) activity to dominate. It is generally believed that the vagal afferent nerve pathway dominates the response to mild and moderate peripheral inflammation, whereas strong inflammatory signals are transmitted to the brain through hormonal mechanisms [34]. The vagus controls and modulates the peripheral inflammatory status by signaling directly to macrophages and microvascular endothelial cells [35].

PERIOPERATIVE REGIONAL ANESTHESIA TECHNIQUES IN TRAUMA

Any technique that is applicable in the elective surgery patient is potentially useful in the trauma patient. Nevertheless, the trauma patient presents additional challenges as a result of the differences in injury, hemodynamic status, and neurologic status. Patients may be intoxicated or have altered mental status from other causes that prevents them from consenting to or cooperating with the initiation of a regional block. The risks and benefits of each technique need to be considered for each individual patient. Only in rare instances does the trauma patient not benefit from a regional procedure at some course of their hospitalization. Although pre-emptive analgesia is preferred, not all procedures need to be preoperative if the circumstances do not permit. The patient can be consented preoperatively for a postoperative procedure.

CENTRAL NEURAXIAL TECHNIQUES

Central neuraxial anesthesia has many advantages and demonstrated benefits, but the contraindications listed next keep many trauma patients from receiving these blocks. Contraindications for neuraxial anesthesia include the following:

- Patient refusal
- Sepsis or localized infection at the desired puncture site
- Severe hypovolemia
- Acute hemodynamic instability
- Obstructive ileus
- Major coagulation disorders or anticoagulation therapy [36]
- Uncooperative patients
- Increased intracranial pressure

The issue of increased intracranial pressure is one that can occur in trauma patients with head injury. If elevated intracranial pressure is present, the concern is that, by suddenly reducing the pressure at the level of the spine, the brainstem may herniate, leading to cardiovascular, neurologic, and respiratory failure. As long as intracranial pressure is not increased, however, the presence of head injury in itself is not considered a contraindication to epidural analgesia, and such patients have been successfully treated [1,37].

Practical problems in trauma patients can come from difficulties in positioning the patient, in particular one with multiorgan trauma or spine injury. The spine must be radiographically clear with no coagulopathy present. The physician must be aware that often the referring trauma physician will "clear" a spine if there is no tenderness present. Before placing a catheter it is prudent to review any relevant imaging studies to evaluate for any injuries to the spine. It is important when placing a neuraxial blockade that the hemodynamic status of the patient is optimized. A unit of plasma expander is helpful in this regard but the potential for hypotension always exists and vasoconstrictors must be readily available.

The possible side effects of central neuraxial anesthesia include respiratory difficulties (especially with thoracic levels of sensory blockade); circulatory effects proportional to the extent of the sympathetic blockade; urinary retention; hyperactive peristalsis; and sphincter relaxation. Most of the side effects can be modified by adhering to safe techniques when performing the blockade and prompt diagnosis and treatment when the undesired effect occurs.

Epidural anesthesia is one of the most effective treatments for pain in trauma patients. Thoracic epidurals are recommended for analgesia of chest trauma [38], abdominal trauma, pancreatitis [39], and thoracic surgery. A thoracic epidural is potentially technically more difficult than a lumbar epidural because angulations of the spinous processes make the entrance to the thoracic epidural space smaller and more difficult to reach. The anatomy of the thoracic spine makes the cephalad and caudal thoracic levels easier to access because the most severe angulation of the spinous processes occurs between T6 and T9.

Lumbar epidurals may be used for orthopedic surgeries and trauma of the lower extremities. There is no indication for lumbar epidural for abdominal or thoracic trauma. With the advent of continuous peripheral nerve blockade, which has advantages even for bilateral injuries over a lumbar epidural, the indications for a lumbar epidural for trauma pain have decreased even more. There are fewer risks associated with continuous peripheral nerve blockade making it a better choice than the lumbar epidural. As technical expertise in the placement of continuous peripheral nerve blockade grows, its use will continue to replace lumbar epidurals for these types of injuries.

Use of continuous thoracic epidural analgesia for ahoracic trauma

There is substantial evidence that multiple rib fractures increase morbidity and mortality, both of which can be decreased with adequate pain relief. The physiologic impact of the severe pain secondary to multiple rib fractures can lead to alveolar collapse, which, along with pulmonary contusions, predisposes the patient to respiratory failure and pneumonia, which are leading causes of morbidity in the already immobilized trauma patient. Flagel and colleagues [40] determined that the number of rib fractures correlates directly with increasing pulmonary morbidity and mortality. Patients sustaining fractures of six or more ribs are at significant risk for death from causes unrelated to the fractures themselves.

Holcomb and coworkers [38] investigated the relationship between age and number of rib fractures and determined that patients 45 or older with greater than four rib fractures exhibit increased morbidity and increased ICU days, ventilator days, and total hospital days. Although thoracic epidural analgesia has not been shown to decrease mortality, ICU, or total hospital length of stay associated with traumatic rib fractures, it has been shown to decrease the duration of mechanical ventilation (when local anesthetics are used in the infusion) and nosocomial pneumonia [41,42]. Intravenous opioid patient-controlled analgesia has been shown to be inferior to continuous thoracic epidural analgesia in improving pulmonary function, modifying the immune response, and providing analgesia [43]. Thoracic epidural analgesia has been recommended as the modality of choice for providing analgesia in the patient with multiple rib fractures whenever possible [44]. The use of epidural block has not become uniformly accepted because of the increased incidence of hypotension, possible complications with thromboprophylaxis, technical problems, and numerous contraindications to placement of a thoracic epidural catheter [41,42]. For those reasons, thoracic paravertebral block has been advocated as an alternative means of providing analgesia for patients with multiple rib fractions [45].

Paravertebral block

Paravertebral block refers to blockade of spinal nerves as they exit the intervertebral foramen. The paravertebral space is a wedge-shaped area between the heads and necks of the ribs. The posterior border is the superior costotransverse ligament, the anterior wall is the parietal pleura, and the base of the triangle is the posterolateral aspect of the vertebra and the intervertebral foramen. Each space communicates with the spaces positioned superiorly and inferiorly. Thoracic paravertebral analgesia is advocated for rib fractures; postthoracotomy pain control; and analgesia after cholecystectomy, nephrectomy, or breast surgery. The standard technique of percutaneous paravertebral space location is by loss of resistance [46]. The patient is paced in lateral position with the side to be blocked uppermost; prone and sitting positions can also be used. Two or three centimeters lateral to the spinous process, at the appropriate dermatomal levels, a short beveled spinal needle or Tuohy needle is advanced at 90 degrees to all skin planes. On contacting the transverse process, the needle is angled superiorly and "walked" 1 or 1.5 cm over the top of the process until loss of resistance to air or saline is appreciated. A bolus of local anesthetic is then given either through the needle or through an epidural catheter. Unlike peripheral nerve blocks, paravertebral block produces anesthesia with strictly dermatomal distribution. Eason and Wyatt [47] first described the use of this block for patients with multiple rib fractures in 1979. Paravertebral analgesia as repeated injections of local anesthetic, continuous infusion, or regular dosing through an indwelling catheter are all effective methods of relieving pain in trauma patients [47–49]. Proponents of paravertebral blocks claim the technique is simple, safe, easy to learn, and has a low incidence of complications [46,49,50].

In a meta-analysis comparing the analgesic efficacy and side effects of paravertebral versus epidural blockade for thoracotomy, Davies and colleagues [51] found that there were no significant differences between the paravertebral block group and the epidural group for pain scores, but the paravertebral block group had a better side effect profile. Pulmonary complications, urinary retention, nausea and vomiting, and hypotension were less common with the paravertebral blockade. In a systematic review of randomized trials of adult thoracotomy, Joshi and colleagues [52] evaluated thoracic epidural, paravertebral, intrathecal, intercostal, and interpleural analgesic techniques with each other and with systemic opioid analgesia. They concluded that continuous paravertebral block was as effective as thoracic epidural analgesia with local anesthetic, but was associated with less hypotension. Additionally, paravertebral block reduced the incidence of pulmonary complications compared with systemic opioid analgesia, unlike thoracic epidural analgesia. In a prospective, randomized comparison of continuous thoracic epidural analgesia versus continuous thoracic paravertebral analgesia in trauma patients with a mean number of five unilateral rib fractures, both methods provided good and comparable analgesia with mean visual analog pain scores with coughing decreasing from greater than 90/100 to 35 to 45/100 within 30 to 45 minutes [53]. There was no difference between the two groups in supplemental morphine requirement, length of ICU stay, and total hospital length of stay, although the incidence of hypotension was increased in the thoracic epidural analgesia group.

Paravertebral block as a regional anesthesia technique can be safely performed on patients distressed with pain and on anesthetized, sedated, or mechanically ventilated patients [50]. If done in the thoracic area, it does not require palpation of fractured ribs and is technically easier than thoracic epidural. It is associated with lower incidence of complications than neuraxial techniques, including urinary retention, nausea and vomiting, and hypotension [51–53]. Possible complications of paravertebral anesthesia are failed block, intravascular injection of local anesthetic, hematoma, pneumothorax, central neuraxial blockade, systemic toxicity, and injury to pleura or pulmonary parenchyma [50]. The few contraindications for the use of paravertebral blocks include sepsis at the entry site or within the chest cavity, tumor in the paravertebral space, patient refusal, and allergy to local anesthetics.

PERIPHERAL NERVE BLOCKS FOR THE MANAGEMENT OF TRAUMA TO THE EXTREMITIES

Single-injection peripheral nerve blocks provide better analgesia, decreased postoperative opioid requirements, less interrupted sleep, and greater patient satisfaction compared with conventional IV patient-controlled analgesia. Peripheral nerve blocks also decrease opioid-related side effects, such as nausea and vomiting, pruritis, urinary retention, constipation, sedation, and respiratory depression [54]. The technique to be used depends on the site of injury and the planned operative procedures, and must always be individualized so that it is appropriate for the specific injury. Based on the nature of the injury and coexisting injuries one approach to the block may have advantages over another; it is important to maintain proficiency in more than one technique. As the anesthesiologist, it is very important to document a neurologic examination of the patient before placement of a peripheral nerve block. It may be prudent to obtain a separate consent for anesthesia that delineates its indications and benefits versus the risks and possible complications. A block can be done in the patent with a neurologic deficit as long as the existing injury is documented. The examination that is done in the emergency room can change by the time the patient reaches the operating room.

Continuous nerve blocks and multimodal analgesia

Continuous peripheral nerve blocks have been shown to decrease pain scores, increase range of motion exercises, decrease hospital stay, and decrease rehabilitation time compared with intravenous patient-controlled analgesia, and have fewer side effects compared with lumbar epidural analgesia [54–56]. The advantages listed previously of single injection peripheral nerve blocks are time limited because the duration of residual analgesia is only 10 to 24 hours, even with long-acting anesthetics, such as bupivacaine. After resolution of the block the pain may be difficult to manage. Continuous peripheral nerve blocks allow prolonged site-specific delivery of local anesthetic and optimal analgesia, and avoid premature regression of the analgesic block [54–56]. Continuous peripheral nerve blocks are superior to periarticular and intra-articular local anesthetic infusion for immediate postoperative pain [55]. The importance of continuous peripheral catheters in the trauma patient cannot be overemphasized. Rarely is the duration provided by a single-injection peripheral nerve block sufficient for pain relief in these patients because their pain generally lasts much longer than a local anesthetic's effective duration. Trauma patients often have multiple sites of injury and multiple operations. A continuous catheter technique provides analgesia for at least one area of their pain. It has been demonstrated that trauma patients may safely have multiple simultaneous continuous peripheral nerve catheter infusions to treat multiple sites of extremity injuries [57]. Many patients need an epidural or paravertebral catheter in addition to peripheral catheters, which significantly decreases the total dose of opioid required for multiple injuries. Continuous peripheral nerve catheters can play a central role in the multimodal approach to analgesia in the trauma patient [58].

Peripheral nerve localization techniques

Both peripheral nerve stimulation and ultrasound may be used to guide needle placement for peripheral nerve localization in the trauma patient and the elective surgery patient. Neither technique has been definitively proved to be superior to the other for increased block success, although ultrasound may potentially decrease the time and number of attempts to complete a successful block [59–61]. Many physicians use a combined ultrasound and nerve stimulation technique. The question of eliciting an evoked motor response across a fractured site causing increased pain is valid but has not been shown to be a contraindication to using peripheral nerve stimulation. If only ultrasound is used, then painful stimulation is not an issue. In certain circumstances, such as existing or newly created traumatic nerve injury where the distal muscles are denervated or do not exist, ultrasound has obvious indications. Plunkett and coworkers [62] demonstrated the effectiveness of ultrasound in such a situation in a wounded soldier needing a continuous supraclavicular block where the nature of the injuries precluded the use of peripheral nerve stimulation.

Peripheral nerve blocks of the upper extremities (and shoulder) for trauma

Suggested regional block locations based on upper extremity injury location are given in Table 1. The anterior or posterior approach to brachial plexus block at the interscalene level and supraclavicular regions may be hampered by the presence of a C-collar in a significant number of trauma patients. This is not an absolute contraindication. Often this is a precautionary measure and reasons for the C-collar can be determined in a cooperative patient. If imaging techniques indicate that there is no damage in such situations, the collar is removed and the head stabilized so that an ultrasound probe can be used to position the supraclavicular block. The authors seldom turn the head for a true interscalene block but opt for a supraclavicular block and have found a "high" supraclavicular block adequate without the need to turn the head. The infraclavicular approach to the brachial plexus is indicated for operative procedures and postoperative analgesia involving the elbow to the hand. The coracoid approach is especially useful for catheter placement because of its deeper location and easy fixation compared with the other approaches. The axillary approach to brachial plexus analgesia is often the least desired in the trauma patient because it requires the most movement of an injured extremity.

Practical problems with peripheral blocks to the upper extremities in trauma patients are that (1) interscalene block can cause Horner syndrome and obscure neurologic assessment, a block of the ipsilateral phrenic nerve can cause loss of hemidiaphragmatic function, and close proximity to tracheostomy or jugular vein catheter sites can increase the risk of infection; (2) infraclavicular and supraclavicular approaches carry the risk of pneumothorax; and (3) axillary nerve block has problems of arm positioning and catheter maintenance. Most extremity injuries are orthopedic in nature but extensive soft tissue trauma can be an indication. The sympathetecomy with regional anesthesia may prove beneficial for revascularization, reimplantaion, or in any case of compromised blood flow with vasospasm from an exaggerated sympathetic response. Although much less common compared with the lower extremity, a radial compartment syndrome can occur. The possibility should be discussed with the surgeon before regional block and, if necessary, a short-acting local

Table 1
Suggested regional block location based on upper extremity injury location

Injury location	Suggested nerve block
Shoulder	Interscalene or supraclavicular block of the brachial plexus
Arm (upper or lower) or hand	Supraclavicular, infraclavicular, or axillary

anesthetic should be used for the surgery itself. In the authors' experience this is more of theoretical interest rather than a true clinical occurrence.

Peripheral nerve blocks of the lower extremities for trauma patients

As with upper extremity trauma, all peripheral nerve blocks and catheters that are useful in the elective surgery patient may be indicated for patients with lower limb trauma (Table 2). Analgesia for the lower extremities may be provided by blocks of the lumbar plexus (femoral, obturator, and lateral femoral cutaneous nerves) by either an anterior approach (femoral perivascular or fascia iliaca techniques) or posterior approach (psoas compartment). The sciatic nerve may be blocked from the level of the sacral plexus to the popliteal fossa by posterior, anterior, or lateral approaches depending on the operative procedure and the ability to position the patient. It is helpful to gain expertise in both anterior and posterior approaches to each of the target nerves.

Lumbar plexus blocks can provide excellent pain relief for the hip and knee joints, femoral neck and femoral shaft, and proximal tibia, and when combined with a sciatic block near complete analgesia or anesthesia can be achieved. Lumbar plexus blocks have been shown to significantly decrease postoperative opioid requirements following knee arthroplasty and for those patients with open reduction and internal fixation of acetabular fracture [63,64]. Peripheral nerve blocks performed preoperatively may decrease intraoperative opioid and inhalational anesthetics requirements during surgery. Acetabular fractures are an exception because the block is often done at the end of surgery because of the nature of the injury and the pain associated with mobilization. The close proximity of the lumbar plexus catheter to the surgical field may be considered a potential contraindication for placing the catheter preoperatively [63].

Chelly and colleagues [63] placed 13 lumbar plexus catheters in anesthetized patients with acetabular fractures at the end of the surgery. They did not experience any complications associated with the use of continuous lumbar plexus technique. The patients were positioned in lateral decubitus position with the operated site up. All lumbar plexus catheters were placed using nerve stimulator and loss of resistance technique. Chelly and coworkers' [63] data demonstrated that continuous lumbar plexus infusion of 0.2% ropivacaine for

Table 2
Suggested regional block location based on lower extremity injury location

Injury location	Suggested nerve block catheter
Acetabulum	Posterior lumbar plexus (psoas compartment)
Femoral neck	Posterior lumbar plexus (psoas compartment) or femoral-fascia iliaca
Pelvis	Epidural
Femoral shaft	Femoral
Knee	Femoral, sciatic
Patella	Femoral
Ankle	Femoral (or saphenous), sciatic
Foot	Popliteal

postoperative pain management reduces morphine requirements by nearly 60% in patients who undergo open reduction and internal fixation of an acetabular fracture. Possible complications of the lumbar plexus technique are epidural block and intrathecal injection of local anesthetic, characterized by bilateral block and hypotension. The cardiovascular consequences can be minimized by the slow injection of local anesthetic mixtures combined with the frequent monitoring of the hemodynamics [63].

Femoral nerve blocks are useful for the management of acute pain from fractures of the femoral neck (hip fractures) and femoral shaft [65,66]. The use of ultrasound might limit the unavoidable pain associated with nerve stimulation in these patients, which otherwise can be treated with remifentanil (0.3–0.5 $\mu g \cdot kg^{-1}$) or ketamine (0.2–0.4 $mg \cdot kg^{-1}$) [67]. Midazolam can be useful in such cases in incremental doses of 1 mg intravenously or 0.015 to 0.15 $mg \cdot kg^{-1}$ infused over 3 to 5 minutes, to produce sedation and amnesia without significant respiratory depression. In patients with femoral neck or femoral shaft fractures, femoral nerve blocks have also been shown to provide superior analgesia and patient acceptance of positioning for spinal anesthesia compared with systemic opioids [68,69]. Continuous femoral catheters in combination with sciatic block provide excellent pain control for the whole lower extremity and even surgical anesthesia for such procedures as external fixation. The choice of an approach to the sciatic nerve should depend on the type of trauma, the ability to position the patient for the procedure, and the skills of the operator. If a combination of catheter techniques is used, the total daily dose of local anesthetic should be adjusted based on catheter location; admixtures, such as epinephrine; drug interactions; and the disease state [70].

The complications from continuous nerve blocks are rare; however, minor adverse effects, such as local inflammation, infection, and vascular puncture, are more common [71,72]. The frequency of infections associated with peripheral nerve catheters remains poorly defined. Recent studies show that 23% to 57% of peripheral nerve catheters may become colonized, but only 0% to 3% results in localized infection. An exogenous source of infection is frequently suspected. Risk factors are duration of the continuous infusion more than 48 hours, the absence of antibiotic prophylaxis, ICU stay, and axillary and femoral locations of the catheter. Although definitive proof is lacking, there is strong evidence that the maximal sterile precautions used for epidural insertion should be recommended to anesthesiologists for continuous peripheral nerve blocks [73]. Practical problems with lower extremity nerve blocks in the trauma patient may arise from patient positioning; catheter maintenance; and interference of the nerve catheter with central, venous, or arterial line placement. Whatever the level of the trauma, continuous peripheral nerve blocks can provide complete analgesia and anesthesia of an extremity avoiding unwanted side effects of opioids.

Advantages of continuous nerve blocks are that they can improve blood flow to the extremity, but because the block is unilateral and postganglionic, they do not cause the hypotension and bradycardia that can result from the bilateral, preganglionic nerve block produced by neuraxial techniques. Continuous peripheral nerve blocks cause no interference with bladder and rectal control and, if placed early, can reduce pain and muscle spasm and allow early mobilization. Finally, peripheral nerve blocks following trauma may prevent the development of chronic pain syndromes.

Other regional analgesic Techniques used in trauma patients

Intercostal nerve block

Intercostal nerve block has been widely used for years to provide analgesia after thoracic trauma and thoracic surgery. Intercostal nerve block is performed posterior to the midaxillary line to ensure blockade of the lateral cutaneous and anterior branch of the intercostal nerve. In cases of chest trauma, intercostal nerve block is performed two to three levels above and below the traumatized zone, because of the overlapping innervations from the segments above and below the fracture site [1,67]. The vascular absorption of local anesthetics is rapid from the intercostals space, and there is a clear risk of local anesthetic toxicity, especially if more than six to eight intercostal spaces are blocked. Repetitive injections risk inducing iatrogenic pneumothorax. The reported incidence of pneumothorax after intercostal nerve block is 1.4% for individual blocks and increases to 5.6% when multiple intercostal nerve blocks are performed simultaneously [74]. A catheter insertion technique in the intercostal space with continuous infusion of bupivacaine, 0.25% 3 $mL \cdot h^{-1}$, has been reported [49]. Unfortunately, the exact incidence of misplaced catheters after intercostal catheterization is not known, but one study reported that only 54.5% of catheters were placed correctly [47]. Another problem with intercostal nerve blocks is that the space for local anesthetic is confined to the intercostal space, which introduces the possibility that the local anesthetic gets injected in the epidural or paravertebral space, or the subpleura. Another disadvantage is that the technique can require multiple painful injections [49].

Interpleural block

Interpleural block arises as a result of injection of local anesthetic between the parietal and visceral pleura (rather than outside the parietal pleura as with paravertebral analgesia) to produce ipsilateral somatic analgesia of multiple thoracic dermatomes [75,76]. This technique lowers pain scores and opioid requirements. Interpleural analgesia provides unilateral analgesia with variable intensity and quality. The more fluid present in the pleural space, which dilutes the local anesthetic, the less likely is the probability to obtain good analgesia. Local anesthetic can also be lost by drains in the dependent chest. With thoracostomy tube in situ, clamping it for 20 to 30 minutes to prevent siphoning away of the local anesthetic is often recommended, but it raises concerns of tension pneumothorax. The interpleural injection of local anesthetic is associated with rapid intravascular absorption. The concern with attaining toxic concentrations and the associated side effects is why some researchers recommend the exclusive use of lidocaine with this technique [77]. Satisfactory results have been reported with injection of 100 mg bupivacaine with epinephrine or 1 mg·kg^{-1} of 2% lidocaine [78].

The efficiency of interpleural analgesia for thoracic trauma compared with other analgesic techniques remains a controversial issue [79]. Epidural anesthesia is superior in providing pain control and pulmonary function is significantly better with epidural than with interpleural analgesia. Although interpleural analgesia is devoid of deleterious hemodynamic effects, there are clear chances for pneumothorax, displacement of the interpleural catheter, and toxicity of local anesthetics. Interpleural injection of local anesthetics can also cause phrenic nerve paralysis or Horner syndrome and may aggravate bronchospasm [80]. Loss of negative interpleural pressure in ventilated patients makes identification of the interpleural space difficult and can result in catheter misplacement, tension pneumothorax, and intrapulmonary catheter placement [81].

LOCAL ANESTHETICS AND ANALGESIC ADJUVANTS FOR REGIONAL ANESTHESIA

Pharmacologic agents suitable for regional anesthesia in the trauma patient include local anesthetics and local anesthetic adjuvant agents, such as opioids, epinephrine, clonidine, and ketamine (Tables 3 and 4). A number of different local anesthetics have been used for epidural anesthesia with bupivacaine, lidocaine, and ropivacaine being the most common. One disadvantage of lidocaine for postoperative analgesia management is its low motor-sensory separation. In trauma patients, who may warrant close neurologic follow-up examinations and the ability to participate with postoperative rehabilitation, a local anesthetic agent with higher sensory than motor blockade is desired. Columb and Lyons [82] established that the minimum effective local analgesic concentration was 0.065% for bupivacaine and 0.37% for lidocaine. Bupivacaine has the advantage of a moderately long duration and preferential sensory rather than motor block; however, it has a high potential toxicity because it can cause cardiac depression, severe arrhythmias, and cardiac arrest from which resuscitation may be difficult, prolonged, and even impossible [83,84]. Ropivacaine has the theoretical advantage of lower toxicity in case of overdose, and its central

Table 3

Doses of opioids for patient-controlled thoracic epidural analgesia along with or without the common local anesthetics bupivacaine (0.0625%–0.125%) or ropivacaine (0.1%–0.2%)

Opioid (concentration)	Dose (mL)	Time Interval (min)	Basal Rate (mL)	Hourly Limit (mL)
Morphine (0.05 mg/mL)	2–3	15–30	–5	7–11
Fentanyl (3 µg/mL)	2–3	10–15	3–5	7–11
Sufentanil (2 µg/mL)	2–3	10–15	3–5	7–11
Hydromorphone (20 µg/mL)	2–3	20–30	3–5	5–11

Table 4
Doses of opioids for patient-controlled lumbar epidural analgesia along with or without the common local anesthetics bupivacaine (0.0625%–0.125%) or ropivacaine (0.1%–0.2%)

Opioid (concentration)	Dose (mL)	Time Interval (min)	Basal Rate (mL)	Hourly Limit (mL)
Morphine (0.05 mg/mL)	3–4	15–30	5–7	8–15
Fentanyl (3 μg/mL)	3–4	10–15	5–7	8–15
Sufentanil (2 μg/mL)	3–4	3–4	10–15	5–7
Hydromorphone (20 μg/mL)	3–4	3–4	15–20	5–7

nervous system toxicity profile is more favorable than others in this class [85]. Ropivacaine solutions of 0.1% to 0.2% seem to be the best concentration range for balance between sensory and motor blockade during continuous peripheral nerve blocks [86–88].

The risk/benefit ratio of using pharmacologic adjuvants should be carefully considered in each trauma patient. Opioids administered in the epidural space exert their central neuraxial effects when they bind to opioid receptors at the presynaptic level in the dorsal horn neurons of the spinal cord. They cause hyperpolarization of the postsynaptic membrane in the dorsal horn neurons, making it more difficult for the neurotransmitter to depolarize. To exert its effect, a drug deposited in the epidural space must transverse a number of membranes and the cerebrospinal fluid before reaching its site of action [89,90]. Epidurally administered opioids have the advantage of producing analgesia without sympathetic or motor blockade, which is an advantage in hemodynamically fragile patients or those who need to ambulate early in the postoperative period. Recent insight into the pharmacokinetics of spinal opioids indicates, however, that the analgesic effect of lipid-soluble opioids is caused in large part by uptake into plasma and distribution to brainstem opioid receptors and systemic effects [91].

In theory, epinephrine should be useful as an adjuvant, but in practice it is used primarily as part of the test dose for intravascular injection. Epinephrine delays absorption of local anesthetics into the systemic circulation meaning that the plasma concentration of the local anesthetic rises less steeply, which reduces the risk of systemic toxic side effects. Concentrations between 2 and 2.5 $\mu g \cdot mL^{-1}$ have no effect on nerve blood flow and is the most commonly recommended dose range [91,92]. The addition of epinephrine to a long-acting local anesthetic like ropivacaine may not increase block duration, but it does help in detection of intravascular injection during the test dose. Epinephrine may also produce analgesia through a α_2-adrenoceptor mechanism. Epinephrine seems to improve analgesia produced by thoracic epidural infusions of bupivacaine and fentanyl or of low-dose ropivacaine and fentanyl (1 $mg \cdot mL^{-1}$/2 $\mu g \cdot mL^{-1}$) after major thoracic surgery [93,94]. Despite the fact that epinephrine seems to be a useful adjuvant in thoracic epidural analgesia, its usefulness in lumbar epidural analgesia is inconsistent [95]. Even in low concentrations, however, epinephrine is considered a possible contributor to peripheral nerve ischemia. Selander [96] performed topical endoneural and intrafasicular injections of saline with various concentrations of bupivacaine in the presence or absence of epinephrine in rabbit sciatic nerves in vivo. Intrafasicular injections inevitably were associated with neuronal degeneration, but endoneurial injections seemed to be associated with degeneration only in the presence of epinephrine at 5 mg·mL^{-1}. Nerves with a generous collateral blood supply may be less vulnerable than those in a watershed area between two tenuous vascular arcades, such as the sciatic nerve. At least for the sciatic nerve, the recommendation is to forgo the addition of epinephrine, especially for the use of long-acting agents, such as bupivacaine.

Clonidine has been investigated as adjuvant in neuraxial blocks. Clonidine may directly prevent impulse conduction and prolong the effect of local anesthetics. It has been primarily used to improve intraoperative analgesia, and to prolong the duration of sensory and motor block during spinal anesthesia [97]. In trauma patients its possible side effects of hypotension, decrease in heart rate, and sedation may limit its usefulness. Clonidine (in dose ranges of 30–300 µg) as an adjuvant to intermediate and long-acting local anesthetics for single-injection peripheral nerve and plexus blocks prolongs duration of analgesia by about 2 hours, but with an increased risk of hypotension, syncope, and sedation [98]. Clonidine (in doses of 1–2 µg/mL) added to ropivacaine 0.2% for continuous peripheral nerve blocks does not provide improved analgesia compared with ropivacaine 0.2% alone and delays recovery of motor function [99,100]. Clonidine seems to offer little advantage as an analgesic adjunct to central or peripheral regional anesthesia-analgesia in the trauma setting.

Ketamine produces central antinociception through a noncompetitive antagonism at N-methyl-D-aspartate receptors. Ketamine may enhance analgesia through various mechanisms, such as an interaction with spinal opioid receptors and α-adrenoceptors [101]. Ketamine (20–30 mg) added to epidural morphine (3.5–5 mg) significantly increased the time to the first request for additional pain medication compared with patients who received morphine without ketamine. At 24 hours after dosing, only four of the patients in the morphine-ketamine group required additional pain medication compared with every patient in the morphine group [102]

RISKS OF REGIONAL ANESTHESIA IN TRAUMA

Treatment of trauma patients is challenging. For example, their injuries may include pre-existing neurologic injuries, their capability to give informed consent may be impaired, and they are not good candidates for deep sedation during block placement because of the possibility of coexisting head injury, and the increased risks of aspiration in the presence of delayed gastric emptying. The goal of regional analgesia is to improve on the analgesia provided by systemic opioids alone, either by reducing opioid requirements and their undesired side effects, or by producing an objective improvement in physiologic status. Whether regional anesthesia is appropriate in the trauma patient depends on the type of the planned operative procedures; the hemodynamic, neurologic, and medical status of the patient; the balance of the potential benefits and disadvantages of the technique; the willingness of the patient and surgeon; available technology (peripheral nerve stimulation or high-frequency ultrasound); and skills of the anesthesiologist. Regional anesthesia is not without risks; one must be concerned about coagulation status, the potential for iatrogenic trauma associated with the procedure, infection-related risks, the potential of local anesthetic toxicity, and the masking effect of analgesia that may delay the recognition of compartment syndrome or of even life-threatening events, such a splenic rupture (Box 1). In addition to analgesia, regional techniques using local anesthetics frequently have a local sympatholytic effect that may be desirable when vasospasm is present or undesirable when it leads to hemodynamic instability. Contraindications of regional anesthesia in the trauma patient include patient refusal, coagulopathy, hypovolemia, fixed cardiac output, localized infection at the desired block site, and sepsis.

Compartment syndrome

Compartment syndrome is an acute medical problem following injury, surgery, or trauma in which increased pressure within a confined space compromises the

---

Box 1: Risks of regional anesthesia in trauma patients

Risks specific to the trauma situation
- Pre-existing hemodynamic instability
- Infection at the site of injection
- Inability to secure the airway, if necessary
- Specific pre-existing medical conditions
- Existing coagulopathy
- Uncooperative patient
- Regional anesthesia masking compartment syndrome

Technique-specific risks
Risks of spinal or epidural anesthesia
- Hemodynamic: hypotension, bradycardia
- Neurologic: headache, back pain, nerve root irritation, epidural hematoma
- Intravascular injection: seizure or cardiac arrest
- Infection: abscess, meningitis

Risks of peripheral nerve blocks
- Nerve injury
- Infection
- Intravascular injection causing seizure or cardiac arrest

circulation and function of tissues in that space. It can occur anywhere that a muscle is enclosed by fascia, but most commonly occurs in an osseofascial compartment of the leg or forearm. When pressure is elevated, capillary blood flow is compromised and the ischemia results in tissue membrane damage and leakage of fluids through capillary and muscle membranes. The resulting edema of the soft tissue within the compartment further raises the intracompartment pressure, which compromises venous and lymphatic drainage of the injured area. Pressure, if further increased in a reinforcing vicious cycle, can compromise arteriole perfusion, leading to further tissue ischemia. Untreated compartment syndrome results in ischemia of the muscles and nerves eventually leading to irreversible damage and death of the tissues within the compartment. Catastrophic outcomes are inevitable if surgical treatment is delayed for more than 12 hours. Full recovery can be achieved if decompression is performed within 6 hours of making the diagnosis [103]. Common causes of compartment syndrome include tibial or forearm fractures, ischemic-reperfusion following injury, hemorrhage, vascular puncture, intravenous drug injection, casts, prolonged limb compression, crush injuries, and burns.

There are classically five "Ps" associated with compartment syndrome: pain, paresthesia, pallor, paralysis, and pulselessness. Pain may be an unreliable symptom, however, because it can be variable. Pain can be absent in established acute compartment syndrome associated with nerve injury or minimal in deep posterior compartment syndrome [104]. The view that analgesia should be withdrawn or an inferior mode of pain control be used to facilitate the diagnosis of compartment syndrome should be discouraged [105,106]. Diagnosing compartment syndrome requires vigilance, a high index of suspicion, performance of serial examinations, and documentation over time. Literature reviews did not find any case reports suggesting peripheral nerve blocks [105] or lumbar epidural analgesia delayed the diagnosis of lower limb compartment syndrome. Karagiannis and colleagues [107,108] in a literature review did not find any evidence of an association of femoral nerve block, femoral shaft fracture, and delayed or missed diagnosis of compartment syndrome. Trauma patients with extremity fractures should be treated with dilute concentrations of local anesthetics to minimize motor block and dense sensory block rather than denying a regional technique for pain control. In such situations the perioperative team (surgeon and anesthesiologist) should maintain a high index of clinical suspicion, followed by immediate assessment and compartment pressure measurement when the diagnosis of acute compartment syndrome is entertained.

Peripheral nerve injury

The fear of complications exceeds their actual occurrence because the actual occurrence of complications related to regional anesthesia is relatively infrequent. This may be attributable, in part, to widespread misperception regarding the role of regional anesthesia in producing neurologic injury. With the primary intent to investigate neurologic complications of regional anesthesia in contemporary anesthetic practice, Brull and colleagues [109] reviewed 32 studies published between January 1995 and December 2005 and concluded that the rate of neurologic complications after central nerve blockade is 0.04%, the rate of neuropathy after peripheral nerve blocks is 3%, and permanent injury after regional anesthesia is rare. The rate of neurologic complications presented in this article [109] may be underestimated because much of the source data relied on self-reporting from anesthesia providers rather than prospective controlled trials. Medicolegal data, however, such as that provided by the American Society of Anesthesiologists Closed Claims Project, may overestimate the occurrence of injury [110]. The rate of serious neurologic injury in a large prospective study was 2.4 per 10,000 peripheral nerve blocks [111], whereas the rate of permanent nerve damage in another study was 1 in 5000 [112].

The American Society of Regional Anesthesia practice advisory on neurologic complications in regional anesthesia [113] states the following:

1. There are no animal or human data to support the superiority of one nerve localization technique (paresthesia, nerve stimulation, ultrasound) over another in regards to reducing the likelihood of nerve injury.
2. There are no human data to support the superiority of one local anesthetic or additive over another with regards to reducing the likelihood of neurotoxicity.
3. Patients with diseased or previously injured nerves (eg, diabetes mellitus, severe peripheral vascular disease, chemotherapy) theoretically may be at increased risk of neurologic injury. Although isolated case reports have been described, clinical experience can neither refute nor confirm these concerns. Careful risk-to-benefit assessment of regional anesthesia to alternative anesthesia and analgesia techniques should be considered.
4. Patients with pre-existing neurologic disease may be at the increased risk of new or worsening injury regardless of the anesthetic technique. When regional anesthesia is thought to be appropriate for these patients, modifying the anesthetic technique may minimize potential risk. Based on moderate amount of animal data, such modifications may include the use of less potent local anesthetic; minimizing local anesthetic dose, volume, or concentration; and avoiding or using a lower concentration of vasoactive additives. Limited human data neither confirm nor refute that these modifications are helpful.

In the early postoperative period, mild paresthesia may be present in up to 15% of patients undergoing peripheral nerve block [114]. Most of these symptoms resolve within days to weeks, with over 99% completely resolving by 1 year [110,115]. From American Society of Anesthesiology Closed Claims perspective, most claims involving peripheral nerve injury were for temporary injury (56%) with half of the deficits believed to be block related. The most commonly injured peripheral nerve structures are, in order, the brachial plexus, the median nerve, the ulnar nerve, and the radial nerve. According to the Closed Claims Database, lower extremity nerve injuries are rare, most likely reflecting the less frequent practice of lower extremity regional anesthesia

[114]. Permanent nerve injury is not completely preventable even in healthy patients receiving competent, standard of care. Peripheral nerve injury associated with regional anesthesia is likely caused by a combination of insults to the nerve's internal milieu. When applied to the trauma patient, it is not ethically or medically justified to withhold a better means of pain control because of fear of neural injury. Thorough documentation of the neurologic examination of the patient and preprocedural discussion with all members of the team (patient and surgeons) about the risks and benefits in the particular situation and the condition of the specific patient should occur before deciding what and whether to use a regional technique in the trauma victim.

Regional anesthesia in the heavily sedated or anesthetized patient

One of the most controversial areas of regional anesthesia practice is whether to perform blocks in patients under heavy sedation or under general anesthesia. Proponents for performing blocks in only mildly sedated patients argue that such patients are able to communicate to the anesthesiologist the sensation of pain and lessen the likelihood of nerve injury. Proponents of performing blocks in anesthetized or heavily sedated patients argue that this practice brings the benefits of regional anesthesia to a wider range of patients. There is no scientifically valid answer to this question. Existing animal and human data suggest the following [113]: (1) the sensation of paresthesia or pain on injection, even if it is sensitive for needle-to-nerve proximity during block, is neither sensitive nor specific for nerve injury; (2) neuraxial and peripheral nerve injuries have been reported in awake patients who experienced no atypical sensation and in those who reported severe pain on injection; and (3) heavy sedation or general anesthesia eliminates patient ability to report abnormal sensation but may or may not impact the actual occurrence of injury.

Placement of a needle or catheter in the subarachnoid space for the purpose of cerebrospinal fluid drainage is frequently performed in anesthetized patients undergoing neurosurgery. In a review of the records of 530 consecutive transsphenoidal surgeries with lumbar cerebrospinal fluid drainage, Grady and colleagues [115] found no cases of nerve injury caused by placement of cerebrospinal fluid drainage needles or catheters in anesthetized patients.

The American Society of Regional Anesthesia recommendations for performing regional anesthesia in anesthetized or heavily sedated patients state the following [113]:

1. The potential ability of general anesthesia or heavy sedation to obscure the early signs of systemic local anesthetic toxicity is not a valid reason to forgo performing peripheral nerve blocks or epidural blocks in anesthetized or heavily sedated patients.
2. At this stage there are no data to support the concept that peripheral nerve stimulation or ultrasound or injection pressure monitoring reduce the risk of peripheral nerve injury in heavily sedated patients or those under general anesthesia.
3. General anesthesia or heavy sedation removes the ability for the patient to report warning signs. This suggests that regional anesthetic or pain blocks

should not be performed with concurrent general anesthesia or heavy sedation in adults except when the physician and patient conclude that benefit
clearly outweighs the risk.
4. Because most reports of injury involve interscalene block in anesthetized
patients, interscalene blocks should not be performed in anesthetized or
heavily sedated patients.
5. Peripheral nerve blocks should not be routinely performed in most adults
during general anesthesia or heavy sedation. The risk-to-benefit ratio should
be considered, however, because it may improve the conditions of select
patients.

Infection

Infectious complications associated with regional anesthesia are rare. The usual
maxims are to avoid (1) performing blocks in patients with sepsis, (2) placing
needles through an obvious skin infection, and (3) the performance of blocks
in infected extremities. Many trauma and critically ill patients, however,
present with a clinical picture of systemic inflammatory response. Fever and
increased white blood cell counts alone (in the absence of positive blood
cultures) do not provide a reliable diagnosis of bacteremia. The combination
of serum markers, C-reactive protein, procalcitonin, and interleukin-6,
however, have been shown to indicate bacterial sepsis with a high degree of
sensitivity and specificity and can guide the decision to place an epidural catheter [67,116,117]. The occurrence of infection related to the performance of
single-shot nerve block is rare, which may reflect the relatively low infectious
risk of sterile needle insertion or the antimicrobial effects of local anesthetics
[117]. There are potentially greater infectious risks associated with the performance of continuous peripheral nerve block techniques. When indwelling catheters are present, it is common for these catheters to become colonized [72,
73,118]. Although catheters are frequently colonized (reported rate between
23% and 57%, primarily with *Staphylococcus epidermidis*), clinical evidence of infection is uncommon (between 0% and 3% for continuous peripheral nerve
blocks, 1:40,000 following spinal anesthesia, and 1:10,000 following epidural
anesthesia) [111]. Risk factors for infectious complications with continuous
peripheral nerve blocks include duration of continuous infusion greater than
48 hours, ICU stay for the patient, axillary and femoral locations of the catheter, and possibly the absence of antibiotic prophylaxis [73]. The risk of infection can be best reduced by using meticulous technique, maximum barrier
precautions, and tunneling the catheter [67,73]. There is no evidence to support
the routine use of preblock antibiotics for single-shot blocks and little to support
the use of preinsertion antibiotics in the case of continuous nerve blocks,
although they do reduce the incidence of colonization [73]. Colonization seems
to be increased with frequent dressing changes [118].

Coagulopathy

The current recommendations of the American Society of Regional Anesthesia
and Pain Medicine should be followed regarding regional anesthesia in the

anticoagulated patients (Table 5) [36]. The benefits of the regional anesthesia should be weighed against the potential detrimental complications [36,66,67].

PREHOSPITAL AND EMERGENCY ROOM MANAGEMENT OF ADULT TRAUMA: REGIONAL ANESTHESIA IN THE FIELD

The primary aim in the prehospital management of trauma remains the stabilization of the vital signs, the diagnosis of life-threatening conditions, avoidance of worsening injuries, and a timely transport to a trauma center. Providing adequate analgesia is often neglected in the prehospital management of the trauma patient. The goal should be early treatment of pain at the point of injury and throughout the continuum of care with a combination of standard and novel therapeutic interventions. Pain control measures should include keeping the patient warm; avoiding shivering; splinting the fractured limb; oxygenation; and the use of appropriate medications locally, regionally, or systemically. Regional anesthesia can benefit patients with trauma limited to a region by providing adequate pain control as an alternative to systemic opioids and avoid hemodynamic instability and respiratory depression in a patient that may be less than optimally monitored at all times in the emergency department.

Some of the single-shot peripheral nerve blocks (eg, femoral nerve block) can be extremely useful to the EMS practitioner. This block, which is simple, safe,

Table 5
The current recommendations of the American Society of Regional Anesthesia and Pain Medicine for regional anesthesia in the anticoagulated patient

Anticoagulant	United States
UFH sc (low dose: prophylactic)	Not contraindicated
UFH iv (high dose: therapeutic)	2–4 h after the last dose/1 h pause before the next dose
LMWH (low dose)	12 h after the last dose/2 h pause before the next dose
LMWH (therapeutic dose)	Relative contraindication or 24 h after the last dose
Fondaparinux	Not indicated
Hirudins (lepirudin) - thrombin inhibitor	Not indicated
Coumadin	INR <1.5
Aspirin	Not contraindicated
Ticlopidine	14 d
Clopidogrel	7 d
Tirofiban/eptifibatide	8 h
Platelet GP IIb/IIIa receptor antagonists	Contraindicated
Abciximab	48 h
Fibrinolytics	Fibrinogen level

Indicated times refer to the times before/after neuraxial blockade or catheter withdrawal.
  Abbreviations: h, hours; INR, international normalized ratio; iv, intravenous; LMWH, low-molecular-weight heparin; Sc, subcutaneous; UFH, unfractionated heparin.

and relatively fast to perform, is extremely popular and has been taught to most physicians in the prehospital setting in France [119,120]. It is a useful pain control measure during the transport of patients with fractured femoral shaft. Providing pain relief from injuries to the foot with an ankle block is also relatively simple. Blocks to the upper extremities may be performed in the prehospital setting, but training is essential. The axillary approach to the brachial plexus is more appealing outside of the hospital. For all blocks in the EMS setting a baseline neurologic examination is required to rule out any adverse neurologic outcomes that may contraindicate or make regional anesthesia unsafe.

The great availability of drugs, personnel, and equipment in the emergency room makes all these techniques even more appropriate for the preoperative treatment of the trauma patient. The emergency room provides a more sterile environment and continuous peripheral nerve block may be considered [121]. The techniques that can be used in the emergency room can be divided into infiltration, peripheral, and central nerve blocks. Analgesia can be achieved by infiltration of local anesthesia into a wound. Irrigation of wounds with local anesthetics has been administered successfully [81]. A modification of this technique is the field block, which is achieved by subcutaneous infiltration blocking of nerves that supply a particular area. Digital nerve block, wrist block, and ankle block have been used in the emergency room for pain treatment in traumatized patients. Patients with fractures to the femoral shaft may benefit from a femoral block while waiting for more definitive treatment [66].

A thoracic epidural should be considered in trauma patients with more than four rib fractures; in those with fewer than four rib fractures intercostal blocks or paravertebral blocks are a better option. The choice of techniques should reflect the assessment of the airway, the possible cardiopulmonary effects in the particular patient, the patient's level of consciousness, the patient's prior neurologic status, the individual physician's success rate for the particular procedure, and the availability of the required safety standards for the selected technique. The monitoring capabilities in the emergency room should be similar to the operating room. In addition, resuscitation equipment and personnel should be available to promptly treat possible complications in trauma patients. After completion of any procedure, monitoring of patients should continue until they are fully awake and resume their former level of function. No anesthetic or analgesic technique should be used unless the clinician understands the proper use of it and can deal with possible complications.

Anesthesiologists, surgeons, and emergency physicians have to interact to accomplish optimal pain treatment to the trauma patient in the emergency room. It remains to be seen how this will affect operating room care. If a patient comes to the operating room with a block performed in the field or in the emergency room how will its duration be determined? Should the block be repeated? What additional technical difficulties arise in placing a catheter in a blocked extremity? As this practice gains in popularity, there is an even greater need to coordinate care. It is the authors' practice to be available

24 hours a day for blocks in the emergency rooms. It is too soon to speculate on the scope of this practice in the future.

SUMMARY

Regional anesthesia techniques are part of the multimodal pain approach to the trauma patient. There are reasons to consider that timely analgesia can intervene in the complex physiologic response to trauma and significantly impact the secondary effects of pain. Although extrapolated from studies of perioperative pain, findings do suggest that there may be a critical period of time during which the secondary effects of painful stimulus may be attenuated or reversed. The duration of this period of reversibility has not been determined and planning for analgesia intervention should occur early. One must exercise extreme caution and sound judgment, however, when performing regional techniques in traumatized patients. Most trauma patients have associated injury and some of them require immediate operations. Highly effective pain relief can mask subtle signs of other visceral injuries, such as splenic and hepatic injury in patients with thoracic trauma. The sympathetic block may unmask or augment hypovolemia. Cardiovascular stability must be established, and abdominal visceral injury must be excluded before contemplating any regional anesthetic technique. Multimodal analgesia, with the balanced use of systemic and regional techniques, has given the best short- and long-term results in the management of pain in the trauma victim. Trauma strikes in variable fashion patients of all ages, with all forms of comorbidity, and is treated with modalities that continue to evolve. By understanding the strength and weaknesses of each technique, the clinician can assess the risk and benefits to individualize pain management for the setting and extent of trauma.

References

[1] Rosenberg A, Grande C, Bernstein R. Pain management and regional anesthesia in trauma. Philadelphia: WB Saunders; 2000.

[2] Wu CL, Fleisher LA. Outcomes research in regional anesthesia and analgesia. Anesth Analg 2000;91(5):1232–42.

[3] Perkins FM, Kehlet H. Chronic pain as an outcome of surgery: a review of predictive factors. Anesthesiology 2000;93(4):1123–33.

[4] Wu CL, Hurley RW, Anderson GF, et al. Effect of postoperative epidural analgesia on morbidity and mortality following surgery in Medicare patients. Reg Anesth Pain Med 2004;29(6):525–33 [discussion: 515–29].

[5] Wu CL, Naqibuddin M, Rowlingson AJ, et al. The effect of pain on health-related quality of life in the immediate postoperative period. Anesth Analg 2003;97(4):1078–85.

[6] Wu CL, Rowlingson AJ, Herbert R, et al. Correlation of postoperative epidural analgesia on morbidity and mortality after colectomy in Medicare patients. J Clin Anesth 2006;18(8): 594–9.

[7] Turner JA, Cardenas DD, Warms CA, et al. Chronic pain associated with spinal cord injuries: a community survey. Arch Phys Med Rehabil 2001;82(4):501–9.

[8] Malchow RJ, Black IH. The evolution of pain management in the critically ill trauma patient: emerging concepts from the global war on terrorism. Crit Care Med 2008;36(7 Suppl): S346–57.

[9] Rivara FP, Mackenzie EJ, Jurkovich GJ, et al. Prevalence of pain in patients 1 year after major trauma. Arch Surg 2008;143(3):282–7 [discussion: 288].

[10] Castillo RC, MacKenzie EJ, Wegener ST, et al. Prevalence of chronic pain seven years following limb threatening lower extremity trauma. Pain 2006;124(3):321–9.

[11] Urquhart DM, Williamson OD, Gabbe BJ, et al. Outcomes of patients with orthopaedic trauma admitted to level 1 trauma centres. ANZ J Surg 2006;76(7):600–6.

[12] Crombie IK, Davies HT, Macrae WA. Cut and thrust: antecedent surgery and trauma among patients attending a chronic pain clinic. Pain 1998;76(1–2):167–71.

[13] Fishbein M. Anesthesia. The new illustrated medical and health encyclopedia. New York: HS Stuttman Co; 1976.

[14] Ring ME. The history of local anesthesia. J Calif Dent Assoc 2007;35(4):275–82.

[15] Robinson V. Victory over pain: a history of anesthesia. New York: Henry Schuman; 1949.

[16] Wagensteen OW, Wagensteen SD. The rise of surgery: from empiric craft to scientific discipline. Minneapolis (MN): University of Minnesota; 1978.

[17] Dunn N, Sutcliffe J. A history medicine. New York: Barnes and Noble; 1992.

[18] Ansbro FP. A method of continuous brachial plexus block. Am J Surg 1946;71:716–22.

[19] Selander D. Catheter technique in axillary plexus block: presentation of a new method. Acta Anaesthesiol Scand 1977;21(4):324–9.

[20] Tuominen M, Pitkanen M, Rosenberg PH. Postoperative pain relief and bupivacaine plasma levels during continuous interscalene brachial plexus block. Acta Anaesthesiol Scand 1987;31(4):276–8.

[21] Pere P, Pitkanen M, Rosenberg PH, et al. Effect of continuous interscalene brachial plexus block on diaphragm motion and on ventilatory function. Acta Anaesthesiol Scand 1992;36(1):53–7.

[22] Borgeat A, Schappi B, Biasca N, et al. Patient-controlled analgesia after major shoulder surgery: patient-controlled interscalene analgesia versus patient-controlled analgesia. Anesthesiology 1997;87(6):1343–7.

[23] Visser V. Epidural anesthesia. Update in Anesthesia 2001;13:39–51.

[24] Bacon DR, Lema MJ. Standing on the promises: the career of Samuel L. Lieberman, MD. Sphere 1989;42:20–4.

[25] Thompson GE. Anesthesia for battle casualties in Vietnam. JAMA 1967;201:215–9.

[26] Jenicek JA, Perry LB, Thompson GE. Armed Forces anesthesiology comes of age. Anesth Analg 1967;46(6):822–32.

[27] Jowitt MD, Knight RJ. Anaesthesia during the Falklands campaign: the land battles. Anaesthesia 1983;38(8):776–83.

[28] Buckenmaier CC III, Shields CH, Auton AA, et al. Continuous peripheral nerve block in combat casualties receiving low-molecular weight heparin. Br J Anaesth 2006;97(6): 874–7.

[29] Army Regional Anesthesia and Pain Management Initiative. The military advanced regional anesthesia and analgesia handbook. 2008. Available at: http://www.arapmi. org/maraa-book-project.html. Accessed June 30, 2009.

[30] Benzon H, editor. Essentials of pain medicine and regional anesthesia. New York: Churchill Livingstone; 1999.

[31] Bach S, Noreng MF, Tjellden NU. Phantom limb pain in amputees during the first 12 months following limb amputation after preoperative lumbar epidural blockade. Pain 1988;33(3):297–301.

[32] Raja SN. Is an ounce of preoperative local anesthetic better than a pound of postoperative analgesic? Reg Anesth 1996;21(4):277–80.

[33] Meissner A, Rolf N, Van Aken H. Thoracic epidural anesthesia and the patient with heart disease: benefits, risks, and controversies. Anesth Analg 1997;85(3):517–28.

[34] Pavlov VA, Tracey KJ. The cholinergic anti-inflammatory pathway. Brain Behav Immun 2005;19(6):493–9.

[35] Bierhaus A, Humpert PM, Nawroth PP. Linking stress to inflammation. Anesthesiol Clin 2006;24(2):325–40.

[36] Horlocker TT, Wedel DJ, Benzon H, et al. Regional anesthesia in the anticoagulated patient: defining the risks (the second ASRA Consensus Conference on Neuraxial Anesthesia and Anticoagulation). Reg Anesth Pain Med 2003;28(3):172–97.

[37] Kariya N, Oda Y, Yukioka H, et al. [Effective treatment of a man with head injury and multiple rib fractures with epidural analgesia]. Masui 1996;45(2):223–6.

[38] Holcomb JB, McMullin NR, Kozar RA, et al. Morbidity from rib fractures increases after age 45. J Am Coll Surg 2003;196(4):549–55.

[39] Bernhardt A, Kortgen A, Niesel H, et al. [Using epidural anesthesia in patients with acute pancreatitis: prospective study of 121 patients]. Anaesthesiol Reanim 2002;27(1): 16–22.

[40] Flagel BT, Luchette FA, Reed RL, et al. Half-a-dozen ribs: the breakpoint for mortality. Surgery 2005;138(4):717–23 [discussion: 723–5].

[41] Bulger EM, Edwards T, KLotiz P, et al. Epidural analgesia improves outcome after multiple rib fractures. Surgery 2004;136:426–30.

[42] Carrier FM, Turgeon AF, Nicole PC, et al. Effect of epidural analgesia in patients with traumatic rib fractures: a systematic review and meta-analysis of randomized controlled trials. Can J Anaesth 2009;56:230–42.

[43] Moon MR, Luchette FA, Gibson SW, et al. Prospective, randomized comparison of epidural versus parenteral opioid analgesia in thoracic trauma. Ann Surg 1999;229(5): 684–91 [discussion: 691–2].

[44] Simon BJ, Cushman J, Barraco R, et al. East Practice Management Guidelines Work Group. Pain management guidelines for blunt thoracic trauma. J Trauma 2005;59: 1256–67.

[45] Karmakar MK, Critchley LA, Ho AM, et al. Continuous thoracic paravertebral infusion of bupivacaine for pain management in patients with multiple fractured ribs. Chest 2003;123(2):424–31.

[46] Karmakar MK. Thoracic paravertebral block. Anesthesiology 2001;95(3):771–80.

[47] Eason MJ, Wyatt R. Paravertebral thoracic block: a reappraisal. Anaesthesia 1979;34(7): 638–42.

[48] Daly DJ, Myles PS. Update on the role of paravertebral blocks for thoracic surgery: are they worth it? Curr Opin Anaesthesiol 2009;22(1):38–43.

[49] Karmakar MK, Ho AM. Acute pain management of patients with multiple fractured ribs. J Trauma 2003;54(3):615–25.

[50] Lonnqvist PA, MacKenzie J, Soni AK, et al. Paravertebral blockade: failure rate and complications. Anaesthesia 1995;50(9):813–5.

[51] Davies RG, Myles PS, Graham JM. A comparison of the analgesic efficacy and side-effects of paravertebral block vs. epidural block for thoracotomy-a systematic review and meta-analysis of randomized trials. Br J Anaesth 2006;96:418–26.

[52] Joshi GP, Bonnet F, Shah R, et al. A systematic review of randomized trials evaluating regional techniques for postthoracotomy analgesia. Anesth Analg 2008;107(3): 1026–40.

[53] Mohta M, Verma P, Saxena AK, et al. Prospective randomized comparison of continuous thoracic epidural and thoracic paravertebral infusions in patients with unilateral multiple rib fractures: a pilot study. J Trauma 2009;66:1096–101.

[54] Richman JM, Liu SS, Courpas G, et al. Does continuous peripheral nerve block provide superior pain control to opioids? A meta-analysis. Anesth Analg 2006;102:248–57.

[55] Capdevila X, Ponrouch M, Choquet O. Continuous peripheral nerve blocks in clinical practice. Curr Opin Anaesthesiol 2008;21:619–23.

[56] Le-Wendling L, Enneking FK. Continuous peripheral nerve blocks for postoperative analgesia. Curr Opin Anaesthesiol 2008;21:602–9.

[57] Plunkett AR, Buckenmaier CC. Safety of multiple, simultaneous continuous peripheral nerve block catheters in patient receiving therapeutic low-molecular weight heparin. Pain Med 2008;9:624–7.

[58] Stojadinovic A, Auton A, Peoples GE, et al. Responding to challenges in modern combat casualty care: innovative use of advanced regional anesthesia. Pain Med 2006;7:330–8.

[59] Tran de QH, Munoz L, Russo G, et al. Ultrasonography and stimulating perineural catheters for nerve blockade: a review of the evidence. Can J Anaesth 2008;55:447–57.

[60] Liu SS, Ngeow JE, Yadeau JT. Ultrasound-guided regional anesthesia and analgesia: a qualitative systematic review. Reg Anesth Pain Med 2009;34:47–59.

[61] Abrahams MS, Aziz MF, RF Fu, et al. Ultrasound guidance compared with electrical neurostimulation for peripheral nerve block: a systematic review and meta-analysis of randomized controlled trials. Br J Anaesth 2009;102:408–17.

[62] Plunkett AR, Brown DS, Rogers JM, et al. Supraclavicular continuous peripheral nerve block in a wounded soldier: when ultrasound is the only option. Br J Anaesth 2006;97: 715–7.

[63] Chelly JE, Casati A, Al-Samsam T, et al. Continuous lumbar plexus block for acute postoperative pain management after open reduction and internal fixation of acetabular fractures. J Orthop Trauma 2003;17(5):362–7.

[64] Morin AM, Kratz CD, Eberhart LH, et al. Postoperative analgesia and functional recovery after total knee replacement: a comparison of a continuous posterior lumbar plexus (psoas compartment) block, a continuous femoral nerve block, and combination of continuous femoral and sciatic nerve block. Reg Anesth Pain Med 2005;30:434–45.

[65] Foss NB, Kristensen BB, Bundgaard M, et al. Fascia iliaca compartment block for acute pain control in hip fracture patients: a randomized, placebo controlled trial. Anesthesiology 2007;106:773–8.

[66] Mutty CE, Jensen EJ, Manka MA Jr, et al. Femoral nerve block for diaphyseal and distal femoral fractures in the emergency department. J Bone Joint Surg Am 2007;89: 2599–603.

[67] Schulz-Stubner S, Boezaart A, Hata JS. Regional analgesia in the critically ill. Crit Care Med 2005;33(6):1400–7.

[68] Sia S, Pelusio F, Barbagil R, et al. Analgesia before performing a spinal block in the sitting position in patients with femoral shaft fracture: a comparison between femoral nerve block and intravenous fentanyl. Anesth Analg 2004;99:1221–4.

[69] Yun MJ, Kim YH, Han MK, et al. Analgesia before spinal block for femoral neck fracture: fascia iliaca compartment block. Acta Anaesthesiol Scand 2009 [published ahead of print].

[70] Rosenberg PH, Veering BT, Urmey WF. Maximum recommended doses of local anesthetics: a multifactorial concept. Reg Anesth Pain Med 2004;29(6):564–75 [discussion: 524].

[71] Wiegel M, Gottschaldt U, Hennebach R, et al. Complications and adverse effects associated with continuous peripheral nerve blocks in orthopedic patients. Anesth Analg 2007;104(6):1578–82.

[72] Neuburger M, Buttner J, Blumenthal S, et al. Inflammation and infectious complications of 2285 perineural catheters: a prospective study. Acta Anaesthesiol Scand 2007;51: 108–14.

[73] Capdevila XM, Bringuier S, Borgeat A. Infectious risk of continuous peripheral nerve blocks. Anesthesiology 2009;110:182–8.

[74] Shanti CM, Carlin AM, Tyburski JG. Incidence of pneumothorax from intercostal nerve block for analgesia in rib fractures. J Trauma 2001;51(3):536–9.

[75] Dravid RM, Paul RE. Interpleural block: part 1. Anaesthesia 2007;62:1039–49.

[76] Dravid RM, Paul RE. Interpleural block: part 2. Anaesthesia 2007;62:1143–53.

[77] Carli P, Duranteau J, Mazoit X, et al. Pharmacokinetics of interpleural lidocaine administration in trauma patients. Anesth Analg 1990;70(4):448–53.

[78] Rocco A, Reiestad F, Gudman J, et al. Intrapleural administration of local anesthetics for pain relief in patients with multiple rib fractures: preliminary report. Reg Anesth Pain Med 1987;12:10.

[79] Shinohara K, Iwama H, Akama Y, et al. Interpleural block for patients with multiple rib fractures: a comparison with epidural block. J Emerg Med 1994;12:441–6.

[80] Shantha TR. Unilateral bronchospasm after interpleural analgesia. Anesth Analg 1992;74(2):291–3.

[81] Thomas DF, Lambert WG, Williams KL. The direct perfusion of surgical wounds with local anaesthetic solution: an approach to postoperative pain? Ann R Coll Surg Engl 1983;65(4):226–9.

[82] Columb MO, Lyons G. Determination of the minimum local analgesic concentrations of epidural bupivacaine and lidocaine in labor. Anesth Analg 1995;81(4):833–7.

[83] Mather LE, Copeland SE, Ladd LA. Acute toxicity of local anesthetics: underlying pharmacokinetic and pharmacodynamic principles. Reg Anesth Pain Med 2005;30: 553–66.

[84] Weinberg G. Lipid rescue resuscitation from local anesthetic cardiac toxicity. Toxicol Rev 2006;25:139–45.

[85] Casati A, Putzu M. Bupivcaine, levobupivacaine, and ropivacaine: are they clinically different? Best Pract Res Clin Anaesthesiol 2005;19:247–68.

[86] Casati A, Vinciguerra F, Cappelleri G, et al. Levobupivacaine 0.2% or 0.125% for continuous sciatic nerve block: a prospective, randomized, double-blind comparison with 0.2% ropivacaine. Anesth Analg 2004;99:919–23.

[87] Seet E, Leong WL, Yeo AS, et al. Effectiveness of 3-in-1 continuous femoral nerve block of differing concentrations compared to patient-controlled intravenous morphine for post-total knee arthroplasty analgesia and knee rehabilitation. Anaesth Intensive Care 2006;34: 25–30.

[88] Ilfedl BM, Loland VJ, Gerancher JC, et al. The effects of varying local anesthetic concentrations and volume on continuous popliteal sciatic nerve blocks: a dual-center, randomized controlled study. Anesth Analg 2008;107:701–7.

[89] Bernards CM, Hill HF. Physical and chemical properties of drug molecules governing their diffusion through the spinal meninges. Anesthesiology 1992;77(4):750–6.

[90] Bernards CM. Recent insights into the pharmacokinetics of spinal opioids and the relevance to opioid selection. Curr Opin Anaesthesiol 2004;17:441–7.

[91] Neal JM. Effects of epinephrine in local anesthetics on the central and peripheral nervous system: neurotoxicity and neural blood flow. Reg Anesth Pain Med 2003;28:124–34.

[92] Heavner JE. Local anesthetics. Curr Opin Anaesthesiol 2007;20(4):336–42.

[93] Niemi G, Breivik H. Adrenaline markedly improves thoracic epidural analgesia produced by a low-dose infusion of bupivacaine, fentanyl and adrenaline after major surgery: a randomised, double-blind, cross-over study with and without adrenaline. Acta Anaesthesiol Scand 1998;42(8):897–909.

[94] Niemi G, Breivik H. Epinephrine markedly improves thoracic epidural analgesia produced by a small-dose infusion of ropivacaine, fentanyl, and epinephrine after major thoracic or abdominal surgery: a randomized, double-blinded crossover study with and without epinephrine. Anesth Analg 2002;94(6):1598–605.

[95] Curatolo M. Is epinephrine unfairly neglected for postoperative epidural mixtures? Anesth Analg 2002;94(6):1381–3.

[96] Finucane B, editor. Complications of regional anesthesia. New York: Springer; 2007. p. 193–210.

[97] Elia N, Culebras X, Mazza C, et al. Clonidine as an adjunct to intrathecal local anesthetics for surgery: systematic review of randomized trials. Reg Anesth Pain Med 2008;33: 159–67.

[98] Popping DM, Elia N, Marret E, et al. Clonidine as an adjuvant to local anesthetics for peripheral nerve and plexus blocks. Anesthesiology 2009;111:406–15.

[99] Ilfled BM, Morey TE, Thannikary LJ, et al. Clonidine added to continuous interscalene ropivacaine perineural infusion to improve postoperative analgesia: a randomized, double-blind, controlled study. Anesth Analg 2005;100:1172–8.

[100] Casati A, Vinciguerra F, Cappelleri G, et al. Adding clonidine to the induction bolus and postoperative infusion during continuous femoral nerve block delays recovery of motor function after total knee arthroplasty. Anesth Analg 2005;100:866–72.

[101] Pekoe GM, Smith DJ. The involvement of opiate and monoaminergic neuronal systems in the analgesic effects of ketamine. Pain 1982;12(1):57–73.

[102] Taura P, Fuster J, Blasi A, et al. Postoperative pain relief after hepatic resection in cirrhotic patients: the efficacy of a single small dose of ketamine plus morphine epidurally. Anesth Analg 2003;96(2):475–80.

[103] Elliott KG, Johnstone AJ. Diagnosing acute compartment syndrome. J Bone Joint Surg Br 2003;85(5):625–32.

[104] McQueen MM, Christie J, Court-Brown CM. Acute compartment syndrome in tibial diaphyseal fractures. J Bone Joint Surg Br 1996;78(1):95–8.

[105] Mar GJ, Barrington MJ, McGuirk BR. Acute compartment syndrome of the lower limb and the effect of postoperative analgesia on diagnosis. Br J Anaesth 2009;102(1):3–11.

[106] Johnson DJ, Chalkiadis GA. Does epidural analgesia delay the diagnosis of lower limb compartment syndrome in children. Paediatr Anaesth 2009;19:83–91.

[107] Karagiannis G, Hardern R. Best evidence topic report: no evidence found that a femoral nerve block in cases of femoral shaft fractures can delay the diagnosis of compartment syndrome of the thigh. Emerg Med J 2005;22(11):814.

[108] Shadgan B, Menon M, O'Brien PJ, et al. Diagnostic techniques in acute compartment syndrome of the leg. J Orthop Trauma 2008;22:581–7.

[109] Brull R, McCartney CJ, Chan VW, et al. Neurological complications after regional anesthesia: contemporary estimates of risk. Anesth Analg 2007;104(4):965–74.

[110] Lee LA, Posner KL, Domino KB, et al. Injuries associated with regional anesthesia in the 1980s and 1990s: a closed claims analysis. Anesthesiology 2004;101(1):143–52.

[111] Auroy Y, Benhamou D, Bargues L, et al. Major complications of regional anesthesia in France: The SOS Regional Anesthesia Hotline Service. Anesthesiology 2002;97(5): 1274–80.

[112] Ridgway S. Perioperative nerve dysfunction and peripheral nerve blockade. Cont Educ Anaesth Crit Care Pain 2006;6(2):71–4.

[113] Neal JM, Bernards CM, Hadzic A, et al. ASRA practice advisory on neurologic complications in regional anesthesia and pain medicine. Reg Anesth Pain Med 2008;33(5): 404–15.

[114] Liguori GA. Complications of regional anesthesia: nerve injury and peripheral neural blockade. J Neurosurg Anesthesiol 2004;16(1):84–6.

[115] Grady RE, Horlocker TT, Brown RD, et al. Neurologic complications after placement of cerebrospinal fluid drainage catheters and needles in anesthetized patients: implications for regional anesthesia. Mayo Perioperative Outcomes Group. Anesth Analg 1999;88(2):388–92.

[116] Bell K, Wattie M, Byth K, et al. Procalcitonin: a marker of bacteraemia in SIRS. Anaesth Intensive Care 2003;31(6):629–36.

[117] Aydin ON, Eyigor M, Aydin N. Antimicrobial activity of ropivacaine and other local anaesthetics. Eur J Anaesthesiol 2001;18(10):687–94.

[118] Morin AM, Kerwat KM, Klotz M, et al. Risk factors for bacterial catheter colonization in regional anaesthesia. BMC Anesthesiol 2005;5(1):1.

[119] Telion C, Carli P. Prehospital and emergency room pain management for the adult trauma patient. Tech Reg Anesth Pain Manag 2002;16(2):221–5.

[120] Lopez S, Gros T, Bernard N, et al. Fascia iliaca compartment block for femoral bone fracture in prehospital care. Reg Anesth Pain Med 2003;28:203–7.
[121] Buckenmaier CC, McKnight GM, Winkley JV, et al. Continuous peripheral nerve block for battlefield anesthesia and evacuation. Reg Anesth Pain Med 2005;30(2): 202–5.

ADVANCES IN ANESTHESIA

INDEX

A

Ablation, aneurysmal, anesthetic management of, 17–18

Acetaminophen
in acute perioperative pain management, 118–119
in perioperative management of opioid-tolerant patients, 36–38

Acute perioperative pain, multimodal therapy for, nonopioid adjuvants in, **111–142**
acetaminophen, 118–119
a2-adrenergic agonists, 127–129
COX-2 inhibitors, 119–121
described, 111–113
gabapentinoids, 125–127
glucocorticoids, 129–134
N-methyl-D-aspartate receptor antagonists, 121–125
NSAIDs, 114–118

Acute stroke, thrombolysis for, anesthetic management in, 20

a2-Adrenergic agonists, in acute perioperative pain management, 127–129

American Pain Society (APS), 25

Analgesic adjuvants, in trauma, 206–208

Anesthesia/anesthetics
for interventional neuroradiological procedures, **1–24**. See also *Interventional neuroradiological procedures, anesthetic management of.*
general. See *General anesthesia.*
local
in perioperative management of opioid-tolerant patients, 42–43
in trauma, 206–208
regional, in trauma, **191–222**. See also *Trauma, regional anesthesia in.*

Aneurysmal ablation, anesthetic management in, 17–18

Angiography, superselective, of AVMs, anesthetic management in, 14–15

Angioplasty, anesthetic management during, 18–20

Anticholinergic(s), for PNOV, 149

Antidepressant(s), in perioperative management of opioid-tolerant patients, 40–41

Antiemetic(s), for PNOV, 145–157
anticholinergics, 149
antihistamines, 149–150
combination therapy, 155–157
dexamethasone, 150–151
dopamine receptor antagonists, 145, 148–149
NK1 receptor antagonists, 153–155
palonosetron, 151–153
serotonin receptor antagonists, 150

Antihistamine(s), for PNOV, 149–150

Anti-inflammatory drugs, nonsteroidal
in acute perioperative pain management, 114–118
in perioperative management of opioid-tolerant patients, 38–39

Anxiety
acute, preoperative, treatment of, 68
during preanesthesia period, 57–63
states of, differential diagnosis of, 62–63
treatment of, 64–69
complementary and alternative therapy in, 69

Anxiety disorders, during preanesthesia period, 57–63

Arterial pressure, monitoring of, 5–6

Arteriovenous malformations (AVMs)
dural, anesthetic management in, 20
superselective angiography and therapeutic embolization of, anesthetic management in, 14–15

Aspirin, in acute perioperative pain management, 114–115

Atherosclerosis, angioplasty for, anesthetic management in, 19–20

AVMs. See *Arteriovenous malformations (AVMs).*

Note: Page numbers of article titles are in **boldface** type.

0737-6146/09/$ – see front matter
doi:10.1016/S0737-6146(09)00019-7

Printed and bound by CPI Group (UK) Ltd, Croydon, CR0 4YY

08/05/2025

01864753-0001